TO ALL
WHO COULD NOT READ
THIS BOOK

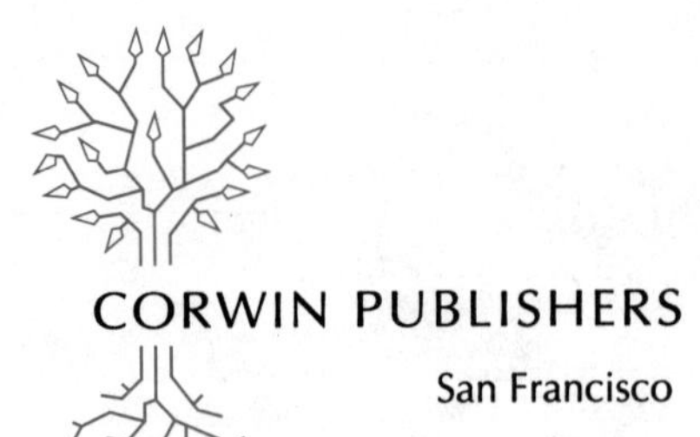
CORWIN PUBLISHERS
San Francisco

Living With AIDS

REACHING OUT

TOM O'CONNOR

WITH

AHMED GONZALEZ-NUNEZ

CORWIN PUBLISHERS, San Francisco 94106

 Published 1987
Printed in the United States of America
92 91 90 89 88 87 5 4 3 2 1

Library of Congress Card Catalog Number: 86–71535
ISBN 0–938569–00–7

ACKNOWLEDGEMENTS

The road to this book was lined with friends, acquaintances, and strangers who gave Ahmed and me constant encouragement and advice—often selflessly braving the many rough drafts and primitive manuscripts in order to help. The list of names is too long for publication. Some persons, however, bear special mention: Ellen O. Setteducati, for her sensitive and sensible editing; Gale Ward, for her conscientious proofreading; and Steve Renick and Chet Grycz at UC Press, for their helpful advice on book design and production. One very special person merits very special thanks: my father, Thomas E. O'Connor, Sr. Without his parental love and understanding—and his financial support—this book would not have gone to press.

ACKNOWLEDGMENTS

The road to this book [illegible] and friends [illegible] encouragement [illegible]
[illegible] editorial [illegible]
[illegible] reflection [illegible] thought [illegible] and [illegible]
[illegible] in [illegible] the list of names [illegible]
[illegible] special thanks to Ellen O[illegible]
[illegible] and [illegible] Work [illegible]
[illegible] and [illegible] OK [illegible]
helpful [illegible] Special [illegible]
[illegible] Thomas [illegible]
[illegible]
[illegible] would not [illegible]

Contents

Tables

Illustrations

Living with AIDS:

Reaching out

Introduction

December 1980 was not the best period of my life. I had broken with my lover, was facing bankruptcy, and had started a new job. And in the midst of all these changes, I got really sick. I experienced bouts of diarrhea, had nightly sweats, and felt constantly tired. My lymph glands swelled, and I slept over twelve hours every day. Finally, I sank into a deep depression. The symptoms continued unabated for months, but the doctors could not explain them.

By June 1982, they had some kind of answer. I was told the results of a blood test that measured my ratio of helper T to suppressor T cells, the on and off switches of the immune system. A healthy individual, my physician informed me, usually has two helper T cells for every suppressor T cell—a 2.0 ratio. My ratio was 0.3. Other gay men my age with ratios of 0.8 and less were dying from a rare pneumonia and cancer *(Pneumocystis carinii* pneumonia and Kaposi's sarcoma). The implications of my physician's words were clear.

I will never forget the feeling in my stomach at that moment. I seemed to be falling down a bottomless elevator shaft. Then I felt myself pop out of my body and, from above, watched myself taking it all in. Everything seemed unreal. "It can't be me," I thought as I left the office. "But then, it is. . . ." The hospital staff were going about their activities with their accustomed calmness. How could everyone remain so cool and unconcerned while I faced imminent death? Didn't anyone understand?

I started a diary as soon as I got home. I wrote down faithfully where I went, what I did, how many vitamins I took, and how tired or energetic I felt, but left out almost every reference to feelings and emotions. In fact, I was feeling a lot of denial, anguish, guilt, and rage about the inevitability of my death.

My illness provided an incentive to find out what I wanted to do with the rest of my life—and a time frame in which to work. The future no longer existed. Only the now remained.

On July 29, 1982, I wrote: "Preparing myself for the worst. On my way back to the office from the Embarcadero,[a] I realized I had been blessed by loving parents, travels, and material comforts. I have had a full and good life." I realized that, whether I lived or died, there was no reason to hurt myself anymore with guilt, fear, and anguish. An invisible force had put its hand on my shoulder and said, "Everything will be all right. Don't fret. Don't worry. It will be okay." I can still remember the bliss of that afternoon. I felt good about myself and my life, and I knew that everything would indeed work out fine.

I could not, however, lie back and wait for grace to bestow a long and bountiful life on me. If I were to live, I had to take the reins of my life and concentrate on what was left rather than on what was lost. Grace would follow.

The next diary entry states, "I will do those things to prolong my life that will not subject my body to misery and pain. Presently studying ways to improve T cell production." Although I lacked research experience, I began studying how to build up my immune system. I did not know where to look or how to discriminate between fact and fiction and consequently spent hours paging through classifieds in the local rags that advertised "healing and personal growth services." My efforts were disorganized. The multitude of options overwhelmed me and slowed my search. I did not know how to reach out. For the next several months I remained passive and read whatever slapped me in the face.

In December 1982 I came down with hepatitis A. When I asked four of my physician friends what I should eat, each had a different opinion. The first told me to eat anything I wanted, the second recommended eating lots of protein, and the third suggested avoiding fats. But the fourth one said candidly, "Why are you asking me? You probably know more about it than I do." I was shocked by this revelation. Apparently, all four physicians had a negligible background in nutrition. Why, even I, from my haphazard reading on the subject, knew we are each a product of the food we eat. How could physicians ignore such a vital fact? Since it was the one neglected area I could directly control, I decided to contribute to my healing through nutrition.

On January 15, 1983, I wrote: "With my body in such a deficient state, I will try to prevent all toxic or nonbeneficial substances from coming in contact with or entering it. The major change must be in my diet. We are indeed what we eat, so the food we consume should be of the highest quality." From then on, I really did hold the reins.

I dived into the study of nutrition believing diet was *the* answer and could greatly change my health. I have since come to realize that there are few simple answers and many paths back to wholeness.

I began my inquiry with *Metabolic Ecology* by Fred Rohe, a book that centers on the recovery of Dr. William Kelly from an inoperable cancer of the pancreas. It offered sound advice and provided me with the hope that even an AIDS diagnosis need not be a death sentence. Most important, it built my confidence. Whenever I was lonely or depressed, I read about people who had survived hopeless prognoses. The stories helped me through evenings like March 23, 1983, when I wrote: "I am very depressed and scared out of my mind about having a monster inside me."[b]

Through further reading, I later understood how people often participate in the onset of disease and why it therefore might help to analyze the roots of such participation. My role in what led to my own sickness thus became clear. I had wanted to show my ex-lover Jon that he was responsible for my hurt after our separation. I had wanted to get even, to have the last word, and the best way to do so was to die. But how could my ex have been responsible for my hurt? After all, my anguish was my own creation and only I could be responsible for it. Finally, it dawned on me that the only person I could really change was myself.

That summer I started working with a hypnotherapist, attended a nutritional seminar in Texas, and began my own reading program on visualization and the thought process. In retrospect, it seems as if these events fell into place like pieces of a puzzle. Having once reached *out* to seek wellness, I understood now that I would find healing only by reaching *within* myself.

Six years ago, I was resentful and unforgiving, had a poor self-image, pitied myself, was unable to maintain long-term relationships, and tended to judge people by how beautiful or ugly they were. Today I enjoy being with myself and other people and look deeper into others to find beauty. Guilt about the past and worry about the future bog me down less. Above all, my life now has purpose and meaning.

Nowadays, I usually feel physically energetic and need only eight hours of sleep most nights. I have not developed any opportunistic infections or body lesions. My helper/suppressor T cell ratio remains the same; it has not deteriorated. The white spots and cold sores on my throat and tonsils are a thing of the past, although the swollen glands persist. They serve as a constant reminder of my need for greater awareness; without such reminders, I could slip back into my old ways. For people who, as I once did, show many of the symptoms of AIDS without developing its opportunistic infections, doctors have finally identified a disease. They call it AIDS-related complex (ARC).

* * *

The American Heritage Dictionary defines health as soundness of body and mind. Conversely, disease, rather than being just physical, involves the whole person: the body, the mind, and the soul. In each of us these three must work in harmony to produce well-being. Without harmony we have disease, and without the whole person working toward health, physical interventions might not succeed. Hippocrates said, over two thousand years ago, "Everyone has a doctor within him. We just have to help him,"

Living with AIDS: Reaching Out is for people who want to do something about their disease but don't know where to start; who see a need to take responsibility over their lives, no matter where they are; and who are willing to participate actively in their healing. It is also intended for healthy individuals who one day might face the threat of AIDS in themselves or their lovers, relatives, or friends. The book deals with the initial part of my journey, and with nutrition and the body. Nutrition plays a vital role in combating AIDS, and a good diet can bring about the quickest and most effective changes in one's health. A second book, *Living with AIDS: Reaching In*, an account of my journey toward mental and spiritual well-being, is in the planning stage.

This book distills information from over 150 books, several dozen magazines and tapes, and various conferences and seminars.

Some information might seem contradictory or repetitious or to have various interpretations. This is because I wanted to present as many views as possible so you could draw your own conclusions and choose your own path. A good deal of the book describes my path toward health, and I hope that what I learned can likewise help you.

I emphasize things you can do for yourself. Doing things for yourself empowers you. Although you should remain open to help from others, feeling that your health depends solely on the intervention of another or on a particular hard-to-get substance will, on the other hand, take power away from you. I try to bring to your attention the harmful and beneficial things in your environment. The more you move away from negative things and surround yourself with the positive, the greater your chances of survival. You may not need to make great changes if you are healthy—although certain changes might always be helpful. If you are ill, however, you will need to look at change squarely in the face. You may want to make immediately those changes you consider harmless, so that you might then have the time to read more about, experience, and validate my other recommendations. Pass over those things you feel might harm you. Listen to your body and let your health be the judge of how deep your changes need to be. Don't look at change only as denying yourself harmful things but as opening up to things that will enhance you. Look at it as loving yourself.[c]

I may sound harsh and severe at times. This is because AIDS is unrelenting in its attack on the immune system and demands a rigorous response. You must be equally uncompromising when confronted by anything that endangers your immunity. And there's another reason to harden yourself: as of November 1986 over 1,500 people in San Francisco alone have already lost their lives to this plague, and nothing but hard resolve will keep this number from constantly escalating.

I wish I could offer you the gift of time: time to look at your life, time to bring about positive changes, time to realize your full potential and enjoy the rewards of life, time enough to see this process as a turning point from which to grow and transform yourself. But only you can give yourself this gift of self-love. Only you can take responsibility for your life. Only you can open new doors and dedicate yourself to your healing. I offer you one saying that has given me great comfort over the past few years: "Live today as if you may die tomorrow, but learn as if you were to live forever."

Part one: Loving the body

CHAPTER 1

Learning about health

Acquired immunodeficiency syndrome—AIDS—is not easy to get. It is almost impossible to catch the human immunodeficiency virus (HIV)[a] associated with the syndrome if one follows simple guidelines for safe sex and refrains from using contaminated needles or blood plasma. What's more, new evidence indicates that most people are able to deal with the virus once it enters the bloodstream. Some other factor or factors must be present for HIV to conquer and destroy the immune system.[1]

If only life were a matter of following simple guidelines, and all disease a question of investigating how pathogens behave in a test tube! But each new obituary, each new diagnosis in a friend, each sign of deficient immunity—real or imagined—in ourselves tell us otherwise. They remind us that, no matter how difficult getting AIDS may be, many of us have in fact caught the HIV virus and are subject to a host of cofactors that might bring about the disease. These daily reminders tell us that many of us will develop immune deficiencies and die.

How radically everything changes when the *us* becomes *me;* the number one becomes too large a number. Numbers, science, and medicine all fail to answer a deceptively simple question: Why me?

The answer is often elusive. It requires each of us to unravel the physical, emotional, social, and spiritual skeins that entangle us in our disease. This book and its sequel describe some discoveries I made in my attempt to unravel my disease. I hope my insight will help you in developing your own.

Most of us are quite familiar with the ravages of AIDS and ARC, especially if we have these conditions. We see and experience their tragedy and ugliness almost every day, and we cannot deceive ourselves: AIDS is likely to be fatal. Yet once we accept this, why should we dwell on death and disease? Deception prevents you from acting, whereas knowledge motivates you to act. Information about AIDS should tell you one of two things: either how to improve your immunity or how to better your life. If it does neither, don't waste time on it. Excessive, unnecessary AIDS data can overwhelm you with hopelessness and despair, but useful knowledge should make life simpler.

For this reason this book contains no lengthy section detailing the sundry symptoms of ARC or the host of opportunistic AIDS infections. Plenty of books about these subjects are available. For an interesting and novel discussion of AIDS, I recommend *A Strange Virus of Unknown Origin (Un virus etrange venu d'ailleurs)* by French AIDS researcher Jacques Leibowitch. For a more personal account, read Barbara Peabody's *The Screaming Room,* the touching and inspiring story of her son's struggle with AIDS.

How do you strengthen your immunity? First, you learn about the immune system and what factors enhance or inhibit its functions. Take, for example, the subject of treatment. All available treatment for AIDS, including conventional medicine, is experimental; there are no tried and true therapies, although there are some that could be detrimental. Your physician might tell you the pros and cons of specific treatments but most likely will lack the time to educate you. That is your job. A well-grounded knowledge of the immune system will be your best counsel. For people with ARC or AIDS, acquiring knowledge often requires great effort and dedication. Even when following the aforementioned guidelines of usefulness, you might run up against much contradictory and confusing data. Don't despair.

Information about the immune system often gets technical. For those of us who paid little attention to science and biology in school, the going can get tough sometimes. Nevertheless, there is no convenient substitute for knowledge; unlike syphilis or tuberculosis, AIDS is a complicated disease. If, like me, you get bogged down easily in scientific jargon and medicalese, find a friend who doesn't and who can explain the terminology. I have tried to define all technical terms as simply as possible in the text. The glossary in the back defines them more extensively. Reference notes are intended to complement your understanding once you have a good grasp of the text. If you feel you're getting nowhere, jump ahead to another chapter, but always come back to where you left off. Any information you acquire about the immune system will prove invaluable. "The more you know about your illness," counsels a booklet from the San Francisco AIDS Foundation,[2] "the better you will be able to make decisions that affect your health."

THE IMMUNE SYSTEM

The immune system is an evolutionary marvel. Every second, its exquisitely complex activities protect us not only from invading microorganisms but also from the air we breathe, the food we eat, and even our own body cells gone wild.

The body's first line of defense is a group of cells that go into action whenever bacteria, viruses, or any disease-causing microorganisms enter the body's tissues. These cell-eating white blood cells, the phagocytes, immediately seek out and engulf the invaders. (See table 1 for an outline of the kinds of white blood cells.) Certain phagocytes, the macrophages, cannot digest invaders on their own. To do so, they need instructions from other white blood cells called helper T cells (The T stands for thymus, the organ where these white blood cells mature). The macrophages secrete a chemical that lures these T lymphocytes to the site of infection. When helper T cells arrive on the scene, they produce another set of substances[b] that allow the macrophages to digest their swallowed victims and mobilize still other kinds of immune cells into action.

Although phagocytes, including macrophages, ingest a wide variety of pathogens and foreign substances overall, each kind specializes in its eating habits. Macrophages differ from other phagocytes not only in diet and their need for helper T cell assistance but also in their form. Their distinctive appearance enables T cells to recognize them, and their contour changes according to what they have eaten so that T cells can also recognize the kinds of pathogen they are carrying.

The recognition process works this way: Whenever a macrophage engulfs an invader, a fragment of the pathogen—an antigen—will remain jutting from the macrophage surface like a key stuck teeth-out in a bar of soap. On its own surface, each T cell possesses a receptor much like a keyhole-and-lock mechanism. The antigen key sticking out from a macrophage will slide into the keyhole structure on a T cell, but only if the keyhole contains the specific lock combination that matches the antigen key. If and only if the antigen key and T cell lock fit together, the helper T cell will release the substance needed by macrophages for digestion, along with substances needed for the mobilization of other immune cells (see figure 1).

Each antigen key has only one lock combination, and only one helper T cell responds to each kind of antigen sticking out from a

TABLE 1
White blood cells

- Lymphocytes
  - T cells
    - Helper
    - Killer
    - Suppressor
  - B cells
- Large granular lymphocytes
  - Natural killer cells
- Other white blood cells
  - Phagocytes
    - Macrophages
    - Other phagocytes
      - Neutrophils*
  - Granulocytes
    - Neutrophils*
    - Eosinophils
    - Basophils

* Classed as both phagocytes and granulocytes

FIGURE 1 Macrophage and helper T cell interaction

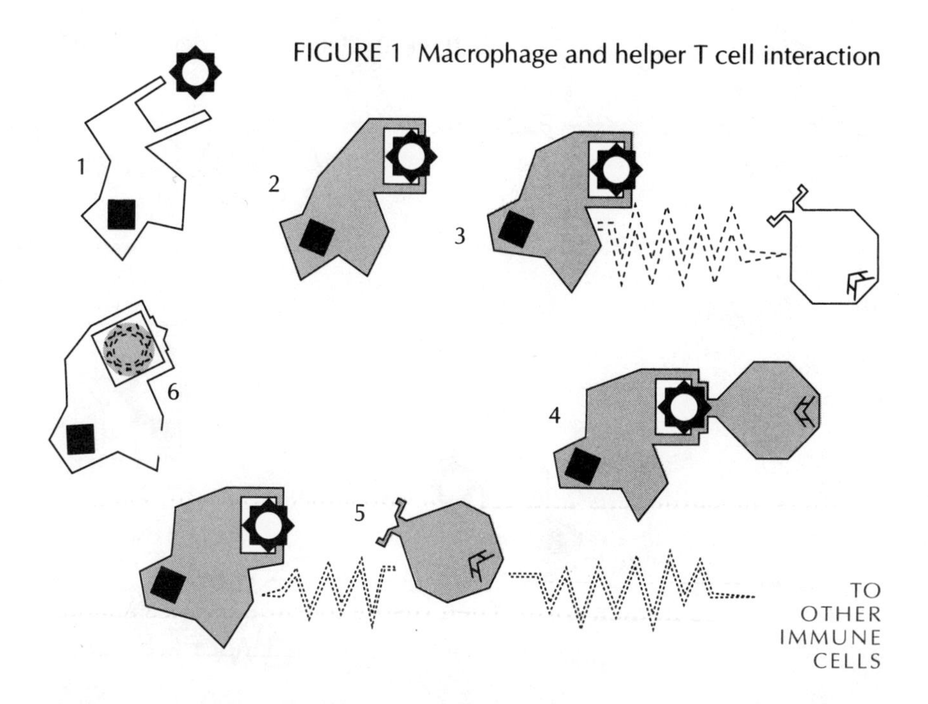

1. Macrophage moves to site of infection, (2) engulfs pathogen, and (3) attracts helper T cell. 4. Macrophage couples with helper T cell, (5) inducing it to secrete lymphokines that will attract other immune cells and permit the macrophage (6) to digest the pathogen.

macrophage. This doesn't mean that one little T cell carries on the battle against a whole army of pathogens: once the helper T cell has been activated by the antigen key, the cell makes many copies of itself. What if an antigen comes along that will not fit into any existing T cell? Luckily, our bodies usually possess about ten million different antigen-specific T cells corresponding to the ten million different protein and polysaccharide combinations that make up antigens. Research indicates that HIV interferes with this lock-and-key mechanism—specifically, with the receptor in the T cell. In this way, HIV disrupts the production of substances that initiate the attack against invading pathogens (see figure 2).

How can HIV run the gauntlet of the macrophages and attack helper T cells? Apparently, most of the time it doesn't. The immune system possesses a series of redundant components that

FIGURE 2 Helper T cell defect in AIDS

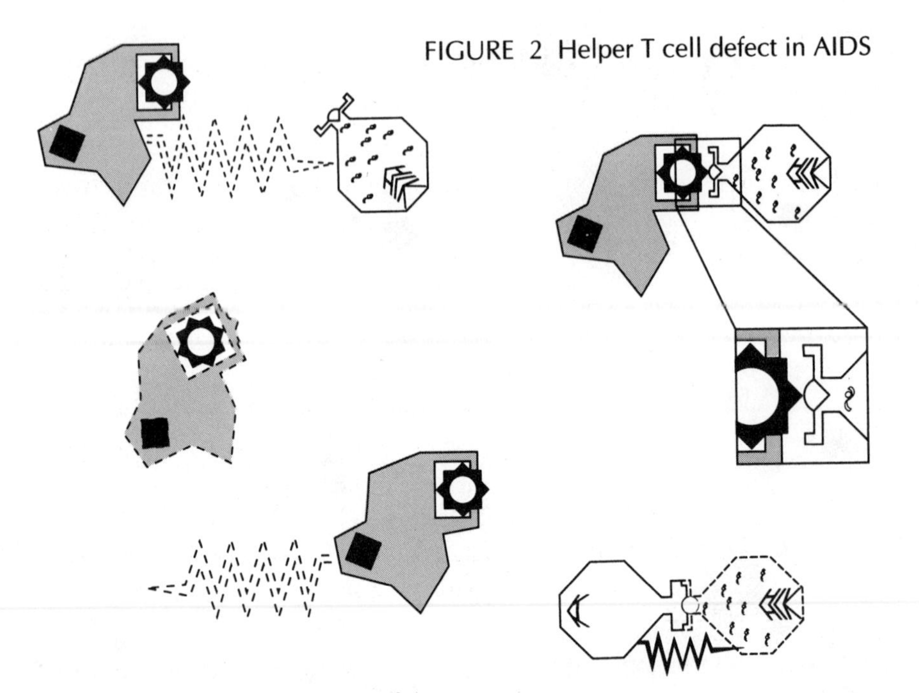

1. After engulfing pathogen, macrophage attracts HIV-infected helper T cell but (2, 3) HIV-induced receptor defect does not permit coupling. 4. Unprimed, the infected helper T cell fails to mobilize immunity and is eventually destroyed. 5. All its efforts to alert helper T cells to no avail, the macrophage (6) eventually dies, unable to digest engulfed pathogen.

often catch what other parts miss. Yet if the immune system is overtaxed because of disease, stress, or environmental factors, even the redundant parts can fail. In such cases, HIV might sneak up on a helper T cell. Since a helper T cell's lock-and-key mechanism is, in a sense, the eyes of the cell, HIV can be compared to an attacker that goes first for the eyes of its victim. HIV grapples on to and disables the lock-and-key mechanism through which a helper T cell senses its world, leaving the T cell helplessly blind. Several lines of AIDS research are looking for ways to prevent this initial onslaught by trying to provide helper T cells with "safety glasses" that will prevent HIV from putting their eyes out.

Helper T cells are crucial to immunity not because they fight pathogens directly but because they call and direct the troops into action. A helper T cell "primed" by a macrophage produces a substance that attracts more helpers and other kinds of T cells to the site of infection and causes them to multiply. Meanwhile, the original helper T cell keeps on attracting new macrophages. These ingest more pathogens and produce more substances that promote the growth of more T cells. The new T cells in turn produce more substances that attract still more macrophages and T cells, and so on in a chain reaction. Increasing phagocytosis and production of substances that lure macrophages and promote the growth of helper T cells eventually defeat the invaders.[c]

Primed helper T cells also activate killer, or cytotoxic, T cells. These cells destroy any infected body cell that shows an invader's antigen. Killer T cells are the commandos of the immune system. They rupture the walls and spill the contents of infected cells in which viruses and certain kinds of bacteria grow. Yet in AIDS, because of the defective lock-and-key mechanism, helper T cells cannot activate killer T cells.

Many opportunistic AIDS diseases are those in which viruses and bacteria lie protected inside infected cells, untouched by the other components of the immune system that still function. Sooner or later a pathogen has to leave one host cell to invade another, and that's when other parts of the immune system come into action. HIV might avoid the hazards of leaving the host cell by making use of the social habits of helper T cells. Helper T cells are geared into action not only by stimulatory substances but also by intimate contact with other helper T cells. Thus, when an infected helper T couples with an uninfected one, it passes HIV on, and the infection spreads.

Once macrophages and helper and killer T cells ward off an invader, the large amount of regulatory substances that these cells produced in the effort trigger into action another kind of lymphocyte, the suppressor T cell. Through cell contact and as yet undetermined substances, suppressor T cells deactivate the army of primed immune cells, thus preventing them from turning against the healthy cells of the body. After suppression ends, a few lymphocytes remain circulating that are keyed to the antigens of the vanquished invader. These memory cells will trigger a quicker immune reaction the next time the same pathogen invades the body.

Normally, there should be at least two helper T cells for every suppressor. The proportion is reversed in people with AIDS or ARC, indicating a low helper/suppressor ratio. In ARC or in the initial stages of AIDS, the ratio is low because there are too many suppressor T cells in action. This low *relative* number of helper T cells is typical in other diseases also and is not necessarily indicative of AIDS. In full-blown AIDS, however, there is a low ratio because not enough helper T cells exist (a low *absolute* number).

Why is the helper/suppressor ratio reversed in AIDS? As HIV infection progresses, the increasing infected helper T cells most likely keep on producing substances that regulate the function of other immune cells. The lock-and-key mechanisms of these infected cells are damaged, however, preventing the cell contact necessary for effective immune regulation. Yet the large amount of regulatory chemicals in the blood tell the suppressors it's time to quiet things down. The infected helper T cells, however, cannot be calmed down. Like blind, deaf, and numb individuals screaming for help, they cannot tell that the suppressors have come to their aid. They will keep on screaming until they die, and the number of suppressors will keep on growing until they turn off other healthy and uninfected helper T cells. Immunity will deteriorate.

A malfunction of suppressor cells brings about autoimmune illness, wherein overstimulated immune cells attack different parts of the body itself. Malfunctioning suppressors are unable to stop immune hyperactivity in illnesses such as rheumatoid arthritis, systemic lupus erythematosus, and multiple sclerosis. The overactive immunity of these diseases might give us a clue to the suppressed immunity of AIDS. Many people with AIDS possess some of the substances that characterize autoimmune diseases—the rheumatoid arthritis and lupus complexes, for example. Both ARC and AIDS might be brought about not merely by viral infection but also by the destructive attack of the immune system upon its master switch: the helper T cell. Once this last attack begins, AIDS becomes an autoimmune disease.

Helper T cells also initiate the production of antibodies by the B lymphocytes, activating them through lock-and-key mechanisms and stimulatory substances.[d] Antibodies are the spies and saboteurs of the immune system. As spies, they bind to the surface of the invader, identifying it for destruction by phagocytes. As saboteurs, they react with the pathogen's toxins and neutralize them. And whenever conditions are right, antibodies can also destroy a pathogen on their own. They initiate on its surface the assembly of a specific sequence of proteins: the complement proteins. When the last of these proteins locks into place, the assemblage explodes, killing the invader. Antibodies perform their job through a lock-and-key mechanism similar to that of T cells. Unfortunately, these accomplished undercover agents function only outside cells and are powerless against pathogens ensconced inside their cellular host. Antibodies do not work against viruses either, whether viruses lie outside or inside cells. Like many spies and saboteurs, antibodies can also forget where their loyalties belong and turn against healthy cells, producing autoimmune reactions.[e]

In AIDS, however, the antibody production is out of sync. B cells produce either too few necessary antibodies or too many unnecessary ones. Some of the antibodies produced in abnormally high quantities may be directed against helper T cells. Thus, a second attack against the helpers may help bring down the absolute number of helper T cells to levels observed in full-blown AIDS.

Whether one develops ARC, AIDS with Kaposi's sarcoma, or AIDS with other opportunistic infections might depend on whether or not, and at what stage, the HIV and autoimmune attacks on helper T cells stop. One particularly promising line of treatment we will discuss later seeks to counteract the autoimmune phase of AIDS.

A note on suntanning and immune suppression: Macrophages might not be the only cells capable of presenting antigens to and activating T cells. Certain skin cells[f] also activate T cells through antigen presentation and indeed could account for a substantial amount of all immune function. Ultraviolet rays that cause sunburn can destroy these important skin cells, severely impairing immune function. Because of such harmful suppression, laboratory mice exposed to severe doses of ultraviolet rays have developed bodywide immune deficiency.[3] Researchers have also found significant reduction of these skin cells in people with AIDS and ARC.[4] For these individuals, as well as for those who want to safeguard their immunity, excessive tanning might be unwise, especially if achieved through sunburning rather than through very gradual exposure to the sun.

In general, helper T cells control other helpers as well as macrophages, killer and suppressor T cells, and B lymphocytes. The defense they provide takes some time to organize, but, once in place, it is singularly effective against many fungi and viruses and some bacteria. In people with ARC and AIDS the defense is ineffective or lacking. There are other immune mechanisms still operating in AIDS, however, and these provide some measure of protection.

Helper-regulated immunity is called specific immunity; the other kind of immunity is nonspecific immunity. When confronted with an unfamiliar pathogen—or a new variation of an old one—specific immunity takes a while to go into action, as I have said. Specific forces need to be assembled, multiplied, and taught how to fight the invader. How does the body cope with the attack, say, when bacteria enter through a wound and the specific forces are still in boot camp? Nonspecific immunity springs into action as soon as an invader breaches protective body or organ surfaces. Because these forces are not antigen-specific, they are quicker to mobilize, although they cannot muster the strength-in-numbers of specific immunity. These forces are indeed the militia of the body, a group of cells always on alert for attack. They are the neutrophils or granulocytes and the natural killer (or NK) cells.

Neutrophils are phagocytes that ingest bacteria, certain fungi, and a lot of debris; they form an important complement to T cell and B cell immunities. Not only are they part of initial defense, but they also constitute the occupation forces. They clean up the battleground and help things return to normal after a T cell–mediated attack. Neutrophils prevent pathogens such as certain fungi from spreading through the body and causing systemic infection. Most neutrophil capability is intact in AIDS patients, a fact that explains why people with AIDS do not catch just any disease. Neutrophils also neutralize the by-products of allergic or hypersensitive reactions. Neutrophils too busy doing this, however, might not have time to help fight off disease. To make things easier for these immune cells, it might be best to avoid all those dietary or environmental substances that would unduly engage them.

The other kind of nonspecific cell, the natural killer cell (not to be confused with the killer T cell), is a kind of civilian commando—a vigilante, so to speak. It destroys cells turned cancerous or infected by viruses and at times seems to circumvent the macrophage/T cell mechanism. Indeed, lack of natural killer cells is the cause of the Chediak-Higashi syndrome, a condition in which patients with normal T and B cell populations are susceptible to recurring infections and have a very high cancer rate.[5] Some investigators report that an increase in vitamin C intake may protect these patients against infections.[6]

Absence of NK cells may account for a newborn infant's susceptibility to the herpes simplex virus. NK activity is also deficient in AIDS patients with chronic herpes infections. NK cells produce alpha interferons. Unlike antibodies, alpha interferons penetrate cell membranes and inhibit viral reproduction within infected cells. Alpha interferon production is normal in people with Kaposi's sarcoma who have no severe infections but is very low in people with AIDS who have other opportunistic infections. In others with AIDS a high level of a particular alpha interferon might indicate continuing immune deterioration.[7] A lively layperson's guide to all the immune components and substances we have discussed is *In Self-Defense* by Steven B. Mizel and Peter Jaret. Table 2 also summarizes these immune components.

The immune mechanisms described above do not exist in isolation from the rest of the body. Evidence is growing of an intimate relationship between the immune and nervous systems. Some researchers have gone so far as to propose that the immune system might be a sense organ. Just as the eyes provide visual and the ears aural information, the immune system might provide molecular data to the brain. This close connection between immunity and the brain is curiously paralleled by the affinities of HIV. In addition to having an appetite for helper T cells, the virus shows an attraction to certain brain cells and may be associated with various brain dysfunctions seen in AIDS. The connection between brain and immunity has also instigated a novel experimental treatment for AIDS that uses substances that affect brain cell receptors to stimulate T cells into action.

Whether or not the immune system is a sensory organ for "molecular touch," it nonetheless seems closely linked to the nervous and endocrine systems that control behavior. All the organs

TABLE 2 Components of the immune system

	MAIN FUNCTIONS	ORIGIN
SPECIFIC IMMUNITY	[One cell, one pathogen; delayed reaction]	
CELLULAR IMMUNITY		
CELLS:		
Macrophages	Ingest pathogens; present antigens to helper T cells	-
T lymphocytes		
Helper	Allow macrophages to digest; prime other T cells	-
Killer	Destroy cancer and infected cells	-
Suppressor	Inhibit helper T and killer T cells	-
Langerhans' cells	Present antigens to helper T cells in the skin	-
Keratinocytes	Produce interleukin-1 in the skin	-
SUBSTANCES:		
Lymphokines		
Interleukin-1	Induces helper T cells into action;	Macrophages; keratinocytes
Interleukin-2	Makes helpers and killers multiply	Helper T cells
Gamma interferon	Keeps macrophages at site of infection and helps them digest; activates killer T cells; makes B cells better at antibody production	Helper T cells
B cell growth factor	Causes B cells to multiply	Helper T cells
B cell differentiation factor	Makes B cells stop multiplying and start producing antibodies	Helper T cells
Alpha and beta interferons	Interfere with viruses in infected cells	Various immune cells
HUMORAL IMMUNITY		
B lymphocytes	Produce antibodies	
Antibodies	Identify pathogens for phagocytes.	B cells
IgM	Produced on first exposure to pathogen; triggers complement proteins	
IgG	Produced on subsequent exposures; triggers complement proteins	
IgA	Functions like IgM and IgG on mucous membranes	
IgE	Participates in allergic reactions	
IgD	Present on B cell surfaces; may help in their differentiation	
Complement proteins	Lock onto pathogens in sequence and implode them	
NONSPECIFIC IMMUNITY	[One cell, many pathogens; immediate reaction]	
Granulocytes	Eat bacteria, fungi, and debris	
Natural killer cells	Kill cancerous cells and those infected by virus	

of immunity show nervous connections to the brain. The part of the nervous system involved in the stress response apparently controls activity in the thymus, the organ where helper, killer, and suppressor T cells undergo their initial training. In fact, the thymus usually shrivels or shrinks in rats kept under extreme stress. Similar connections exist in the bone marrow, where white blood cells are produced, and in the spleen, where many white blood cells collect to exchange information and engage in phagocytosis.[8, 9]

The hormone epinephrine, or adrenaline, is partly responsible for the stress response and is also one of the chemical messengers of the nervous system. Epinephrine decreases helper and increases suppressor T cell activity, thus putting a damper on the immune response. That's why too much stress isn't good for you. Other substances produced by the nervous system might stimulate immunity. The endorphins and enkephalins produced in the brain after strenuous exercise, for example, enhance helper T cell activity. The nervous system produces hundreds of such substances, called neurotransmitters, and white blood cells possess surface receptors for many of them. Macrophages have receptors for all.

These neurochemical and nerve fiber connections between the central nervous system and the immune system provide evidence, however tentative, that we might have access to immune control through the hardware of the brain, and therefore possibly through its software, the mind.

STRESS

The brain prepares the body for stress by sending alarm signals through the sympathetic nervous system. This subdivision of the central nervous system increases heartbeat and blood flow and stimulates glandular secretions. The presence of sympathetic nerve fibers in various immune organs or tissues suggests that the sympathetic system also controls immunity during stress reactions. Although researchers have discovered that the stress response generally suppresses immunity, they have yet to work out exactly how and when such stress-induced immune suppression leads to illness.

What is stress? If by this question we are asking which factors create stress for you or me, there is no one answer. Although stress implies a kind of tension or pressure, what is stressful for one individual might not be for another, and vice versa. In discussing stress, then, it is easier to start with those nervous, hormonal, and immunologic responses that are common to all individuals. We shall call these objective and measurable body changes *the stress response* in order to distinguish them from the subjective and variable pressures generally called stress.

The body needs the stress response for survival because that's how it reacts to any threat—real or imagined, external or internal. An organism responds to threat in one of two ways: actively, by fighting or running away from it, or passively, by tolerating it. Variations on these fight-or-flight reactions help the organism adapt to a changing environment. More specifically, the biological stress syndrome, called the general adaptation syndrome (GAS), has three stages: alarm, resistance, and exhaustion. In response to stress the body first shifts into high gear for action, then goes into intense activity, and finally shuts itself down to rest. The first two stages help the body adjust to the increased demands of a stressful situation (table 3 details physiological changes in these two stages). The final stage helps the body recuperate after intense activity.

You are walking in a city park and a mugger approaches you. Almost instantly your sympathetic nervous system goes into action. It stimulates the adrenal medulla to produce large quantities of the hormones epinephrine and norepinephrine that shift

TABLE 3
The Stress Response

Accelerated pulse
Activation of blood-clotting mechanisms
Cessation of digestion
Dilation of the pupils
Enlargement and hyperactivity of the adrenal cortex
Increased blood pressure
Increased breathing rate
Increased muscle tension
Increased perspiration
Increased production of cortisol
Release of stored sugars and fats into the bloodstream
Shrinkage of the thymus gland

Adapted from Hans Selye, *Stress without Distress,* and from the Bob Hope International Heart Research Institute, *Start Taking Charge: Adapting to Stress.*

your metabolism into high gear.[g] At the same time, the sympathetic nervous system inhibits your immune response so that all energies will be directed to the situation at hand. The alarm mechanism also stimulates your pituitary gland, the control center of most hormone production in your body. Pituitary secretions trigger the adrenal cortex to produce cortisol.[h] This steroid hormone increases the efficiency of your glucose metabolism, which provides you with the extra energy you need to confront the mugger. It also inhibits tissue inflammation, thereby curtailing any possible slump in blood flow and oxygen delivery. All this increased efficiency, however, has a price: cortisol also inhibits the action of the macrophages, lymphocytes and white blood cells necessary for maintaining immunity.[i]

Now you are ready for the fight-or-flight confrontation with the mugger. You start to sweat, your pupils dilate, your heart races, your blood pressure climbs, and the sugars and fatty acids in your blood increase. Your body is primed to do more than is normally expected of it. The mugger, however, decides you're not worth it, slips away, and leaves you all strung out. You hobble to the nearest bench and collapse. That night you come down with a cold.

If your encounter with the mugger had been followed by physical exertion, it would have done you little harm. If you had fought or run away, all the released hormones and chemicals would have been used as intended. Muscles would have been worked out and tension and waste products released. During the last stage of the stress response, exhaustion, those primary neurophysiological changes would have subsided quickly. Your tired-out body would have then fallen into deep relaxation and eventually returned to normal.

Whether you're the type who flees from or fights muggers, you most likely don't run into them daily. The stress response is usually triggered by events we can neither flee from nor fight. They might represent either real or imagined dangers, but your neuroendocrine system cannot differentiate between them. A mugger in the park, a monster in a dream, a work deadline, an argument with a relative, or a good dose of rush hour traffic will all produce the same response: the production of powerful hormones and chemicals that rev you up for action.

In the modern world, several factors prevent us from avoiding stressful situations or from acting out and nullifying the stress response. Modern stressors are rarely physical, concrete, or avoidable. (You can run away from a bear in the woods, but how do you run away from a deadline?) Fighting *and* fleeing are usually considered unacceptable behaviors in our society. Stress often builds up because it cannot be directed toward any specific target. Moreover, our lives have very little strenuous physical activity that will make the stress response subside. The biochemical changes produced by stress—especially those that lower immunity—become chronic and potentially detrimental to health.

So the way to avoid damage to your health is to avoid stress, right? Wrong! There is no way (or reason) to avoid all stress because stress is the result of everything we do or come in contact with. Hans Selye states, in *Stress without Distress:* "Biological stress is the nonspecific response of the body to any demand made upon it."[10] The body strives to maintain a delicate equilibrium between external forces and internal functions. But no matter whether it causes pain or pleasure, everything we come in contact with alters this equilibrium or homeostasis. The body will then try to compensate for the new factors and search for the elusive middle ground it favors. This urge toward balance—often sensed as a vague, inexplicable, uneasy feeling—is the essence of stress. This kind of stress—or *eustress,* as Selye calls it—is both unavoidable and necessary because it forces the body to adapt to the unceasing changes in life. Without it, we would be hard put to survive.

TABLE 4 Signs of distress

Dry mouth and throat	Talking too fast
Sweating	Proneness to errors
Heart palpitations	Feelings of unreality
Headaches	Desire to run away
Nausea	Tendency to be startled by small sounds
Indigestion	Trembling or sighing
Queasiness	Grinding the teeth
Stomach cramps or knots	Biting the lips
Weakness or dizziness	Stroking moustache or beard
Fatigue or weariness	Twirling or twisting the hair
Nightmares	Biting fingernails
Insomnia	Wagging the legs
Depression	Clammy hands
Irritability	Clenched fists
Hyperactivity	Rocking back and forth
Floating anxiety	Frequent need to urinate
Ready tears	Over or under eating
Inability to concentrate	Oversleeping
Confusion	Chain smoking
Stuttering or other speech difficulties	Alcoholism and drug dependence

Adapted from Hans Selye, *The Stress of Life*, and from the Bob Hope International Heart Research Institute, *Start Taking Charge: Adapting to Stress.*

Indifference toward life might reduce stress, but only death will free us from it.

Unlike merely biological stress, the kind of stress that increases susceptibility to disease—and that Selye calls *distress*—is subjective in nature. This harmful stress reflects "the perception of individuals that their life circumstances have exceeded their capacity to cope."[11] In a given stressful situation, certain people will thrive and others will wither. Individuals who thrive on stress have been found to be hardier, that is, able to make the most of a situation; individuals who wither under stress, on the other hand, feel they have lost control—they have given up. (See table 4 for some of the common signs of distress.)

Animal experiments support the theory that stressful situations become harmful when control is lost. For example, Canadian researchers implanted cancer cells in two groups of mice. Both groups received electric shocks, but one was given the chance to escape before the shocks while the other was not. The cancer rate was higher in the mice who received the inescapable jolts.[12] Other experiments have shown that a similarly induced sense of helplessness in rats depresses their immune functions. Mice subjected to various types of inescapable stress appear more susceptible to infection by viruses, bacteria and parasites.[13]

An experience that prompts an individual to give up—a change in a relationship, for example—triggers a sense of helplessness: the person feels let down, left out, or deprived. This helplessness reinforces the person's perceived lack of power, bringing about hopelessness. The individual feels incapable of meeting self-imposed standards, no matter how realistic these might be, and gives up.

Giving up is a result of feeling both let down and unable to meet life's demands. The giving-up complex explains why many men show depressed immune function and higher death rates as long as one year after a spouse's death. Such bereaved men often feel unable to cope with life; life becomes a source of distress. Although the giving-up complex itself does not cause disease, a predisposition to physical problems and illness often rides the rear of its emotional train.[14]

In gay men the emotional train is often overloaded beyond capacity. We have to cope not only with life's regular stresses—which can translate into dangerous distress—but also with the stress of being homosexual in a society that actively and often ruthlessly condemns homosexuality. Coping with this last source of stress is the essence of the gay experience, though there may be many coping styles with various degrees of success. For those who choose to remain in the closet, the stress of being discovered is frequent and intense. For those who have fully come out, the stress of being homosexual is diminished but will occasionally come into full force—as, for example, when the Supreme Court decides that what you do in your bed with a consenting adult friend is the business of the state and the police. But for many the stress of being homosexual is not so clear-cut.

Many of us have come out by moving to the gay ghetto of a big city only to return to the closet when we visit our parents or confront our employers or straight friends. Some of us have come out of the social closet—everyone we value knows—but remain in the emotional closet. We cannot experience our sexuality as being totally natural. We have not fully examined what being homosexual, let alone becoming a better person, means. Many of us reveled in the new-found sexual freedom of the seventies while the self-hate tapes of our childhood and adolescence continued to run.

Denial of our personhood abounds in the coping styles so commonly observed in a gay bar. There, we seek to forget our problems and any negative feelings that might remind us of them. As a result of the denial and low self-worth programmed into us, we often turn to drugs, alcohol, compulsive sex, and improper diets, thereby depriving our bodies of adequate sleep and rest. What's more, today, for those of us who want no soup, life seems to have served us a second cup. As if the stresses of society's or our own homophobia weren't enough, we now have to deal with the often inescapable stress of AIDS. The constant uncertainty and anxiety about getting AIDS can often be unbearable. I have often felt as if I were in a concentration camp, waiting for my turn. Other gay men feel the same.

A pilot study of people with AIDS conducted during 1982 by the University of California in San Francisco uncovered several frequent stress-related themes. Although coping styles varied, they often included denial—that is, plodding ahead despite one's emotions—and avoidance of so-called negative feelings such as anger. Many of the people under study experienced stressful events during the year before diagnosis or expressed guilt about their homosexuality or about previous sexual activity (those who didn't sometimes were doing better immunologically). Others had felt difficulty in fully coming out to parents or employers.[15] Of course, none of these factors caused AIDS in these men; there might be no such thing as an AIDS-prone personality. But when considered singly or in combination with the helplessness and hopelessness felt about the disease, they add up to extreme distress. Such emotional strain could have opened the way for more tangible AIDS cofactors—use of drugs and alcohol; poor nutrition; parasites, fungi, and viruses—that could have sent immune function into a downward spiral. In a sense, AIDS could be seen as the ultimate stress-induced shutdown of immunity.

What should you do about the stresses of AIDS and of being homosexual in a homophobic society? First, accept the reality of AIDS. I know it's a bitch, but it's here. Try to do something about it by helping others and thus yourself. Physical chores like grocery shopping for a bedridden friend can help you work stress out of your system. Second, be honest with others about your emotions. Remain kind and considerate, but be sure to let others in on what's going on. If you cannot communicate your feelings to someone, write them down in a letter, which you can deliver or not as you see fit. Finally, if you're afraid people will know you are gay, then all the more reason to come out! It is the fear of being found out that is stressful. Coming out is like a visit to the dentist. Put it behind you and it will no longer haunt you. Let people react to your gayness however they wish to react. In the end, those who really care about you probably won't even bat an eye. Most likely they have known all along.

MIND, BODY, AND HEALTH

Through the stress response, emotional strain temporarily suppresses immune function. Chronic emotional stress could eventually erode a person's hardiness and open the way for immune dysfunction and illness. We can conclude that by controlling emotional stress we can also influence immune function and health beneficially. The theory is simpler than the practice, however. No one fully understands the nature of thought and emotion, much less how complex mental and emotional processes interact with the immune system. Yet progress is being made. Psychoneuroimmunology, the emerging branch of medicine that studies the relationship between mind, brain, and disease, is steadily confirming what we have always known intuitively—that the mind does influence health and disease.

Although this information in a way confirms Norman Vincent Peale's gospel of positive thinking, wellness is not only a matter of correct thought (if this were the case, I would have circulated a list of "right thoughts to think" instead of writing this book). Analytical thoughts occur on the surface of the mind. They are a reflection of those deeper processes[k] that determine the chronic attitudes and emotions that in turn may influence our health. Trying to control mind and brain—and, ultimately, immunity—through analytical thought alone would be like trying to stop water from boiling by blowing on it while the heat is still on. In other words, thinking that you feel fine while you hold, deep inside, an anger carried over from childhood is not as effective as reaching in and feeling and looking at the root of that anger so that, eventually, you will be able to think, "I feel fine." Like water falling on a stone, positive thoughts eventually erode chronic emotions, yet positive thoughts can often be too slow. Reaching into the deeper processes of emotion—while still thinking positively—can offer a quicker way of changing the chronic mental states that affect our health.

Like stress, emotions have both objective and subjective components. These components, however, are so intimately related as to be inseparable. Everything occurs at the same time during emotional response. When we are angry, for example, our heart beats faster and our blood rushes, our face muscles tense into a scowl, and we feel uncomfortable, all at the same time. Although emotions do not occur in any one place in the brain, they do have physiological, behavioral, and subjective components associated with specific brain locales. The physiological component—increased heart rate and blood pressure, for example—can be associated with the hypothalamus, a small region of the brain that controls the body's hormone production. Behavioral aspects of emotions—such as a scowl or menacing posture—are controlled by the limbic system, a complex neural network that includes the hypothalamus. The subjective aspect of emotion—the perception of anger, for instance—occurs mainly in the neocortex, the outermost area of the brain where conscious thought and volition originate. The instantaneousness of a surge of anger after an insult tells us how closely these three areas are connected and how quickly they feed back to one another.

The hypothalamus is both a gland that secretes hormones and a bundle of nerves that acts as one of the brain's master switches. It maintains homeostasis, or the internal equilibrium of the body, by controlling body temperature, thirst, hunger, water balance, and sexual functions. Most important, the hypothalamus relays signals that control involuntary functions like heartbeat and digestion, and translates many nervous impulses into blood chemicals that control hormone production throughout the body. For example, your hypothalamus controls the sympathetic nervous activity and pituitary secretions that trigger the fight-or-flight reaction during an encounter with a mugger. Damage to the hypothalamus results in suppressed immune function.

The neocortex of the forebrain processes stressful situations and compares them with past experience. The limbic system relays this information to the hypothalamus, where it is translated into emotion-inducing hormones. By connecting the neocortex and hypothalamus in this way, the limbic system is responsible for the expression of emotions. Without the limbic connections our emotions would be out of control or inappropriate. The limbic system also governs the expression of instinct and motivation, thus controlling the survival activities of the body: food procurance, self-preservation, procreation, and the perception of pain and pleasure. (Figure 3 illustrates the interaction between neocortex, limbic system, and hypothalamus.) Although specific correlations between forebrain or limbic system and susceptibility to disease are difficult to pinpoint, several studies indicate a possible connection.

People with an unusual disorder called alexithymia are incapable of verbalizing even the strongest of emotional experiences, especially the so-called negative ones. Besides often being unaware of their emotions, these individuals seem predisposed to physical illness. Alexithymic personality traits have been found among people with certain autoimmune disorders such as rheumatoid arthritis and systemic lupus erythematosus as well as among many individuals with cancer or infectious diseases such as tuberculosis. Researchers speculate that alexithymia might be caused by faulty connections between the forebrain and the limbic-hypothalamic network, or by a severed link between the left and right hemispheres of the brain. At any rate, researchers believe that emotions and stress reactions when felt but unexpressed may seek alternate expression through illness. In a possibly corresponding way, chronic suppression or denial of negative emotions as a way of coping with life is often found in people with AIDS.

By tightening or loosening control over our emotions, we can suppress or enhance them. Conscious or unconscious impulses from the forebrain may override activity in the limbic system or

FIGURE 3 Physiological Basis of Emotion

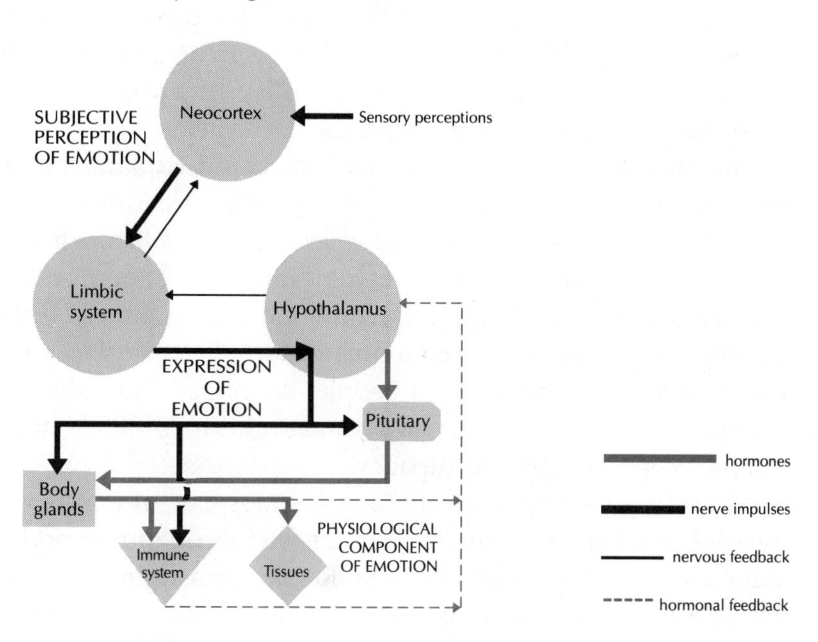

hypothalamus. We can therefore suppress or enhance not only emotions but also less tangible behavior patterns whose expression is rooted in these brain structures. Motivation, for example, is basically a matter of seeking a reward or pleasure and avoiding punishment or pain, activities that are controlled in animals by two small limbic regions. Nerve fibers to and from these two limbic areas come together in the hypothalamus. A person often perceives this pleasure/pain motivation, along with its sociocultural embellishments, as *purpose.*

It is not surprising, then, that inhibition of motivation may lead to certain immune irregularities and disease. The "inhibited power-motivation syndrome" exists in individuals who feel great need for power but have little interest in family and intimate friendships. Such people exercise enormous self-control and often suppress their hostility. When their need for power is frustrated, these individuals show lower concentrations of salivary immunoglobulins, greater susceptibility to upper respiratory infections, and increased epinephrine in the urine.

Similar biopsychosocial mechanisms could explain the higher statistical incidence of illness among low-status minorities and individuals caught in status inconsistencies (e.g., an M.B.A. who takes a job as a bartender or a gay man who cannot make the mental transition between an executive daytime job and nighttime activities among the leather crowd). Depression might also play a role in immune suppression in such people: depressed individuals have large amounts of stress-related hormones in their blood, and measurably impaired immune capacity.

Minor emotional or motivational states can often also cause physiological change—just putting oneself through the motions of emotion can sometimes be enough. Researchers at the University of California in San Francisco found that actors who relive a past emotional experience or merely mimic emotions have the same involuntary heart rate or skin temperature reactions as if they were experiencing the real thing. Such mimicry might even have an indirect effect on immune function.

Experiments with mental imagery that creates pictures in the mind to attain a desired effect (like the destruction of cancer cells by lymphocytes) show that thymus activity increases during a positive visualization but decreases during a negative one.[16, 17, 18] The body doesn't seem to distinguish between the real and the imagined. As a result of the hopelessness and helplessness associated with AIDS, many people with the disease are too quick to visualize the details of forthcoming immune deterioration. One wonders to what extent this activity amplifies immune deficiency.

Science has confirmed our long-held belief that the mind affects the body. Certain emotional and motivational states can cause subtle neurological changes, which in turn may affect the way the immune system works. The neurochemical changes produced by distress and misdirected emotion seem to involve a swing away from the internal equilibrium that the hypothalamus strives to maintain. Like a tower with a weak structural support, a person in internal disequilibrium cannot withstand the onslaught of external agents of disease. That is the nature of susceptibility.

With this in mind, we should now define health positively as the balance among the interior physiological, mental, and spiritual and the exterior biological, social, and environmental forces rather than defining it negatively as the absence of disease.[19] This definition allows us to see how, for example, the disappearance of AIDS-related opportunistic infection alone does not in fact guarantee health. The complex interactions among these forces make the equilibrium of health dynamic. This equilibrium fluctuates around a center the way a scale balances on its fulcrum. On any given day, a perfectly ordinary person will feel the usual aches and discomforts that are signs of the perfectly ordinary balancing act of health. Even the most perfect of persons cannot attain perfect health.

Conversely, our positive definition of health implies that even someone with an imperfect immune system can attain a healthy internal equilibrium. Where the balance is struck doesn't matter as long as it indeed happens. To establish equilibrium one must avoid unbalancing factors such as immunosuppressive therapies, alcohol, drugs, and poor diet while engaging in activities that counterbalance a radically off-center immune system and strengthen the fulcrum of one's existence: oneself. I will discuss many of these rebalancing activities in later chapters.

DISEASE AS MESSENGER

Seeing health as an always sought but elusive equilibrium brings you a new perspective on disease. Disease is no longer an enemy that noisily intrudes upon your daily pleasures; rather, it is a messenger whose gentle initial warnings turn into shouts if ignored. Through disease, your body directs your attention to a forthcoming equilibrium crisis, one that might have not only biological but also psychological and spiritual roots.

I have talked about physical, or energetic, connections between mind, brain, and body. These links are not random processes. A hormone molecule, for instance, has a specific shape that is recognized by those cells upon which the hormone acts. All interchanges in the equilibrium of health possess similar order and organization, and thus, they convey *information.*[l] Health is the optimum exchange of information necessary for equilibrium between the body, brain, mind, and spirit[m] as well as between the individual and the environment. Figure 4 illustrates the different organizational levels present in an individual. Health is the amount of connectedness existing between these levels.

Disease, on the other hand, is disconnectedness, a nonoptimum flow of information among the organizational levels of an individual. Conventional medicine, for example, views bacterial or viral infection as *the* disease, but information theory regards it as part of a larger process. In this wider definition, psychosocial or genetic factors disrupt the normal discourse between nervous and immune systems, increasing susceptibility or worsening predisposition to outside agents. The idea of cause moves to the background. (In fact, in diseases like rheumatoid arthritis, cancer, or AIDS, where pathways to illness are often too numerous and intertwined, the concept of cause can often hinder.) Healing thus becomes more than merely treating symptoms. It involves discovering the relationship between the individual's disordered components and the adaptations to changed physical, mental, and spiritual circumstances that the symptoms reveal. Relationships between data can be called meaning. By trying to discover the disordered relationships that lead to illness, we are seeking meaning in disease.[20]

Disease can have meaning, but that doesn't imply that it is just the bodily manifestation of mental conflict, because the complex interaction between biopsychosocial factors makes such a view too simplistic. It does mean, however, that we must investigate all the factors that Western medicine has traditionally avoided. *Dis-ease* is your body's way of telling you that, by eating poorly, getting inadequate rest and exercise, being unable to cope with anxiety or stress, or holding on to beliefs and attitudes that prevent satisfying emotional experiences, you haven't treated it as well as you should have. Such maladaptive behavior is often the result of an all-too-common indulgent self-blame and lack of self-love. By this reasoning, AIDS is a disease caused by too little love rather than by too much sex.

In looking for meaning in your disease, however, you needn't blame others or yourself, or feel guilty about past actions. This is where I see the idea of cause as fruitless. Was it my drug abuse, compulsive sex life, poor diet, or self-hate that brought about my illness? I don't know, and it really doesn't matter. What matters is the message of my disease: that I need to take better care of myself now. Of course, while searching for meaning, you do find reasons for what you did, and you must look at those squarely to avoid guilt. I found I used compulsive sex to fill in for the love I thought I needed from others. But most important, I found I needed the love of others in order to feel whole.

Disease does not scold. It is, in fact, rather indifferent. Garrett Porter, a child who recovered from brain cancer using directed imagery, talks about responsibility and guilt in his book, *Why Me?*

FIGURE 4
Organizational levels in the individual

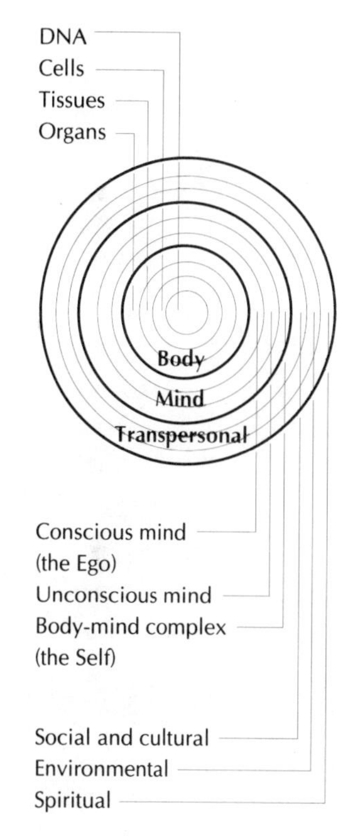

Redrawn from Alastair J. Cunningham, "Information and health in the many levels of man," *Advances* 3(1):32, Winter 1986.

> The idea that we can assume responsibility for the course of our illness suggests to some people that patients are being accused of causing their cancer, that guilt might be aroused by such an idea. Of course no one chooses to have cancer or causes their body to become cancerous in any conscious way. But the way our bodies unconsciously respond to stress may be, and probably is, a contributing factor in every stress-related illness. This is *good* news. It means that there is something we can do to affect it in a positive way.[21]

Disease can be seen as a call for personal transformation through metamorphosis. It is a transition from the death of your old self into the birth of your new. This centuries-old view, held equally by the ancients and the so-called primitive societies, has been strengthened by Carl Jung's work in psychoanalysis. Because of the meaning it could convey, illness is not a conscious weakness but an unconscious strength. In our culture, however, where generally feelings are given little attention and emotional needs ignored, the message of illness assumes even greater importance.

Illness is frequently the only way a person can satisfy unfulfilled needs. The love and care lavished on the ill can sometimes be a banquet for the lonely or love-hungry. Illness becomes a respite from problems we cannot solve or face, as when one catches the flu before an important deadline at work. This kind of relief from stress is seen in people who, after months of worry, are finally diagnosed with AIDS.

Disease can often be

- a way to vent suppressed hostility, usually toward ourselves;
- a means to influence someone else in our favor;
- a release from responsibility to ourselves and to others;

- an attempt to replace something or someone we have lost;
- an attempt to escape from inadequacy, real or imagined;
- a physical expression of emotional struggle;
- an escape from an unbearable situation;
- a temporary surrender of the will to live; or
- a form of slow suicide.

Because illness allows us to postpone or avoid underlying problems, it can also be a trap. One has a greater stake in staying sick when illness becomes the preferred mode of solving problems.

One way to avoid this entrapment is to listen to disease and open ourselves to the changes it can bring. Illness can help us

- override social conditioning;
- express our feelings;
- do away with too high expectations, our own or those of others;
- pay attention to our true needs and meet them openly for the first time ;
- throw away nonessential problems;
- accept care, attention, and love from others;
- modify undesirable habits;
- regroup and strengthen our psychological energy;
- learn more about ourselves and our fundamental values;
- rethink our understanding of health and sickness;
- re-examine the basic premises of our life;
- rebuild a stronger body; and
- gain incentives for growth.[22, 23]

Growth never ends.

Once in a while, disease hits me over the head again. It reminds me of my continuous need for transformation, balance, awareness, and growth. I am human and frail. I have my moments of pessimism and despair, and I cease to believe in and fail to love myself. I do stupid things and even repeat my mistakes, yet my body is always there to alert me, to say, "Hey, cool it! Whoa!"

My disease has been a demanding teacher that has guided me—sometimes with a heavy hand—toward what I need to do. I now do things not so much because of ARC but because I want to grow and realize my full self. How ironic it is that we often have to face death to learn about life. How beautiful, too. My disease is one of the best things that has happened to me; it has pulled me out of a quietly desperate life toward one full of love and hope.

Do not ignore the message of disease! If you do, your body will probably repeat its warning with greater severity and intensity until its final shout. Maybe that finality is the message intended for you. That's fine also, but you will never know what course to take if you don't listen to your illness.

Allow yourself the introspection granted by illness. Be gentle with yourself. If you respond to the message of disease, meet the demands of adaptation, and educate yourself to recognize and satisfy your true needs, you will reach a new level of awareness, and you will have taken a major step toward learning about yourself, your body, and your immunity, and toward reconnecting yourself to health.

CHAPTER 2

Nurturing health

HOPE

Few things in AIDS are as tragic as the hopelessness the disease can bring. Most people see no outcome to AIDS but death. Yet AIDS is not a hopeless disease. Neither hopelessness nor helplessness has to be a part of any disease at all. In fact, these attitudes often precede and hasten a number of fatal diseases. None of us can live long without hope, yet finding it can be difficult when we face AIDS.

Where should we seek hope for AIDS? Not in the six o'clock news. Television's message is one of endless hopelessness: no hope for treatment, no hope for cure, and no hope for an end to the deaths. Television presents what people like, and people like to be scared. The news draws on AIDS hysteria and feeds it back to already hyped viewers. For TV, AIDS is just another docudrama. Unless you believe they will contribute to your mental health, avoid the news and the so-called AIDS specials, and seek your information elsewhere.

Unfortunately, TV and the other news media are not our only sources of hopelessness. They take their cue from medical authorities whose well-intentioned but grim opinions can squelch hope in even the strongest optimist. Many doctors believe no hope is better than false hope, one that is later cruelly shattered by reality. But how can hope be false? By its very nature, false hope, like false truth, false beauty, or false good, cannot exist.

Malpractice suits, however, do exist, and offering no hope is often a doctor's surest way to avoid them. "According to the malpractice law," physician Robert F. Cathcart III states, "if you predict the worst, you're covered; if you're optimistic and you fail, you get sued."[1] A healthy amount of caution need not result in the bleak, untherapeutic attitude so common in medical circles today. Instead of saying, "This disease is serious. Most people don't live past eighteen months," a physician could say, "We don't really know how the disease will progress. There are several treatment avenues to explore, and we will certainly do our best to help you deal with the disease and keep a good quality of life." What your physician says often tells more about his or her attitude toward life than about the disease itself. At all costs avoid doctors who don't believe there's at least some hope for a person with AIDS.

Remaining staunchly pessimistic is like hiding your head in the sand. No matter how devastating, almost no disease in the world has proven 100 percent fatal, and AIDS is no exception. A small but growing number of people with AIDS have lived—and are still living—much longer than the predictions of their doctors. There are those who say these PWAs (persons with AIDS)[a] are *yet* to die of the disease. But when you find yourself living and enjoying life three or four years beyond your predicted time of death, that *yet* objection becomes a matter of mere words. Any of us might die in that period of time, and no one can foretell whether death is as close as an accident tomorrow or as far away as an old person's bed. This uncertainty allows us to look at the future any way we please. You can expect life just as easily as you can expect death.

Hope and a positive attitude are matters of choice, of seeing the glass half full rather than half empty. I do not for a moment suggest that you cheerlead yourself into an illusion of wellness, which is the kind of denial found in many participants in the San Francisco biopsychosocial AIDS pilot study. A positive attitude calls for a realistic, hard look at what is as well as the most optimistic assessment of what can be. Such an attitude toward AIDS begins only when you realize the disease is likely to be fatal. But you must go beyond this realization and recognize that although life will give you no guarantees, it will constantly offer you new possibilities. Failing to take this step toward hope, many people lie down and wait for death. Their tragedy rests not in dying (for there are those for whom death is a new opportunity) but in failing to live while alive. Surrendering your will to live by giving up and waiting passively for the end can be a last-ditch attempt to control and deny death by trying to have the last say about its time: "I will die now, when I want, and not later, when death wants."

Hopelessness can be alluring and comforting for some of us. Since life with AIDS can be so uncertain, we often grab on to the reassuring guarantee of death after AIDS. That's why so many gay men feel an initial relief when diagnosed. Immune deterioration spurs many people to make changes early on. But some of us interpret this signal to mean only that the disease is near and unavoidable. Our emotional life is thrown into chaos. The certainty of death can end one's emotional turmoil, so the idea of hope—the possibility that death might not happen after all—could raise a disquieting specter.

Why do some people cling adamantly to hope while others do not? Several studies suggest that hopelessness and lack of self-worth go together. One study found that 76 percent of subjects who felt hopeless about their cancer suffered from low self-esteem, usually a result of a stressful childhood occasioned by a broken home, abuse, or lack of closeness to their parents. "Why should I hope?" was a frequent theme. "The last time I did and opened myself up, I was let down. I will never go through that pain again."[2] Deep inside, these people were waiting to die because they could not live with themselves.

The message that "gay is no good," drummed into us as we grew up and still lurking in our minds, makes this kind of self-hatred too frequent among gays. Loving ourselves as gay people—let alone just as people—is often no easy task.

BEATING THE ODDS

Learning self-love and forgiveness is the first step toward strengthening hope and nurturing your health. "You have to forgive yourself first," says Los Angeles bodybuilding contestant and AIDS veteran Louie Nassaney; "then forgive the rest of the world, including your family. A lot of people have a lot of parental guidance they just don't agree with. They blame their parents for what happened in their life, and that's no way to get anywhere in this world. *You've got to do the work.*"

When Louie was diagnosed with Kaposi's sarcoma in 1982, he expected his doctors to save him immediately. Seven months of interferon treatment gave him very unpleasant side effects. Then the doctors wanted to try chemotherapy and radiation. Louie said no; friends who had undergone radiation and chemotherapy had died. Instead, he changed his diet, engaged in exercise and bodywork methods, and turned to the self-affirmation, meditation, and guided imagery techniques of Louise Hay, the director of the Love Yourself, Heal Yourself Center in Santa Monica, California. Louie also sought, and got, the support of family and friends.

"I cleaned up all the garbage," Louie says. "I talked a lot about death and about my personal friends who were dying. [Louise] said that was okay, that's part of what's going on." Louie's particular visualization consisted in "erasing" the purple lesion of his sarcoma as if it had been just pencil marks on his skin. Six months later, the doctors confirmed that his sarcoma had disappeared. Louie became a participant in the Los Angeles Superman Contest, a bodybuilding pageant in which he was runner-up. When I saw him at a San Francisco healing service last August, I would not have known he had AIDS. Those who had set their eyes on this beautifully muscular thirty–year–old man were also surprised when he told them about his disease. "My personal view is that the AIDS virus doesn't like people with AIDS to go and put energy into themselves and work out. When I go to the gym and do aerobics, I'm not being lazy and letting it grow. The virus might still exist in my body. But it's been three years now, and see how I look."[3,4]

San Francisco playwright and composer Dan Turner refused to crumple when he was diagnosed with Kaposi's sarcoma in February 1982. Dan remembered how depression and a belief that he would not get well had prolonged an earlier bout with hepatitis. "When I was told I had cancer," Dan says, "I reflected on that experience. I knew I could win. And I knew if I got into the same negative head trip again, it would kill me."

Believing that emotional expression through music, his lifelong avocation, would help lower stress, Dan started writing a musical after giving up his word-processing job and going on disability. To bolster his immunity Dan now works in his garden, practices transcendental meditation, has used acupuncture and Chinese herbal medicine, and employs the visualization techniques developed by well-known cancer therapists O. Carl Simonton and Stephanie Matthews Simonton.

Dan is a Catholic, so he uses the image of the doubting Thomas in his visualization. "I put my hands on the wounds of Christ," he says, "and feel the blood of Christ go through my hands, into my body, and eliminate all my toxins. The blood of Christ is such a powerful image if it's part of your faith." The week-long course of interferon shots Dan gives himself every third week does not seem to have produced serious side effects. He hasn't had any new sarcoma lesions since April 1982.

Although Dan became an activist and spokesman early in the fight against AIDS, he rose to national fame when a photograph in an AIDS article in the June 1986 issue of the *National Geographic* magazine showed him working out on a Nautilus machine. "People have to know they have an option," says Dan. "You can focus on living in the present moment, or you can get wrapped up in the horrors of the future and let those burden you. If you blame everything on AIDS and become obsessed with it, you can create a powerful monster within."[5]

Because stories about AIDS successes do not usually make the news (understandably, quite a few long-term survivors avoid publicity), the idea that one can survive the disease despite lack of a medical cure or effective treatment fails to reach many with AIDS. You do not have to go public in order to help spread hope, however. If you were diagnosed with AIDS four or more years ago and wish to participate in confidential survivor studies, you or your physician can write to the organizations listed under AIDS Complimentary Therapy in appendix H.

All AIDS treatment, conventional or not, is experimental. There are alternatives, however, to immunosuppressive drug and radiation treatments. The most widely known alternative has been developed by former National Institutes of Health researcher and physician Russell Jaffe in Vienna, Virginia. Dr. Jaffe's protocol uses a therapeutic diet, vitamin C, and several herbal preparations to bolster immunity. It includes conventional treatment where unavoidable—sulfa drugs or pentamidine for *Pneumocystis carinii* pneumonia (PCP), for example—but rejects immunosuppressive cancer chemotherapy or radiation treatment.

Jaffe's program also includes visualization techniques like those of the Simontons and Louise Hay. The program is one of self-healing. Although self-healing programs do not suggest that a person with AIDS carry all the responsibility for recovery, they operate on the idea that only the PWA can spark into action the biopsychosocial components of the self that promote healing. This method was once employed by the old-style family doctor, who was well aware of the self-healing aspect in all recovery. Jaffe's program also recommends small self-healing support groups as antidotes to the isolation and self-worthlessness brought about by the disease.

Dr. Jaffe's results are impressive. Of the nineteen people who started treatment between September 1982 and September 1983, eighteen were still alive in 1986. Of these people, six had Kaposi's sarcoma alone, five had had PCP, and eight had had both KS and PCP at the start of the program. All had begun therapy with helper/suppressor T ratios below 0.2. In 1986 the group average ratio rose to 0.8, with several individuals showing 1.8, only two-tenths below the value for a healthy person. More important, during treatment all group members developed an increased sense of well-being and a positive outlook on life. Self-healing, however, is not a one-shot deal; it is demanding and complex, and the program is equally rigorous.[6] "Health is easier to maintain than it is to acquire, just like the other significant possessions in our lives," says Jaffe. "If we make the investment in health, tangible reward is probable."[7] For an implementation of the Jaffe protocol by Oakland physician Keith D. Barton, see appendix A.

DEATH

Many people with AIDS or ARC show no progress despite their perseverance. Sometimes the disease cannot be reversed, and death then becomes an acceptable alternative. There comes a time in our lives when we feel we either have attained our goals or shouldn't struggle any longer to do so, when our desire for peace is greater than the happiness we derive from survival. At such times, death liberates.

Death is a natural process in which all of us sooner or later must participate, and we shouldn't feel guilty or defeated when we switch from fighting the disease to accepting death. But in accepting death we should approach it without anger or bitterness. It is sad that many people have died from AIDS hating and blaming themselves for having gotten the disease, bitterly accusing their gay brothers and sisters of abandoning them, and resenting the medical community for not curing them. What a terrible burden to bear as you leave this world! Freeing yourself from obligations has little to do with material matters such as debts, wills, and the disposition of your possessions (although these could be attended to, if the time and desire exist). But it has everything to do with *trying* to leave this world loving yourself and loving others. To die this way is never a failure. It is to die in a state of hope and grace.

Recurring symptoms or deterioration might be asking you to investigate two alternatives: dying or living. Even taking an honest approach to this question, you might find it difficult to choose between preparing yourself for death or working back towards health. This ambivalence and confusion is natural. If death haunts you, go inside, be introspective. Perhaps exploring and even visualizing the possibility of your death will bring you a measure of comfort. It is perfectly normal to wonder what your death will be like, how it will come about, if you will feel pain, and whether you want to be conscious. Do not shun such questions. Facing things is the essence of living.

THE WILL TO LIVE

After exploring your death, you might find yourself reaffirming life all the more. You have rekindled your will to live by being imaginative and creative about your death.

The will to live is a powerful biological and psychological force that operates unconsciously. It is perceived as a sense of connection with the rest of the universe and as being part of a higher order, often referred to as spirit. It is also a vital force that enhances your body's ability to fight disease. Some societies, such as some native American, Australian aborigine, and African tribes, believe that a person succumbs to disease because his or her spirit has been taken away. Many doctors today would agree with this observation. "[The will to live] is not a theoretical abstraction," says Norman Cousins, "but a physiologic reality with therapeutic characteristics."[8]

To be human is to engage in a struggle between the will to live and the will to die, a pull between our own creative and destructive forces, with love, hope, and freedom on one side and self-hate, hopelessness, and despair on the other. We can express our will to act, our will to propel ourselves forward, either creatively or destructively. When we express our creative energies fully, no room is left for destructive forces to operate. But when our creative forces are blocked by emotional entanglement or suppression, the destructive forces become unleashed and endanger our health.

Unlike animals, we possess few instincts that tell us what to do. We live mostly by choice, and during the twentieth century many of the traditions that once guided these choices have been lost. As a consequence, we often don't know what to do with our lives and live in what psychiatrist and concentration-camp survivor Victor E. Frankl calls the "existential vacuum." Our lives seem empty.

To ease this unbearable boredom, we resort to satisfying obsessions for money, possessions, and power. We turn to alcohol and addictive drugs and mindlessly pursue sexual pleasures. Self-destruction seems preferable to ennui.[9] (How many have committed suicide out of excruciating boredom?) When all these material pursuits lose their appeal—as they must at one point or another—we're back to the initial emptiness. Without meaning in our lives we become hopeless, and not knowing what to do we feel helpless. We give up on living.

Existential despair in gay men often results from the fear of aging. Many of us therefore fill our existential vacuum with an exclusive concern for physical beauty that we believe is at its best during our twenties and thirties. The forties signal the end of this beauty for many of us. Hair starts to thin out or gray, wrinkles appear, the body goes to pot, and life loses its meaning. How many times have you heard "I shall never live to be 40"? "AIDS is the perfect answer to check out at that age," says Louie Nassaney.

The existential vacuum need not exist. We *can* get back in touch with our will to live by trying to be a part of the rest of creation and seeing ourselves as part of a greater scheme of things. For some people this greater order might be God—the higher power personified. For others it might be the realization that things in the universe are interrelated in a way that defies explanation—a conceptual higher power.

When you wake up in the morning, try to feel grateful for your participation in the scheme of things. Give thanks for your food, for the rain and the sun, for the cold and the warmth, for your life. Whether or not you believe in a higher order doesn't matter. What does matter is the beneficial effect of giving thanks, which every once in a while reminds you that life is worth living. If you don't remind yourself of this or if you habitually start your day thinking how miserable it will be, you might eventually forget why life is worth living and decide to leave it.

MEANING AND PURPOSE IN LIFE

It is natural to ask why your disease happened to you because in doing so you are trying see how it is woven into the fabric of your life. You are trying to assign meaning to your disease. But in asking this question you risk falling into the trap of blaming rather than coping.

You might blame your parents for the inevitable mistakes they made, your friends for abandoning or failing to understand you, or the medical community for not coming up with a cure or treatment. If you are religious, you might even blame God for allowing your illness to exist. But most likely you will blame yourself and find many things in your past to feel guilty about. Your past is over, however; you cannot go back and do it again. Laying blame is often an unwillingness to live in the present. As long as you ask, "Why me?" to blame someone or something, you are avoiding your current reality.

Another way to avoid the present is to hold fate responsible for the way things turn out. Such a fatalistic view of life comes swathed in pseudoscientific argument nowadays, as when people say that surviving AIDS depends solely on whether you're infected by a "weak" or "strong" HIV virus or got "good" or "bad" genes from your parents, on whether you had your tonsils removed when you were a child, or on any such happenstance. Whether or not these events have any bearing on survival is beside the point. What matters is that by proclaiming yourself the innocent victim of circumstance, you are abandoning your free will. People—especially those with AIDS or ARC—who claim that surviving the disease is a question of a lucky draw are usually saying, between words, that they will eventually pick a losing number.

A productive inquiry into the past should first ask, "What did I do?" and then focus on "What can I do about it now?" "What can I do?" implies responsibility, the recognition that you are the one who can best solve your problems. You must also recognize your limitations, however, and know when to seek support from others. Responsibility means admitting that problems do not go away unless they are worked through, sometimes painfully. By facing your pain, you make freedom and healing possible. Blame makes you feel guilty and depressed, but responsibility brings control back into your life and strengthens your will to live. Its benefits can also compensate for the pain.

To acquire meaning, our lives may need restructuring. We often suppress or reject our creative selves. Have you ever found yourself wishing for a freer life or wanting to abandon a nine-to-five routine so you could really do what you wanted? If you have, you may have once suppressed a vital part of your identity. Somewhere in life's journey, you forgot what you wanted to be when you grew up. Go back and rescue this forgotten self from that old toy chest. Dust it, oil it, wind it up, and listen again to its tune. You might be prompted to turn your life around, as Dan Turner did when he turned to music. And you might also turn back to health by revitalizing your creative self.

"What reason do I have for living now that I have AIDS? Why should I plan things I will never live to do?" I realize these are tough questions. Life can seem rather short after an AIDS diagnosis. Then again, we have no crystal ball with which to foretell the future. Life can be equally short for everyone. The future exists only in our minds, and seeing it as meaningless or purposeless will only make life more difficult. The question "What reason do I have for living?" can be turned to your advantage. Use it to find out what you really want from life so you can reorder your priorities. Your distress about life might mean you have been living for the wrong reason, not that you have no reason for living.

Death visualization can serve as an aid to reorganizing your life.[b] Start by finding a quiet, comfortable place where you can relax your body and quiet your mind. Then visualize a peaceful and painless death. See yourself leaving your body and observe those you have left behind. Review your life, both its good and its bad moments. Now that you can no longer speak, what would you want to say to those who were close to you? Now that life is over, what would you do differently if you could do it over again? Now that there is no way to turn things around, what do you regret not doing or saying? Live your death in all its intensity. Get in touch with your feelings, and tune in to your emotions as you answer these questions.

Not all is past; you have been given a reprieve and can come back again. What are the things you must do this time around? Re-establishing priorities may become easier after you do this several times.

Meaning and purpose in life are reinforced by concrete goals. Purpose is a fixed horizon that we never reach but that gives us a general sense of direction in life. Goals are the passing landmarks that tell us we are indeed moving. The excitement of achieving positive goals can help spark the will to live and mobilize our healing energies. Setting goals can make us aware of our needs, clarify priorities, and reinforce meaning in our lives. Moreover, goals are excellent tools for change and often can provide very powerful reasons for staying around. Goals commit us to life.

It takes practice to determine which goals are proper for you. You should write down your goals, because unwritten goals remain vague and are usually ineffective. Written goals can be analyzed, refined, and changed. This doesn't mean you should keep laundry lists of goals (unless you are indeed the laundry list kind). Goals might be written as part of a journal or diary. For starters, write down what your death exercise taught you about making changes in your behavior. Ask yourself, "If I die in one week, how do I want to live until then? What are the things I want to do that I am not doing now?" Ask the same question giving yourself a month, three months, a year, and three years to live. Whether or not you will, in fact, live this long doesn't matter. Just come up with the goals.

Weekly and monthly goals should be quickly accomplished and provide immediate benefits. Long term goals basically say we are willing to work to be here in the future. Goals should be concrete, preferably things you can observe or experience—learning to draw, increasing the size of your chest, or visiting the Parthenon. Be realistic. Don't commit yourself to more than you can do, or you might be setting yourself up for failure. ("See, I told you I couldn't do it.") Be sure that by being realistic, however, you do not limit yourself. Realism can be an excuse for no growth, and then it defeats the purpose of goals. Remember your childhood dreams. These visions turn goals into plans worth living for. Above all, your goals should be challenging and balanced. They should meet all your physical, emotional, and spiritual needs.

While writing down your goals, include what you will gain or lose by achieving them.[c] This is the time to analyze the enjoyment you get out of harmful habits and to decide which beneficial activities could replace them. Review your goals and revise them as needed. Abandon any that do not turn out to be realistic. Remember, you should always plan plans and never plan exact results. Things rarely turn out the way you envision them, but they can come close.

We achieve goals through actions. Only activities, not goals, are doable, so figuring out the specific actions that will take us to our goals—especially the long-term ones—can be helpful: breaking down a large task into smaller actions makes it less formidable. Rewards can also help you accomplish things. Make sure you reward yourself each time you attain a goal.

Visualization, creative imagery, or directed imagination can also help you accomplish goals. You visualize every day but are probably not aware of it. There are many ways to do creative visualization. The gist of it, however, consists in finding a quiet place, relaxing your body through deep breathing, and trying to live in your mind the goal you want to accomplish. Let's say you want better health. Affirm your goal with something like "I have a healthy body that is strong, energetic, and well defined" while you picture yourself with a muscular body, running up a hillside. Your vision might not reflect the truth about your current physical condition, but it reflects the truth of what you want to be. Try to include as much detail and emotion as possible in your visualization. Smell the grass, hear the birds singing and your heart beating, taste the sweat running down your face, see the bright blue sky and the puffy white clouds. You could even have your friends cheering you on to the summit. Your visualizations don't have to be as vivid as dreams, but they should involve as many of your senses as possible.

The subconscious cannot distinguish between real or imaginary experiences; it will say "yes" to either an actual or a visualized uphill run. Visualization will not only help your body's relaxation mechanisms to mobilize your immunity but will also help dissolve the blocks to your creative energy and reprogram the deep processes of your mind.

CHANGING THE BALANCE OF YOUR LIFE

Health is optimum communication between the physical, emotional, and spiritual parts of your self. In this ideal state all your different parts constantly balance each other. To bring the balance of health back to your life, you should consider all the various techniques I have described in this chapter: accepting death, dealing with the possibility of survival, nurturing your hope and your will to live, loving yourself and others, finding a new meaning and purpose for your life, and setting goals to accomplish your newly found priorities. These things represent a good amount of work and might require support from others or professional help. Once this balance is re-established, it will feed back into and enhance the things that helped bring it about. You will find goals easier to accomplish, your life will acquire an exciting purpose, and you will love yourself and life more and more.

Self-examination and visualization can also help you identify the major causes of stress in your life so you can recognize when distress reaches dangerous levels. With such knowledge, you can create a stress management program to regain the equilibrium of health. This program might involve simple exercises, but it will not be easy. It will not produce instant results. Re-establishing equilibrium puts you in contact with change, and change is not quick, effortless, or painless.

If we do not let go of the old—especially the guilt and the blame—life does not go forward. All change involves giving up a part of yourself, letting an old life die in order to be born into a new. Thus, change can entail the denial, isolation, depression, anger, and bargaining we go through in accepting death. Change might make you feel worse before you feel better. Don't despair; keep going.

Change also involves confusion. Every housekeeper knows that one must first disorganize a closet before rearranging it. A similar process happens when you go through life changes. Many of us, however, get stuck in the temporary disorganization of our lives and fail to rearrange things. Things pile up, the mind becomes cluttered, and soon there's such a mess that the task of putting things back together becomes overwhelming. We give up. In this way, confusion can provide us with a good excuse to stop all change.

Whenever you feel overwhelmed by change, stop looking at the totality of your task. Find the smallest task you can handle and do that. Then do another, and so on. Soon you will find things suddenly clicking back into place, and you will have acquired a new outlook.

Besides giving in to confusion, there are other ways to avoid change. You can escape to an earlier form of behavior (as an alcoholic does when going back to drinking), deny you need to change or find many "good" reasons for not changing, or blame your inability to change on some other thing or person. All these excuses may give you temporary relief, but in the end they will prove to be blind alleys.

A good stress-management program requires several positive changes. Illness often begins after an increase in stress. Reducing that load speeds recovery. In managing stress you should first avoid sources of stress you can control, such as alcohol, drugs, harmful additives and toxins in foods, and other environmental offenders. A child who was born without any immunity whatsoever survived for twelve years inside a plastic bubble that protected him from hostile bacteria, viruses, and noxious chemicals. Although we cannot actually live in a plastic bubble, we can do many things to avoid opportunistic infections until our health is normalized, through either self-healing or future medical discoveries. Of course, some stresses you won't be able to avoid. You can, however, develop strategies to cope with stress and engage in activities such as relaxation and exercise that will counteract stress and boost your immunity.

Another stress-management tool is entertainment. Temporarily distracting your mind can be more relaxing than complete rest and will go a long way toward increasing your strength. It can also be lots of fun. Vary your entertainment. The best entertainment involves the greatest number of senses—sight, touch, hearing, and smell, for example. It also allows you to participate or at least expands your potential to enjoy life. Try going to a funny movie,[d] listening to great music, looking at works of art, enjoying the outdoors, or doing whatever moves or excites you as long as it keeps you from getting bogged down in the humdrum of life.

Constantly watching the tube, however, more often than not contributes to dullness. Commercial television in this country panders to the tastes of an imaginary audience. Its programming appeals to a mythically average person living a mythically average life in a mythically average community; it therefore appeals to nobody in reality. When you watch TV indiscriminately, you are often just filling the vacuum of your life with white noise, masking one meaninglessness with another, and placing control of your life in the hands of a TV programmer who knows and cares little about you. If you must watch TV, try public television. Unlike commercial TV, it allows you to participate in activities that may not normally be available to you—ballet, opera, concerts, theatrical performances, nature expeditions. Turning the set on and off for specific programs can help you overcome TV addiction and regain control over your life. If you feel you need TV for company, try cultivating friendships. Talking can help you not only to break TV's spell but also to bring fears and frustrations down to manageable size.

Managing stress involves preparation and re-education. Although you cannot always avoid stress, you can often prepare yourself so that stress will be less deleterious when it arrives. A great deal of stress vanishes when we accept that we cannot control certain things. We must learn we cannot change or control others, only ourselves. Try to see the world as your mirror. When you find yourself trying to control another, first find out what needs change in you. Understanding your needs and rhythms can also help you adjust to stress, but you shouldn't use your habits as an excuse for avoiding the pain of growth ("That's not *my* way of doing things!"). Self-knowledge puts you in charge and makes you less susceptible to control by people or circumstances. Finally, you can try neutralizing harmful responses to stress. Breathing, exercise, meditation, and other activities that exhaust the fight-or-flight response help turn distress into eustress. Yet to bring about a lasting change you must act at a deeper level and alter your way of thinking. You must allow hope, love, and positive expectations to enter your life.

And so we return to where we started, for all the things we have discussed feed into one another. Without health you will not be able to deal with stress and will have little room for hope, love, and the will to live. And without hope, love, and positive expectations you won't be able to handle stress, and your health will be impaired. Changes in one area of ourselves will bring about changes in other areas. That's why we need to look at the totality of ourselves. No single approach can be effective in AIDS or ARC. We must combine spiritual awakening, self-knowledge, meditation, exercise, nutrition, vitamins, and conventional and alternative therapies in a comprehensive program that will lead us back to health.

⁂ ⁂ ⁂

I consider the following books almost compulsory for anyone interested in the ideas discussed in this chapter:

- *The Will to Live* by Arnold A. Hutschnecker;
- *Man's Search for Meaning* by Viktor E. Frankl;
- *You Can Heal Your Life* by Louise L. Hay;
- *Getting Well Again* by O. Carl Simonton, Stephanie Matthews-Simonton, and James L. Creighton

(also listen to the tape *Healing and Believing: Learning to Trust the Universe.* It updates many of the book's ideas);

- *The Road Less Travelled* by M. Scott Peck; and
- *Beyond the Relaxation Response* by Herbert Benson.

Were I limited by time and health to reading only a few books, I would choose these above any others. Other valuable books and tapes are listed at the end of this book under Suggested Reading. Tapes are often more convenient and can be useful tools for learning relaxation, meditation, and creative visualization.

If you want even more information on the themes discussed above, I suggest you read *Human Options* by Norman Cousins, *You Can Fight for Your Life* by Lawrence LeShan, *Overcoming the Fear of Success* by Martha Friedman, *Creative Procrastination: Organizing Your Own Life* by Frieda Porat, *Setting Goals* by John Renesch, and *Realize Your Potential* by Robert J. McKain, Jr.

CHAPTER 3

Others and your health

FRIENDS, FAMILY, AND SUPPORT GROUPS

We are all social beings. No existence can be more painful than loneliness, no punishment more cruel than exile. Without the presence and reassurance of others, our individuality often wavers and flickers—and we die. Nowhere is this more apparent than in AIDS. Hundreds of people with AIDS have been abandoned by friends, family, and society, exiled to cold hospital wards, and sentenced to bitter deaths. Only an exceptional person could turn disease into healing under these conditions. Even if you were to start the journey back to health with enthusiasm, lack of support from those closest to you could eventually erode your perseverance.

The love of friends and family can be crucial to your survival. Indeed, friends and family can often carry the ball for you when disease weakens you and carry it until health returns. New Jerseyite Mike May was diagnosed with PCP in February 1986. By the end of March, he had become concentration-camp thin and had developed painful herpes lesions and a consuming fungus throughout his body. He had nightly sweats and constant fever; he couldn't eat and his strength was gone. "I knew my death was imminent," Mike says.

Luckily for Mike, a friend in Israel didn't. She had learned about a treatment for AIDS developed by the Weizmann Institute of Science in Rehovot, Israel, and promptly informed Mike about it. It was AL 721, a natural substance derived from egg-yolk lecithin (AL 721 is not yet available by prescription in the U.S.; we will discuss this substance in a later chapter). "I took a leap of faith," Mike mentions. "I had nothing to lose." Still convinced he was going to die, Mike wrote goodbye letters to all his friends and boarded an El Al flight to Tel Aviv in April. Or rather, he was boarded into the flight, as he was not in the best condition to travel. Mike had to be strapped to a wheelchair all the way to Israel; his mother and his lover helped him along. "I don't know how I endured that long flight, " he says. "The three of us were planning how to deal with a corpse so far from home."

Mike underwent treatment for two and a half months. There was no improvement the first week, but during the second Mike's diarrhea abated. His appetite improved and he began to eat. His strength returned. He returned to the States in June—without wheelchair, fevers, herpes sores, or fungus and with increased weight and an increasing helper T cell count. Although he is still convalescing, Mike May has no symptoms today. The shock of being alive kept him silent until recently. "When you've been to Auschwitz and survived, I think you never get over it. I had had to let go of my plans, my loves, my hopes, my career, my possessions, and life itself." Mike himself acknowledges that he wouldn't be alive today had it not been for a caring friend in Israel, a loving mother, and a supportive lover.[1]

Mike's friends and family were not only loving and supporting. They refused to give in, even when Mike wanted to, and offered him an alternative to death. Allowing alternatives and providing choices are the key characteristics of a support group that enhances the chances of survival. For a long time researchers wondered why in very close-knit, loving families people diagnosed with cancer often died sooner. Shouldn't love and support have the opposite effect? Not if they're the wrong kind of love and support. Researchers found that people often died sooner in those families that bought into the fatal prognosis. Their love often came with the trappings of a prisoner's last meal and their support with the sympathy a doctor often lends when he or she feels that no more can be done for the patient. Love and sympathy were poured on so thickly that the dying family member sometimes expressed a wish to die more quickly to liberate the family from the ordeal.[2] You do not need this kind of love from friends and family.

The love of your family and the support of your friends should strengthen your resolve to bring about your healing. If this is not the case, try educating your loved ones. Have them read Stephanie Matthews Simonton's *The Healing Family.* If your close ones are beyond education or if they abandon you, look for a support group that shares your philosophy about health. The world has plenty of loving people to offer. By the way, if your family abandons you or disapproves of your lifestyle or philosophy, make sure you grant power of attorney to a trusted friend who knows and will follow your treatment preferences. Unwanted family may turn up at an unwanted moment and run the show *their* way and not yours. If property is at stake, make sure all your legal arrangements are airtight.

If you are sick and alone, abandoned by uncaring family and friends, various community organizations and groups can offer you help and support. Good support groups can provide you with love and care, yet, as we said of friends and family, you must make sure these groups offer the kind of love and support you need. Not a few organizations dealing with AIDS have bought into the notion that the disease is invariably fatal. A support group that sells the idea of reconciling you with impending death might make that death very impending indeed. Avoid any group that doesn't offer you alternatives. Any group more concerned about pet research projects, about keeping up with the medical or academic Joneses, or about its public image rather than about the people it should serve is not the group for you either.

Look for service organizations with a holistic outlook on healing (you can find some of these in appendix H under AIDS Complimentary Therapy, Information Groups). These may direct you to appropriate support groups in your area or, if none exist, help you organize your own. I cannot emphasize too much the importance of the right support groups. Had the kind of support groups in which I now participate existed when my illness started, these last seven years could have been easier. A hug, a hand, even a word would have made a world of difference during the inevitable moments of loneliness or despair. Luckily, my love of books turned me toward research. My investigations buffered the loneliness and eventually put me in touch with others doing the same out there. Even so, joining others earlier could have made my own efforts more effective. Though I learned a lot by having to step and stumble by myself, I wouldn't go at it alone nowadays. You will find that in joining a good support group, you will participate in the healing of others and thus accomplish your own more pleasantly and effectively.

PHYSICIANS AND OTHER HEALTH-CARE PROVIDERS

If you have AIDS or ARC, visiting your physician could be one of your frequent activities. Physicians and other health-care providers are crucial in helping you improve your health. Yet you must always remember that they are far from omnipotent. As far as AIDS goes, some even consider themselves impotent. It is tempting to place yourself in your physician's hands and expect to be cured or treated with no effort on your part. But to anticipate such magic is to look for trouble. By accepting blindly what an expert thinks you should do about your health, you lose power of choice and add to the helplessness that is harmful to your will to live.

Before AIDS came along, we expected doctors to fix almost everything that went wrong with us. Modern medicine had been very successful in treating many infectious diseases that baffled pre-twentieth-century doctors. Some physicians encouraged this complacent, "fix-me" attitude in order to make us "easier" patients. A patient who followed doctor's orders without questioning made the doctor's job simpler—and more pleasant. The fix-me attitude was reinforced almost daily by pharmaceutical companies pandering the notion of "a pill for every ill" through ads and commercials (contributing thus to this country's licit and illicit drug addiction problem). Yet after the advent of AIDS, we crashed from the high of our expectations and awoke to a stark reality: there are no quick fixes in health. Some physicians now consider the fix-me mentality not only unreasonable and unfair—because it grants godlike duties along with godlike powers—but also unlikely to lead to recovery.

Alone, your doctor cannot bring you health. Your physician may have the knowledge and expertise to help you shift your health back toward center, but only you can start the process and keep it going. Thus, your relationship with your doctor should be based on trust and cooperation. Your doctor shouldn't be a father or mother who tells you what to do, but a knowledgeable friend who offers advice and belongs to the wider support system that furthers your health.

CONVENTIONAL MEDICINE

Like the rest of us, physicians have diverse intellectual capabilities and educational backgrounds. Not all doctors are equally knowledgeable, even in their own areas of expertise. Modern medicine, like any other human endeavor, is not invariably effective. "Regular medicine," says physician Andrew Weil in *Health and Healing,* "is on very shaky grounds in attempting to treat such problems as acute infections associated with viruses, nutritional and metabolic diseases, chronic degenerative diseases, allergies and autoimmune diseases, cancer, 'psychosomatic disease,' and mental illness." We might add AIDS as number one on this list.

Because of a growing reliance on harmful drugs, technological gadgetry, and invasive techniques, regular medicine can often be risky and expensive. Many diagnostic tests are often needlessly invasive[a] and are used by doctors who feel they must cover all bases as protection against malpractice. Yet overreliance on ultrasophisticated, costly testing may also reflect reluctance on the part of some doctors to cultivate the art of diagnosis and to accept the consequences of medical decisions. Excessive testing can be counterproductive. "Doctors often end up treating abnormalities in test results rather than people," says Weil. "This possibility is very real, especially since abnormalities will usually turn up if enough tests are done."

Despite these shortcomings, however, regular medicine can be most effective in treating common, serious conditions like acute trauma, acute medical and surgical emergencies, and acute infections caused by bacteria, protozoa, some fungi and parasites, and a few other organisms. Yet although conventional medicine is very good at handling crises like these, it is still ineffective in preventing the diseases that really concern us today and in maintaining the optimum quality of health.[3] For further reading about the abuses of conventional medicine in the U.S., I suggest Robert S. Mendelsohn's book *Confessions of a Medical Heretic.*

ORTHOMOLECULAR VERSUS TOXOMOLECULAR MEDICINE

Aware of the shortcomings of modern medicine, a growing number of physicians are using the less invasive and more biologically sound methods of orthomolecular medicine. Orthomolecular medicine posits that predisposition to disease and much disease itself result from various chemical imbalances or deficiencies that can be corrected by restoring these substances to their proper levels in the body. Since vitamins and minerals are often a major source of these imbalances, orthomolecular treatment is likely to include—but not restrict itself to—vitamin and mineral therapies.

Nobel biochemist Linus Pauling, the discoverer of the function of vitamin C, coined the word *orthomolecular*, to describe therapies that use the "right molecules"—those molecules the body needs to function. Others have labeled the methods of conventional medicine "toxomolecular," that is, using toxic or poisonous molecules. Many drugs have the potential to push the body into a greater chemical disequilibrium and start the downward spiral of ill health that leads to death, a potential that is actualized too often in AIDS. Many chronic degenerative diseases, such as rheumatoid arthritis, certain kinds of schizophrenia, and severe allergies, have responded to orthomolecular treatment. Vitamin C therapy and other orthomolecular treatments also seem to have had some success in the treatment of AIDS.[4]

HOMEOPATHY

Although what we have been calling conventional medicine is the only kind of medicine taken seriously by most Western societies, it is not the only kind available or the only kind that works. During the early nineteenth century, German physician Samuel

Christian Hahnemann became dissatisfied with the medical practices of the time—such as bleeding with lancets or leeches and violent intestinal purging with heavy-metal salts—and laid down the foundations of homeopathic medicine in his book *Organon of Medicine*.

Homeopathy (from the Greek roots meaning "like the disease") maintains that the body gets rid of disease through symptoms and that therefore substances to be prescribed should be those that elicit in healthy people symptoms similar to those of the disease. Though conventional medicine makes some use of this homeopathic principle in treatments such as vaccinations and allergy desensitizations, homeopaths feel that regular medicine, or allopathy (meaning "other than the disease"), prescribes drugs with no or very little logical relationship to symptoms.

Homeopathic medicine also holds that the same set of symptoms in two individuals do not necessarily point to the same disease. (If we were to include spiritual and emotional factors as part of the symptoms, then no disease would be the same for any two people.) Those collections of symptoms that regular medicine calls "hepatitis," "gastric ulcers," or "AIDS" thus hold no meaning to a homeopath. These diseases won't even be mentioned in a homeopathic diagnosis, so expect your first visit to a homeopath to be rather different from a visit to the usual doctor. Through a long series of questions the homeopath will try to uncover the pattern of symptoms peculiar to you. Some of these questions will be obviously related to your symptoms and some will not. Others may seem outright strange ("Do you love your mother? Are you happy?"). When the pattern becomes clear, the homeopath will prescribe remedies according to the "like cures like" principle mentioned above.

Homeopathic remedies are a source of controversy. Hahnemann believed out of religious conviction that the "spiritual" essence of a substance, not its material constituents, was effective against disease. After experimenting with dilutions, he became convinced that the more extensively diluted a dose was,[b] the better it helped the body fight disease. This is where homeopathy and conventional medicine come into conflict. Some homeopathic preparations are so extensively diluted that, according to the laws of chemistry, they should not contain a single atom of the original substance! Homeopaths claim, however, that the energetic shakings homeopathic remedies are subjected to between successive dilutions leave an "imprint" of the original substance in the end product. This "imprint," they say, persists long after the original substance has disappeared. Despite this somewhat animistic explanation, some extremely diluted homeopathic remedies seem to work, perhaps by eliciting a strong placebo response.

OTHER HEALTH-CARE PROVIDERS

You should work closely with a physician, but you can also look into what alternative therapies might offer. There are several therapeutic methods, such as traditional acupuncture, Chinese herbal medicine, and contemporary chiropractic, that can complement conventional treatments well. Acupuncture, for example, has at least improved the well-being and overall quality of life in several people with AIDS. (We will discuss several of these alternatives at greater length in chapter 15.) Whenever appropriate, you should explore and use all healing modalities. Some of the work done in integrating conventional, complementary, and alternative approaches in cancer therapy may be useful to those seeking a similar approach to AIDS. *Integral Cancer Therapy* by Michael Lerner offers an overview and evaluation of methods and centers that use such integrated cancer therapies (the pamphlet is available through Commonweal, listed in appendix H under Alternative Cancer Therapy).

TABLE 5 Choosing among alternative therapies

1. Rely on statistics rather than on claims. A practitioner should be able to show you some sort of data on the effectiveness of a particular therapy. Data can always be shared in anonymous form.
2. Does the practitioner advise you about the risks as well as the benefits? A practitioner should allow other options even if they conflict with the practitioner's philosophy. A macrobiotic nutrition counselor might, for example, condemn vitamins, as "unnatural substances," while a physician might fail to mention diet because of lack of knowledge about nutrition.
3. What are practitioners doing to lower the costs of particularly elaborate and costly treatment? Where there are only claims of the effectiveness of expensive treatment, don't start paying until your lab tests improve.
4. Always maintain an open mind about alternatives. Only results and not theories matter. Accept or reject only after investigation.

Adapted from Health action: Solid advice from a reader with ARC, *New York Native*: 19, 31 March 1986.

THE HOLISTIC APPROACH

Whether your primary-care physician is an allopath, an orthomolecular doctor, or a homeopath, he or she should see you as a unique individual whose health is a balance between physical agents on the one hand and emotional, social, and spiritual factors on the other. In other words, your doctor should have a holistic approach to healing. Rather than focusing on just the disease and its symptoms, a physician with a holistic healing approach should aim at restoring the whole person to health. In any disease it is essential to alleviate symptoms—for symptoms, after all, are what make illness undesirable and uncomfortable—yet in AIDS or ARC we are headed for trouble if we try to fix symptoms through treatments that do not stop or, worse, that speed up the underlying deterioration of immunity. The immune system is too complex for simplistic remedies. Only an attitude that considers the whole person can have a chance at success.

A holistic approach and holistic practice are not necessarily one and the same. In their reaction against a too-rationalistic orthodox medicine, many self-styled holistic doctors have swung to the other extreme and adopted an anti-intellectual, antiscientific attitude. These physicians rant at the excesses of conventional medicine—radiotherapy and chemotherapy are two favorite and often deserving targets—while they themselves indulge in indiscriminately trying anything labeled natural or homeopathic. They reject anything conventional medicine comes up with, often just because it came from the "allopaths."[c] But we cannot close our minds to some of the solutions of conventional medicine. Avoid those who have run so far into left field they have lost sight of the ball. Beware of guruism. Any type of orthodoxy can be lethal in dealing with AIDS, whether such closed-mindedness comes from holistic practitioners, homeopaths, allopaths, or those psychopaths who want to quarantine us out of society.

True holism encompasses a lot, indeed, too much. No single person can be an expert in everything. Thus, every physician or alternative health practitioner we deal with will be a specialist to a degree. You will probably have to work with several physicians and other health-care providers. Your primary-care physician should be strongly rooted in a specific tradition yet open to learning from others and willing to utilize other methods when appropriate. Your primary-care physician should encourage independence and help you develop a truly holistic approach to your health because you are the only one who can mobilize the totality of your self. I strongly recommend Andrew Weil's *Health and Healing*, a very entertaining book that describes and critiques the various types of medicine—conventional, homeopathic, holistic—practiced in the West today.

THE ROLE OF THE PHYSICIAN

Wrong decisions can kill patients, so doctors are under great pressure to be right. They are understandably cautious. Sometimes, however, fear of being wrong can limit: some doctors do not want to consider any approaches besides those they learned as students. Many of these physicians stand at the opposite extreme from the anti-intellectual and antiscientific holistic practitioners. For them, nothing is true unless repeatedly demonstrated by extensive double-blind and reputedly unbiased research. They have substituted the sound intuition and common sense of the old family doctor with the cold logic and rationale of the laboratory researcher. Watch out for doctors who have abandoned healing in order to defend a system of belief.

Doubtful and unverifiable methods are unacceptable in treating disease, yet conventional medicine can't be the sole judge of what's verifiable and acceptable. While orthodox medicine insists on scientifically rigorous testing for alternative therapies, it doesn't seem to apply that golden method to itself. According to a report from the U.S. Congressional Office of Technology Assessment, just around 20 percent of all standard medical procedures used in 1978 had been proven effective scientifically.[5] Many doctors fail to see this beam in modern medicine's eye when they criticize alternative therapies. "Individual experiences, especially in cases of recovery or cure," says Norman Cousins, "are suspect. The adjective used to describe these experiences is 'anecdotal.' Few words in the medical vocabulary carry more connotations of scorn and even contempt."[6] Be wary of doctors who call others what they would never call themselves.

Orthodox physicians have seen all new and unestablished therapies as quackery at first—even those that later become respectable, like psychoanalysis. To be sure, quacks and charlatans abound—people that pretend medical knowledge in order to make money from your pain or misery. Warnings against these creatures render you a service. Yet warnings may also indicate a mind closed to people honestly dedicated to their methods who, no matter how unorthodox their methods seem, instill in patients belief in the possibility of a cure. Your physician should be open to this kind of practitioner.

A physician—or any other health-care provider, for that matter—should minister to *you* and not to your disease. Your doctor shouldn't treat you as just another patient. A physician should adapt theory and treatment uniquely to you, consider the role of stress and emotions on your disease, remain open-minded and compassionate, and be a source of encouragement and support. Your doctor should also demystify your condition by providing up-to-date, understandable, and *usable* information. He or she should defuse your anxiety by helping you discover sources of distress and suggesting ways to handle them. Unfortunately, some doctors feel it is their job only to diagnose, prescribe, administer treatment, or operate and not to educate or counsel. Any doctor worth his or her pay, however, knows that all he or she can do is summon and amplify the healing abilities residing in you. The truly skilled physician makes healing a cooperative venture with you, the patient. If yours doesn't, then you should go elsewhere.

One of the traditional and most important roles of a physician is to reassure you as a patient. Your doctor needs to know how to deal with the conscious or unconscious fears that a new diagnosis or new symptoms could bring about. Panic after diagnosis, if unresolved, can often aggravate disease.[7] Your doctor should be able to speak freely about the "seriousness" of disease without closing the door to hope. No matter how adverse your condition, your doctor should feel you have the potential to survive your disease. If you asked most doctors whether or not you could survive any disease, they would say yes no matter how they felt. How could they say otherwise? But actions and feelings, not words, are what count here. Rely on your own feelings. If you feel your doctor is open to the possibility of success, stay with him or her. If you sense futility or hopelessness in your physician, look for someone with more faith.

There are several things only physicians can do because of training or licensing requirements. Your doctor can

- provide a diagnosis for your symptoms;
- administer prescription drugs;
- evaluate tests that monitor therapy;
- treat parasites and opportunistic infections;
- attend to medical emergencies, such as broken bones, spinal injuries, poisonings, and cardiac and respiratory failures; and
- recommend a course of vitamin and mineral supplementation best suited to your condition.

A doctor, however, has no business prognosticating the time and manner of your death. Physicians are no better at predicting the future than any of us. The death statistics some of them are so fond of are of little use to you as an individual and are best left to insurance companies who need them to calculate how much to charge for a policy.

CHOOSING A PHYSICIAN OR HEALTH-CARE PROVIDER

Selecting a physician or health-care provider may well be the most important decision of your life. A good start is a referral from a source you trust: a friend, another health-care professional, or a professional association (see appendix H for addresses). There's no shortage of physicians or practitioners. The *New England Journal of Medicine* recently reported there will be a surplus of 40,000 to 50,000 doctors in the United States within the next decade.[8] It's a buyers' market. You can afford to be choosy, especially if you live in a major metropolitan area, so don't hesitate to interview more than one practitioner. When you do, ask for the names of other patients to whom you can speak. Don't go for the first physician you speak to; get the best one for your needs.

Choosing a physician or health-care provider is like interviewing any applicant for a job. If you feel uneasy about talking to a physician, bring a friend who can help you ask questions. Does your candidate have a back-up to take calls during sickness, absence, or vacation? Is he or she affiliated with a hospital? Are there any admission problems in emergencies? How do you contact him or her after regular working hours? What other health professionals are part of his or her practice? Ask about educational background, experience, and credentials.

Knowledge about nutrition is essential in dealing with AIDS or ARC, cancer, and heart disease. Because of lack of training in the subject, however, many doctors ignore nutrition. You may prefer to choose these not as your primary-care physicians but as peripheral specialists. I would be more comfortable if my physician were a member of the American Holistic Medical Association, the Orthomolecular Medical Society, the American Society for Clinical Nutrition, the American Institute of Nutrition, or the American College of Nutrition or were certified by the American Board of Nutrition.

Your doctor should also communicate well with you and show compassion. Does your candidate use a lot of jargon? Does he or she listen well and answer your questions satisfactorily? Do you feel he or she cares about you? Do you see this physician as a friend and ally, or do you feel like a depersonalized subordinate because of the way he or she treats you? Treatment will be ineffective if it doesn't include care or concern for you.

Make sure your physician's philosophy about health care matches yours. As we discussed before, your doctor should be open to new information—remaining constructively critical where necessary—and be willing to consult with those alternative practitioners you employ.

DEALING WITH YOUR PHYSICIAN

Once you have decided on your primary-care physician, you cannot simply hand yourself over as if you had fulfilled your part of the bargain. The relationship between you and your physician should be one of cooperation. It implies an involvement of more than one.

Make a list of your current symptoms before you visit your physician or any other practitioner. Note when the symptoms began, what you think may have brought them about, and what you have done to relieve them. Don't forget any medications or drugs—prescription, over-the-counter, or recreational—you have been taking. If you are seeing several health-care professionals, make sure each knows you are seeing the others. The need for consultation may arise.

Many of us grew up in awe and fear of medical authority. Yet doctors are in no way our superiors; they're only regular people who happen to possess knowledge and skills that we don't. Deifying your doctor will only make the cooperative healing effort more difficult. If you are intimidated, take a friend along who can help communicate your concerns clearly and courteously.

Your doctor should be able to speak your language in an honest and caring way. Make sure you understand. Ask questions. An important part of a physician's job is to demystify illness. Don't be afraid to ask repeatedly for clarification. Always ask your doctor why he or she recommends a specific course of treatment. Ask for reading material on the subject. Your doctor should inform you about suggested treatments and alternatives and explain how these can fit your life. Your thoughts, feelings, and fears may sometimes determine a choice of treatment. Be sure to share these with your doctor. Don't be a "good" patient if that means being passive, accepting, and unquestioning.

Rather than assuming a take-it-or-leave-it attitude, your physician must be willing to negotiate alternatives. A unilateral decision by your doctor is unacceptable, except in emergencies. Taking the power of decision away from you will make you helpless in the face of your disease and may help worsen your condition. Whenever any form of radical treatment is suggested, be it radiotherapy, chemotherapy, or surgery, go elsewhere for second, third, and even fourth opinions. If your physician isn't willing to discuss and negotiate a course of action acceptable to both of you or if he or she ignores your emotional needs and doesn't care for your playing an active role in your health, then you need to get a new physician.

Your faith in your doctor and your doctor's faith in you are essential to healing. "The physician must have the complete confidence in his healing system or ritual," physician Irving Oyle writes in *The Healing Mind,* "and the patient must trust that the physician knows what he is doing. If either aspect of this inner belief is missing , the healing process is adversely affected."[9]

CHAPTER 4

The hard choice of drugs

There are some remedies worse than the disease.

PUBLILIUS SYRUS, first century B.C.

Some drugs are often beneficial, and a few, including some of those used in the treatment of AIDS, are essential. Yet no matter how beneficial or essential they might be, all drugs are potentially toxic. You should not take them casually. Your physician should advise you of a drug's side effects and whether the drug's therapeutical benefits outweigh these. Know what you are taking. Ask your doctor or the pharmacist for the literature accompanying a prescribed drug. For prescriptions that have none, if your condition permits, get a copy of the *Physician's Desk Reference* (PDR) and read about the drug and its effects. Neville Hodgkinson's *Will to Be Well* discusses the drawbacks of drugs and invasive procedures in modern medicine and suggests some alternatives to these. Even though you will probably follow your doctor's advice, the choice of treatment is always yours. You can exercise that choice judiciously only if you keep yourself well informed.

PRESCRIPTION AND OVER-THE-COUNTER DRUGS IN AIDS

AIDS intensifies the side effects of some drugs. Sixty percent of all AIDS patients, for example, often can't tolerate sulfa drugs. These drugs would normally produce nausea, vomiting, headaches, and loss of appetite; in those with AIDS the drugs also cause fever, skin eruptions, and reduction of white blood cells.[a] Bactrim and Septra, the most effective drugs against *Pneumocystis carinii* pneumonia (PCP), are sulfa drugs (or, more properly, sulfonamides).[b] As such, Bactrim and Septra may reduce white blood cells and thus further suppress immunity. Some physicians therefore prefer to treat PCP with pentamidine, a drug used against African sleeping sickness. Pentamidine is not without side effects either. It can cause kidney failure, temporarily low blood pressure and painful abscesses wherever there is an infection.[1, 2] An aerosol formulation of pentamidine new on the market goes straight to the affected lung areas and is said to produce fewer systemic side effects.

Azidothymidine or AZT, approved by the FDA for people with AIDS who meet the manufacturer's distribution criteria, seems to be the first drug to limit the progressive immune deterioration of AIDS. The drug works by a ruse: it poses as a substance that the HIV virus needs for replication. When it takes AZT in, the virus cannot make further copies of itself, and the spread of the infection is stymied.[c] AZT doesn't kill the nonreplicating virus, however. If treatment were stopped, the dormant virus in other cells could start to replicate, re-instating immune deterioration.

Because some of the body's own cells might also accept AZT and die, the drug is toxic. Twenty-five percent of all participants in the initial trials developed anemia (from red blood–cell deficiency) and required multiple transfusions. Some of these people—the literature is unclear as to how many—experienced reduction in neutrophils. Both side effects reversed when the drug was discontinued. The benefits of AZT may outweigh these serious disadvantages, however. Only 1 person of the 145 under AZT, compared to 16 out of 137 under placebo, died from opportunistic infections during the initial trials.[3,4]

Would I consider AZT if I had pneumocystis pneumonia? Probably. As things now stand, there's a three in four chance that I would react well to the drug, a much better chance than that of survival under PCP. Yet because the full range of the drug's side effects when tested in a large population have not yet been released, my approval of AZT would remain tentative. I would consider some of the other substances discussed below before any AZT treatment. Even if Burroughs Wellcome decides you merit an ongoing AZT prescription—for theirs is the power to do so—the drug can cost around $1,000 a month. Money can become a decisive factor.

Despite its side effects, AZT at least does what no other drug has accomplished in AIDS: it slows down the fatal progression of the disease. Other chemotherapy used in AIDS might sometimes even be counterproductive. The treatment of Kaposi's sarcoma, for example, is a cauldron of controversy. Most oncologists advocate immunosupressive radiotherapy or chemotherapy for their KS patients, yet other doctors and researchers insist that treatment of KS lesions might not be necessary, especially if the lesions don't threaten vital organs or the person's appearance. They maintain that treatment aggravating immune deficiency is often unacceptable.

Whether Kaposi's sarcoma is a true cancer or not, it consists of cells that have multiplied excessively and can often be controlled by drugs that prevent cell division: the cytotoxic, or antimitotic, drugs. Yet cytotoxic drugs are not selective.[d] Besides killing the unruly KS cells, they also kill normal cells such as those of the immune system and the bone marrow. They are all immunosuppressive. The most common cytotoxics used against KS are vinblastine (trade name Velban) and vincristine (Oncovin), both derived from the poisonous Madagascar periwinkle.[e, 5] Because these drugs can impair the production of granulocytes, they deprive people with AIDS of the only functional immune cells they possess. Cytotoxic drugs can also breach the intestinal wall, allowing fatal bacteria to enter the body.

Chemotherapy can indeed be effective against KS, yet it can be equally effective against the patient. Some of the clinical drug reports sound like the old surgeon's joke: "The treatment was a success but the patient died." Many PWAs seem to die not from the sarcoma being treated but from subsequent opportunistic infections that a riddled immune system cannot handle.[6]

Ironically, radiotherapy or chemotherapy may not be at all necessary against certain kinds of KS lesions. When present only on the skin of people with no other opportunistic AIDS infections, Kaposi's sarcoma often refrains from spreading throughout the body. A 1985 pilot study of men with this type of KS who elected little or no medical treatment concluded that these men were no worse off for their lack of treatment than the average person under treatment for KS. Indeed, some seemed to be better, showing higher helper/suppressor T cell ratios than expected for people in their condition.[7] One is left to wonder whether this type of immunosuppressive therapy has contributed to the particular aggressiveness of the sarcoma that spreads so extensively in some PWAs. Medical literature is ominously silent on the subject.

Some nonimmunosuppressive cytotoxic agents, mainly plant extracts, might be effective against KS. Among them are podophylin—used against venereal warts—and some of its derivatives, and extract of periwinkle, a plant to which folk medicine attributes astringent properties. In homeopathic dilution, periwinkle seems to be relatively harmless compared to its derivatives vinblastine and vincristine.[8]

Kaposi's sarcoma has also been treated with the interferons that cells produce to protect themselves against viruses and certain pathogens. Of all patients in several interferon tests, at least 50 percent showed alleviation of symptoms, while 20 to 30 percent achieved substantial improvement.[9] Interferons are orthomolecular substances, yet they can produce side effects such as fever, malaise, and headaches.

One of the most promising drugs in the treatment of KS is dinitrochlorobenzene, or DNCB, a substance slated for controlled clinical studies by the University of California Medical Center in San Francisco./ DNCB is a common chemical that causes a poison-oak-like reaction in people with normal immunity. In people with KS or AIDS-associated diseases, DNCB stimulates the development of T cells, as San Francisco dermatologist and former Stanford researcher Bruce Mills discovered.[10] DNCB may work by normalizing the high levels of antibodies produced by B cells. As explained previously, these antibodies could attack and kill T cells, thus contributing to the immune deterioration of AIDS after HIV infection has run its course.

Demand for DNCB, as well as for other drugs lacking institutional approval, has fostered the rise of "guerrilla clinics" in major U.S. cities (see Project Inform, listed under AIDS Complimentary Therapy, Information Groups, in appendix H). Several physicians in San Francisco, Berkeley, Los Angeles, San Diego, and New York use DNCB as well. Physicians and guerrilla users report not only the disappearance of KS lesions—which, according to anecdotes, may even peel or fall off—but also clinical improvement in those with either KS or other opportunistic infections. Table 6 shows Dr. Mills's classification of AIDS and ARC patients according to blood immunoglobulin levels and response to DNCB treatment. DNCB therapy is inexpensive (the major expense is that of the blood lab work), easy to administer (requiring basically a Q-tip and a sterile adhesive pad), and relatively safe. A few persons show a more severe skin reaction than expected, but the reaction subsides when the DNCB solution is diluted further.[8]

DNCB seems to work by somehow changing T cell protein receptors to which harmful anti–T cell antibodies bind, thus stopping the autoimmune attack that results in immune deterioration.[11] This line

TABLE 6 AIDS/ARC response to DNCB

CATEGORY	RESPONSE
GROUP I	
Immunoglobulin levels not too high (near upper normal range of 1,480)	In three to six months, excellent and often dramatic: Helper/suppresor T ratio improves Helper T cells within normal value Hemoglobin normalizes Lupus and rheumatoid complexes disappear. KS lesions generally disappear Well-being and energy return
GROUP II	
"Reasonable" immunoglobulin levels	Does not respond as quickly or as well as Group I. May need antiviral
GROUP III	
Immunoglobulin equal to or greater than 3,000	Too many antibodies. Lab tests often unreliable. May need a year of DNCB treatment to reduce antibody levels
GROUP IV	
End-stage AIDS	Though DNCB may raise T cells, it is too late to save life.

Source: Adapted from John S. James, "DNCB AIDS/ARC Treatment," *SF Sentinel* 16(20), 26 September 1986. An article about Dr. Bruce Mills's work with DNCB.

of research opens another promising avenue of treatment for AIDS: preventing the HIV virus from infecting a cell. In order to enter a cell, HIV needs to bind to a receptor protein on the cell membrane. Any substance that prevents the virus from attaching to a receptor will also block the virus from infecting the cell. This is how AL 721 also may have worked in reversing the progress of Mike May's disease.[12]

AL 721, derived from egg-yolk lecithin and safe for consumption, is a mixture of three lipids shown effective in reducing HIV infection in the laboratory.[h] These phospholipids replace the cholesterol in the cell membrane and make the membrane more fluid. Because receptor proteins sway back and forth freely in such a fluid membrane, a virus has a hard time attaching itself to them and fails to infect the cell. The fluidity of cell membranes decreases with aging, as does immune competence. The U.S trials of AL 721 in humans involved restoring immune function lost due to aging.[i]

Even though AL 721 showed excellent in vitro action against HIV as early as 1985, the first controlled trials of the substance's effectiveness against AIDS may start as late as May 1987 in the U.S. The company holding the patent for AL 721 in this country, Praxis Pharmaceuticals, is said to be vacillating between obtaining drug approval from the FDA and marketing the substance as a food supplement. Although recently relaxed approval criteria for AIDS drugs and the endorsement of AL 721 by the National Instititutes of Health could speed up things, FDA drug approval might take years. In the meantime, AL 721 could be made in any kitchen "lab" by anyone with a working knowledge of chemistry and the necessary equipment. And because AL 721 consists of ingredients found only in food—it's basically processed egg lecithin,[j] an essential dietary substance—it could be sold legally as a food supplement provided no medical claims were made. When asked why AL 721 wasn't being used in the U.S. for treating AIDS,

Mike May's Israeli physician answered: "The Americans don't like our treatment. It's too simple."[13, 14]

In animal studies AL 721 also proved useful in alleviating withdrawal symptoms and preventing relapses during morphine and alcohol dependency treatment.[15] Again, the substance seems to work by changing the nature of the receptor proteins to which opiates and opiatelike substances attach. These opiate receptors are found not only in brain cells but also in the cells of the immune system—a discovery that emphasizes the interdependency between brain and immunity. Because of this interdependency, if a substance that can re-energize immunity can also alleviate drug dependency, couldn't a substance used in treating drug addiction help restore an immune system that has crashed?

Naltrexone, the trade name of the drug trexan used to treat heroin addiction, has been under clinical testing for effectiveness against AIDS and ARC during the past year and a half. Although the results of the study have not been released, the drug holds promise. The initial study was double blind: neither doctors nor patients knew who received the drug and who the placebo. After three months, however, all patients were placed on the drug. This is the pattern now apparently followed in AIDS research whenever a drug might turn out to be a winner.

Naltrexone temporarily blocks immune-cell receptors to opiumlike substances that act as immune stimulators. These substances are the endorphins also produced during moderately strenuous exercise. When immune cells find their endorphin receptors thus blocked, however, they increase the number and the sensitivity of the receptors on their surfaces and begin producing more endorphins on their own. When the Naltrexone blockage wears off, a greater amount of endorphins are circulating in the blood than would normally be available.

The greater amount of endorphins, the greater number of endorphin receptors on a cell's surface, and the greater sensitivity of these receptors to the action of available endorphin all stimulate an immune cell into action for a much longer period than would normally be possible. Apparently this kind of immune "revving up" somehow neutralizes the effect of the high number of suppressor T cells found in people with ARC and some people with AIDS. A reduction in the abnormally high levels of a special kind of alpha interferon indicates whether Naltrexone is working. Naltrexone may produce harmful side effects at high dosages, yet the very small amounts used in AIDS and ARC treatment are mild and present no danger.[16] Many other drugs are being used in the treatment of opportunistic AIDS infections, as antivirals against HIV, or as immune enhancers. Several of these drugs are not currently available in the U.S. through FDA-approved channels. Appendix B presents a partial listing of these pharmaceuticals.

What about vitamin C? Increasing evidence shows that vitamin C is essential for proper immune response. Clinical studies demonstrate that large doses of vitamin C in human subjects—over 18 grams per day—can increase antibody, lymphocyte, and interferon production, kill bacteria or prevent its growth, detoxify bacterial poisons, and assure phagocytosis. Very large amounts of vitamin C administered in a 1982 study to people with AIDS inhibited the immunosuppressive substance secreted by some of their white blood cells. Physician Robert F. Cathcart III, the leading expert on the vitamin C treatment of viral diseases, studied twelve of his own AIDS patients and about ninety people with AIDS taking high doses of ascorbate—50 to 200 grams per day. He concluded that vitamin C helps suppress the symptoms of the disease and reduce the incidence of secondary infections. Cathcart's observations are limited, however, so controlled studies are necessary. Cathcart, Linus Pauling, and physician Ewan Cameron are still looking for an institutional sponsor for such studies. Cathcart's article on vitamin C AIDS treatment has been reprinted in appendix C.

Lack of interest in vitamin C stems partly from a lack of knowledge in the medical profession about vitamins in general. Jane or Joe Doctor often knows only as much about vitamins as what Jane or Joe Bloe learns in a college biochemistry course. And even that is later forgotten by the physician as the complexities of medical practice increase. True, interest in vitamin therapies is on the rise, especially among younger doctors. Yet many physicians still refuse even to consider that vitamins may have therapeutic value. The mere mention of the word *vitamin* may sometimes bring about a total shutdown of logical and objective processes in many a medical mind.

So we see that researchers Frederick and Martha Siegal, authors of one of the first popular AIDS books, talk on one page about the need for carefully controlled trials for new AIDS treatments and totally reject on the next the value of vitamin C in AIDS for the most unscientific of reasons: an "impression . . . [based on] so many AIDS patients who have tried 'megadoses' of this vitamin, without apparent benefit." These so-called megadoses turn out to consist of 10 to 15 grams per day, less than the 18 grams thought necessary for immune enhancement and considerably less than the amount used by Cathcart in the treatment of his AIDS patients. The Siegals, no doubt very conscientious about their own research, then add insult to injury by stating that such flimsy evidence constituted a "negative clinical trial." AIDS research needs only a few of these negative clinical trials to turn into a blind and fruitless pursuit.[17]

Antibiotics can often be a problem for people with AIDS. A relatively simple infection will sometimes need an antibiotic, and afterward a patient that was doing relatively well will all of a sudden develop an opportunistic infection that fails to respond to treatment. "If any patient (with or without AIDS) has superficial candidiasis," says physician Donald B. Louria, an expert in fungal infections, "is treated with antibiotics, and has indwelling vascular catheter, systemic candidiasis is likely to occur."[18] Although candida infection isn't at all simple, its treatment could illustrate how antibiotics may reduce an individual's resistance to disease.[k] Often, however, one again has to accept the possibly deleterious side effects of a drug over the fatal consequences of an opportunistic infection.

Not all antibiotics are used judiciously; in fact, they may be among the most misused drugs in the U.S. Indiscriminate use of broad-spectrum antibiotics—certain penicillins and tetracyclines, for example—for even the most trivial of infections is making many people so antibiotic-sensitive, and bacteria so antibiotic-resistant, that the drugs often cease to be effective.[19]

Antibiotic-resistant bacteria present other problems. Many large bacteria populations contain individuals resistant to antibiotics. By killing nonresistant bacteria, antibiotics allow the resistant ones to multiply. What's more, the survivors can pass on to other bacteria the ability to resist the antibiotic.[l] A prolonged hospital stay increases the chances of someone with AIDS catching resistant bacteria that will pass this resistance to other pathogens in the body. "I would be willing to predict," Louria says, "that not only will salmonella infections be reported with increasing frequency but also that . . . initially susceptible salmonellae will become broadly antimicrobial-resistant and then they may even cause intrahospital epidemics."[20] By reducing the normal intestinal flora that competes with harmful bacteria, antibiotics may also foster the overmultiplication of resistant pathogens. Remember that antibiotics are not cure-alls but toxic substances that, wrongly used, may cause greater havoc than the original illness they were to treat.

The familiar phrase "take aspirin and call me in the morning" reflects a current reality: the misuse of over-the-counter drugs.

Aspirin isn't the harmless substance it is thought to be. It is a toxic drug. At least one child dies every day from aspirin poisoning in the U.S. Aspirin is the most common single poison used in suicide, yet it is easily available and widely used for even the most transient of symptoms. Aspirin could be unsafe for anyone with deficient immunity. The drug works by inhibiting the action of two hormonelike substances that cause inflammation, fever, and pain: prostaglandins PGE2 and PGE2-alpha. The same aspirin pill that rids you of flu symptoms may also suppress your immunity further. Aspirin also inhibits prostaglandin PGE1, necessary to lymphocyte formation.[m, 21]

Our experience with AIDS tells us that chronic pain as well as any other chronic symptom may indicate serious illness. Pain killers, antihistamines, and fever and cough medicines often mask symptoms, preventing early detection and treatment of disease. And who knows what effect these drugs might have on an already taxed immune system! You needn't seek martyrdom through pain, yet you shouldn't rely on over-the-counter medications either. If you do use them, I recommend you read *Over-the-Counter Pills That Don't Work* by Joel Kaufman and others. Be sure to consult your physician about all these remedies.

The pharmaceutical industry would like us to believe that there's a pill for every ill. Drug advertising plays upon our wish for quick and easy remedies to our problems. In 1981, for example, the makers of Tylenol, Anacin, Bayer, Bufferin, and Excedrin spent $150 million in advertising. The kind of medicine Madison Avenue prescribes through advertisement results in excessive consumption of over-the-counter remedies, worth up to $10 billion dollars a year,[22] and in 30,000 deaths each year from legal drug misuse, as revealed by recent U.S. Senate investigations.[23]

The FDA knows this. Its experts have found that only one-third of the ingredients in all over-the-counter remedies are safe and effective. Why then does the FDA allow these unproven and unsafe drugs to remain on the market? Maybe because they make too much money for their manufacturers. Under pressure from these billion-dollar industries, the FDA fails to implement its findings, violating drug laws that prohibit medications with unproven and unsafe ingredients from being sold to consumers.[24]

Over-the-counter consumers are not the only target of Madison Avenue leechcraft. Drug companies invest millions in advertising to doctors. The quality of ads in medical publications is frequently top-of-the-line, sometimes more entertaining than the text. A physician whose practice permits little time to keep up-to-date may sometimes come to rely too much on the pharmaceutical representative's information about new drugs. And like the rest of us, some doctors may tire of too slow a result and opt for the quick fix of needlessly toxic drugs. Sadly, a few physicians cannot think of anything else. The steadfast efforts of drug companies, all those billions of dollars and years of advertising, have turned some doctors and many patients into legal junkies.

RECREATIONAL DRUGS AND ALCOHOL

Candy is dandy, but liquor is quicker. — OGDEN NASH

My advice on the use of alcohol and the so-called recreational drugs could be very short: DON'T! But because these substances unfortunately form too large a part of our lives, we need to discuss them in greater detail.

Some of my recovering-alcoholic friends, however, have expressed worries about explanations of alcoholism. They say such explanations might provide the alcoholic with another excuse to drink (the "poor li'l oppressed me" line). I agree with and applaud their good intentions, yet I believe that anything that I say, or fail to say, will provide that wanted excuse for the alcoholic who isn't done drinking. After all, there are people drinking or using drugs because they feel their drinking or drug abuse dooms them to acquire AIDS! Nonetheless, for gays with no drinking problems—a 70 to 80 percent majority—learning about the social roots of alcoholism in our community is essential to understanding AIDS. Both illnesses reflect underlying problems we need to address: our poor self-image and the distress it brings into our lives. AIDS and substance abuse feed into each other.

Alcoholism among gays is about three times the national average. Between 20 and 30 percent of all gay men and women are alcoholic or at risk of turning alcoholic.[25] Homosexuality, however, doesn't automatically imply alcoholism as anti-gay groups would have us believe. A gay man or woman has a greater chance of turning to the bottle than the average American, not than the average straight person in the U.S. Alcoholism among gays can be brought into perspective by comparing it with alcoholism among other minorities: native Americans, Chicanos, and Harlem Puerto Ricans, for example. High rates of alcoholism are not uncommon among the disempowered.

In addition to coping with the stresses of daily living, gay men and women have to deal with the added stress of living in a society that spurns their existence. The stress that arises out of the conflict between daily life and homosexuality often can't be resolved. Every gay man and woman clearly remembers what it was like to grow up gay. The oppression of family, the ridicule of friends, the intolerance of society, and above all the self-doubt were often too painful. For some of us, coming out of the closet was almost a spiritual experience. It often transformed our soul—our innermost self—and allowed us into the circle of the select, a fellowship of those who had survived the same ordeal.

Yet for many of us, the closet remains comfortably near no matter how open we say we are. We step back into the closet as we see fit—when we go to work, when we visit family and friends, or when we're threatened by the straight world out there—and in these days of AIDS the closet often does look temptingly inviting. We need the closet to shield us from the unresolved pain of those growing-up years. Yet, paradoxically, shielding ourselves from pain brings a new kind of pain altogether: the pain of denial. It hurts to deny our self-worth and dignity as gay men and women; thus, some of us turn to alcohol, drugs, and even sex in order not to feel that pain.[26]

Alcohol and drug abuse have physiological and genetic roots as well. Research indicates that children of alcoholics may inherit genes that code for an inordinate ability to metabolize alcohol. Most of us generally shut down after a few drinks. We get either drunk or sleepy and get a hangover in the morning. The person at risk of alcoholism doesn't. During the early days of drinking, the alcoholic-to-be may drink everyone under the table and not even look drunk. After the honeymoon with the bottle is over, however, the alcoholic's metabolism does what a normal person's can't do—switch from glucose to alcohol for energy. Turned on to alcohol, the alcoholic's body will demand it as fuel when energy is low. The symptoms of alcohol withdrawal are those of very low blood sugar: headaches, dizziness, tremors, nervousness, and depresssion. Just as the symptoms of low blood sugar go away dandy with candy, those of alcohol withdrawal do so quicker with liquor—only to come back again and again until drinking stops altogether. For the recovering alcoholic, consuming sugar and dietary stimulants like caffeine may be playing with fire. Symptoms of sugar or caffeine lows may feel too uncomfortably close to the urge to drink. A whole-foods diet low in sugars, stimulants, and additives and high in complex carbohydrates and vegetables could make life easier for the recovering alcoholic.[27]

Inheriting a metabolic trick gene from an alcoholic parent doesn't guarantee becoming an alcoholic. Children of alcoholics know the ravages of alcohol firsthand and often will not drink. They sometimes become "dry drunks," however—people who but for a lack of desire and willingness to drink are psychologically identical to alcoholics.[n] Alcoholism may be higher among gays not because of a higher absolute population of alcoholics but because of a higher proportion of "wet drunks" to "dry drunks." That is, because of the way society has structured gay life, more potential alcoholics who would have otherwise remained "dry" are exposed to alcohol or drugs and turn to them.

Gay life existed for years only in the gay bar; it still is so in many towns today. More than a locale, the gay bar was the only territory a community of gay men and women could claim as their own. Pickups were only incidental; those could be procured elsewhere with more success. The bar was the place to meet friends, to exchange news and gossip, and to feel safer from the threat of the streets. Unlike other kinds of bars, the gay bar became an institution, a way of life, a vital tradition that gave us a sense of community until gay life blossomed on its own. Unfortunately for those at risk of alcoholism, the gay bar was also a place where you drank. For some , the bars provided an eagerly sought occasion to drink. For others, what started as a half-hearted attempt to conform ended as too real a need for the bottle. Although the gay bar as institution gave cohesiveness to our numbers in those early days, it also reinforced the scapegoat role society demanded from us: that of the drunk, and unhappy, homosexual.

Alcoholism or substance abuse, however, is not a matter of choice. "Substance abuse," say two leading San Francisco drug-abuse counselors, "is not a weakness but rather a chronic and progressive disease for which there is hope."[28] Both the current AIDS epidemic and the ongoing epidemic of substance abuse reflect, as

TABLE 7
Substance Abuse Assessment

1. Emotional, social, relationship, employment, legal, or other difficulties that can be linked to the use of alcohol or drugs
2. Loss of control of frequency or amount of use
3. Preoccupation with drugs of choice or alcohol
4. Self-medication with drugs or alcohol for anxiety or sadness
5. Drinking or using drugs while alone
6. Rapid intake of drugs or alcohol
7. Protection of drug or alcohol supply—stocking or hiding supply
8. Tolerance to large quantities of alcohol
9. Withdrawal symptoms
10. Blackouts

Excerpted with permission from Faltz and Madover, "AIDS and substance abuse: Issues for health care providers," *Focus* 1(9):1, August 1986.

we have said, an underlying psychological and social illness in our community. And both epidemics feed into each other. Intravenous drug use is one of the risk factors in AIDS; the virus is transmitted not only by the use of shared needles but also by sexual contact between infected IV-drug users and their partners. Alcohol and drugs also cloud judgment, increasing the probability of unsafe sex practices that contribute to the spread of HIV. More directly, alcohol, marijuana, amphetamines (speed, crystal or crank) and cocaine are immunosuppressive. Several studies have also linked the use of amyl or butyl nitrites (poppers) to the incidence of Kaposi's sarcoma in gay men.

In fact, according to noted medical statistician and physician Cesar Caceres of Washington, D.C., AIDS is primarily a disease of substance abuse. Dr. Caceres maintains that improper statistical classification of AIDS data by the Center for Disease Control in Atlanta has led to improper conclusions about the disease. The CDC risk categories for AIDS are hierarchical and mutually exclusive. Thus, a homosexual IV-drug user will always go into the "homosexual" and not into the "IV-user" category. This misclassification hides the fact that IV-users represent over one quarter of all AIDS cases. Moreover, Dr. Caceres maintains that reports from the field hold that "half of those with AIDS use as many as five street drugs in a year, that 93 percent smoke grass, 97 percent use poppers, around 68 percent take some form of amphetamine, and 70 percent take one or more drugs intravenously."[29]

"The CDC has refused to collect data on drug use," he adds. "We know also that there are articles the CDC hasn't cleared for publication, and those in reference to oral drugs have been held for two years at least."[30] Habitual drug use, as well as heavy drinking, may play a major role in in furthering susceptibility to AIDS, Dr. Caceres believes, and the withholding of drug-use data by the CDC not only conveys the wrong impression that all gay men are equally at risk[o] but also prevents the high-risk gay drug users from adopting the one measure that may reduce their chances of developing AIDS: staying off immunosuppressive substances.

A diagnosis of AIDS or ARC can trigger bouts of heavy drinking or drug use in substance abusers. Increased use might cause further immune deterioration that leads to more drinking and using and so establishes a fatal downward spiral of abuse and immune deterioration. The lack of control a substance abuser often experiences can lead to detrimental helplessness and hopelessness. Abuse of alcohol and drugs can also interfere with AIDS treatments, resulting in deterioration or lack of progress.

How can you tell whether you have a substance abuse problem? Some say that if you think you have this kind of problem, then you probably do. This criterion, however, leaves the door too open for those who do not want to confront their addiction. Table 7 details a series of factors that, when considered along with the amount, frequency, duration, and last time of use, can help you determine whether indeed you could be a substance abuser.

If you feel you have a problem and are concerned about AIDS or ARC, you should

- stop using alcohol and drugs, and if you can't, at least cut down;
- seek professional help for substance abuse;
- reduce stress through meditation, exercise, hobbies, and the support of a group or of friends;
- learn to "get high" without drugs;
- get plenty of sleep and rest;
- consume a whole-foods diet low in sugars, stimulants, and additives and high in complex carbohydrates and vegetables;

- center your life around activities other than going to the bars;
- restructure your goals and priorities to live a happier, healthier, and more satisfying life.

Two books that can be of great value if you are trying to overcome substance abuse are *Detox* by Phyllis Saifer and Merla Zellerbach and *Eating Right to Live Sober* by Katherine Ketcham and L. Ann Mueller.

Part two: Nourishing the body

CHAPTER 5

How food affects people

In this second part of the book I have placed particular emphasis on nutrition. Although I consider spiritual consciousness the most important aspect of our lives, diet is where we can make the quickest and most beneficial changes.[a] For those of us who have less than perfect health, an improved diet can give us the precious months or years needed to change other areas of our lives.

Nutrition can be a major stress factor, and yet it is the easiest to control. Because so many foods and dietary patterns are fuel for distress, diet modification can be a powerful tool in lessening the burden of harmful stress. Like the interplay between disease and distress, the interaction between disease and nutrition is synergistic. Poor nutrition lowers resistance to disease, and disease in turn aggravates existing nutritional deficiencies. The strength of our minds, spirits, and emotions and the state of our bodies' health likewise influence one another.

To say that we are what we eat is not merely to repeat a tired phrase. Indeed, there are foods that will wreck us emotionally and alienate us from the peace we can feel within. Paying attention to what we consume will help us conquer what consumes us.

For thousands of years the diet of our ancestors consisted

mainly of unprocessed plant foods and occasional animal protein. Any changes in daily diet took place slowly, allowing people time to adapt to new foods. In the past fifty years we have changed our diet drastically, switching to one based on animal products, sugars, fats, highly processed foods, and a multitude of frequently toxic additives. Because this change was so quick, our digestive organs have failed to adapt. They still work best with the diet for which they evolved—one centered around whole plant food—which is why our bodies are currently rebelling and screaming for help. Our daily aches and pains tell us to stop our newfangled eating habits and go back to the older, healthier, nontoxic diet.

Our current eating habits are the product of affluence, the bounty of American farms, and the activities of the food industry. So effectively has the food industry lobbied government, the medical profession, and the public that we believe our diet to be the best in the world because of its abundance and diversity. Yet our diet remains a far cry from being well balanced. We eat an abundance and variety of the wrong foods.

The health of consumers is not foremost in the minds of food lobbyists, and as the products their industry introduces become a greater portion of our diets, more regulation of nutritive content may become essential. We have been sold on convenience, and for convenience we let ourselves be poisoned, slowly and quietly. We are sacrificing our health for the smooth, creamy, easy-to-apply, and ready-to-eat concoctions that we place on our tables. How much time are we really saving when we eat prepared, prepackaged, ready-to-go foods that place a lien on our future?

The United States Senate Select Committee on Nutrition and Human Needs has strongly suggested that the major causes of death and disease in the United States today are related to what we eat.[1] The rest of the nation may be complacent enough to let the toll of cancer, heart disease, arthritis and a myriad other diseases rise, but some of us cannot afford to wait. For those of us with compromised immunity, every extra day a positive diet change gives us will be a bounty.

Give food a chance.

COMING TO FOOD IN AMERICA

Before my disease, I never gave food a chance. In fact, I rarely gave any thought to the adequacy of my diet. This was America; just living here assured me I was well fed. Malnutrition was a problem only in places like India or China, not in the good ol' U.S. of A, or so I had been told from childhood on. It didn't matter that practically everything I ate came out of a bottle, can, or box. TV commercials assured me that milk was the most perfect of foods, that frozen or canned vegetables and fruits arrived at my table at the peak of perfection—little of them wasted or spoiled—and that the white bread and breakfast cereals fortified in X different ways would wondrously provide me with all necessary vitamins and minerals. If they didn't, no worry; a single pill taken daily would. Not only was this type of food allegedly more nutritious, it was supposedly cheaper and, best of all, freed Mom from the drudgery of cooking and gave her more time to take care of me. It didn't matter that every couple months I had an ear infection, a strep throat, or a cold. TV and the grown-ups said my diet was good, and one never questioned these infallible sources of information. At least I didn't, until I was old enough to be sent to Vietnam. My change in attitude toward authority had little to do with food, although, as I recall, we were fed a meat-and-potatoes diet well suited, perhaps, for German winters but totally unsatisfactory for a tropical climate. I soon realized that the army, like its diet, was out of touch with reality. Never again would I trust authority so blindly.

After returning to the U.S., I gorged myself on cakes and pastries to add weight to my lanky 6'1" frame and quickly went from 136 to 160 pounds. Then I read Adele Davis and Carlton Fredericks, whose books convinced me that one could not possibly get enough proteins or vitamins from the average diet. So I went on a cheese-and-egg eating binge to insure that I would, and, just as in childhood, I got lots of colds; in addition, I was constantly tired. But I never questioned my diet until my doctor told me I had high blood cholesterol. Although Adele Davis's books had warned me there was something very wrong with the American diet, I decided Mom knew best; and since Mom baked the most scrumptious fresh bread every night, I put all doubts aside temporarily. For the next ten years, my diet varied according to who my roommates or what my finances were or what article I had read most recently in the evening newspaper.

I never studied up on nutrition until I came down with hepatitis A and read *Metabolic Ecology* by Fred Rohe. In describing the regime that physician William Kelley followed to treat his inoperable cancer of the pancreas, the book details a series of lifestyle changes, dietary alterations and massive vitamin and mineral supplementation. A computer analysis in a Texas nutrition seminar on the Kelley program recommended that I reintroduce into my diet the meat and animal products I had practically given up. It alerted me to the dangers of highly processed and fractured foods but at the same time suggested a plethora of costly dietary supplements. For several months, I spent between $300 and $500 a month on various supplements, including about 30 grams of daily vitamin C (this high dosage produced no ill effects and might have been the one factor in the program that altered the course of my disease). While my pocketbook was protesting against the monthly drain, my body was sending messages that some of the foods recommended, especially the meat and animal products, did not sit well with it. Something seemed to be lacking.

It was then than I came across macrobiotics and Michio Kushi, its primary exponent in the U.S. Mr. Kushi's dietary regimens were linked to dramatic reversals of fatal cancer prognoses. Writing about macrobiotics, he suggested a diet of basically unprocessed vegetable foods and no vitamin or mineral supplements. My body seemed to agree almost instantly. Whenever I ate a simple meal of, let's say, rice, broccoli, and soup, I did not feel as tired or as sick as when I ate meat and fried or processed foods. Unfortunately, I had great difficulty reading Mr. Kushi's *Book of Macrobiotics*. Much of the book seemed too esoteric, so I abandoned any further inquiries into macrobiotics and went back to my simple vegetarian meals while continuing to research nutrition.

In August 1984 I was reintroduced to macrobiotics by a group of people with AIDS in New York who felt their health was improving with such a diet. Today, after more than two years, I too can attest to the benefits of a modified macrobiotic diet. Because of my continued inquiry into nutrition, however, I was able to analyze many of the claims of macrobiotics in a more scientific and empirical light and tried whenever possible to relate macrobiotic claims to the latest findings about the causes of viral disease, cancer, and AIDS. Many of the tenets of macrobiotics withstood such a test, and others did not; I chose accordingly. My findings became the bedrock on which I laid my path to wellness. I will now share my discoveries with you.

ACHIEVING DIETARY BALANCE

My diet excludes several foods common in the average American diet. Although there are several reasons why I am selective, my main concern is nutritional balance. The foods I eat allow me to achieve dietary balance without fuss or strain.

I usually avoid foods that make this balance harder to achieve.

For most adults, a balanced diet should ideally possess a protein-to-carbohydrate ratio of between 1:6 and 1:8—one part of protein to six or eight of carbohydrate, as in human milk. If we draw a line and place high-carbohydrate foods on the left and high-protein foods on the right, it will look something like a seesaw, with human milk at the center as the fulcrum.

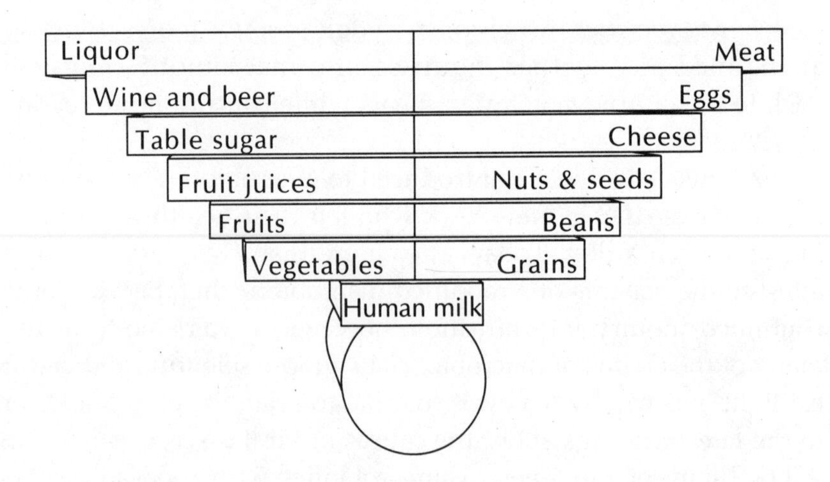

Choices made from the far left or far right can upset the balance much more easily than those made from the central area.

Our bodies strive to maintain the balance, or homeostasis, represented by the protein-to-carbohydrate ratio of human milk. If we ingest a food high in protein but low in carbohydrate, such as meat, the body goes out of balance and often will crave the opposite kind of food, a concentrated carbohydrate with no protein, such as table sugar, to re-establish balance. Thus, cravings for one particular food often signify we've had an excess of another food on the opposite end of the diet seesaw.

The farther from the center we move in one direction, the farther we must move in the opposite direction to achieve balance. This has nothing to do with will power; it is the law of opposites. As in the typical American diet of animal proteins and refined carbohydrates, homeostasis may be achieved by eating at the extremes, but we will feel the ups and downs of the seesaw while we search madly for such a balance. It is easier and less stressful to achieve balance by choosing most of our foods from those in the center.

Where in the seesaw we get our foods from will affect how we think, feel, and act. A centered diet will give us a centered disposition and a feeling of calmness and self-control, whereas a diet from the extremes will often produce extreme thoughts and behavior, with feelings of depression, anxiety, fear, and disorientation. Mind and body are inseparable, so when food affects the body, it can have a positive or negative effect on the mind and spirit as well.

CHAPTER 6

The elements of nutrition

CARBOHYDRATES

Many people think carbohydrates are bad for them. When they hear the word *carbohydrate,* they think of pastries, cookies, and white bread and therefore believe all carbohydrates are fattening. They are right in thinking pastries, cookies and white bread are bad but wrong in believing all carbohydrates will make them fat. What's fattening is eating the wrong kind of carbohydrates, those that are typically highly processed. In fact, certain carbohydrates—the *complex* carbohydrates—are our most efficient source of energy because they do not produce the toxic by-products that occur when the body burns fats and proteins.

To meet its most important need—the need for energy—the body will first use carbohydrates and then fats. If the carbohydrates and fats in our diet do not provide enough calories, the body will then turn to proteins and finally to its own tissue if dietary proteins are still inadequate. What's more, in severely low-carbohydrate diets, the body will break down fats faster than it can eliminate their toxic by-products, possibly causing dehydration, sodium loss, and a deadly accumulation of ketone bodies.[a, 1] To prevent this process, carbohydrates are not only beneficial but also necessary.

There are two broad categories of carbohydrates: sugars, and polysaccharides such as starches and cellulose. Sugars are divided into the simple sugars, or monosaccharides, made up of a single molecule, and the double sugars, or disaccharides, made up of two molecules. Glucose, fructose,[b] and galactose are the three simple sugars of dietary importance.

Glucose is the carbohydrate that circulates in the blood and the only sugar used by the cells for energy. It is found in some fruits such as berries and grapes and in vegetables such as sweet corn and carrots. Glucose is less sweet than table sugar. Fructose, on the other hand, is much sweeter than table sugar. It is found in honey, ripe fruits, and some vegetables. Galactose comes only from the breakdown of lactose, the double sugar in milk.

Like simple sugars, double sugars are water soluble and vary in sweetness. They are split into their component simple sugars by gastric juices and digestive enzymes. The three disaccharides that concern us are sucrose, lactose and maltose. Sucrose, table or refined sugar, is *the* sugar in cane and beet sugar and in molasses and maple syrup and is made up of glucose and fructose. Lactose, or milk sugar, is composed of glucose and galactose and is found in milk. Maltose consists of two glucose molecules and does not occur appreciably in foods except as an intermediate product of starch breakdown. It is produced, for example, by malting and fermenting grains.

The second broad class of carbohydrates are the polysaccharides, complex structures that consist of many—sometimes up to 2,000—simple sugars strung together. Complex carbohydrates are not sweet and are not all equally digestible. Humans can digest starches, for instance, but cannot digest the cellulose, hemicellulose, pectins, gums, and mucilages that make up the fiber in their diets. By the way, although fiber yields no nutrients, it is hardly useless. Fiber slows the rate at which simple sugars enter the bloodstream and provides bulk, which stimulates bowel movement and reduces the time food remains in the colon.

Cooking is the first step in the digestion of complex carbohydrates such as starches. Our salivary glands produce an enzyme, salivary amylase, that breaks down only those starches that have been cooked. How well the salivary amylase digests these starches depends on how well we chew the food, how well it is mixed with saliva, and how long it remains in the mouth. If we gulp our food down, very little digestion takes place. On the other hand, if we chew the food slowly and carefully, the amylase will do a substantial amount of its work in the mouth.

Starch digestion stops when gastric acids neutralize the salivary amylase and resumes after the food has passed from the stomach into the duodenum. At this point, pancreatic amylase breaks down both cooked and raw starches into double sugars; further down in the small intestine, other enzymes break down these double sugars into simple sugars. Because they have been gradually broken down into progressively smaller units, starches slowly and evenly release their glucose molecules into the bloodstream, thus providing a steady supply of energy that will last usually until the next meal. The simple sugars in a meal, however, enter the bloodstream rapidly and immediately and, if consumed more than moderately, will produce the roller-coaster mood swings of blood-sugar imbalance.

The last station of digestion is the liver, which converts fructose and galactose into glucose. Some of the glucose is then converted into glycogen, the carbohydrate the body uses to store energy. Although the body's glycogen reserves are limited, they can be maintained at a maximum level by a diet rich in carbohydrates. A high-protein, low-carbohydrate diet produces fewer glycogen stores, whereas a high-fat, low-protein, and low-carbohydrate diet will result in the poorest glycogen reserves. So if you want to keep your energy high, you should maintain a diet high in complex carbohydrates from whole grains, vegetables, and beans.

Storage of glucose by the liver is only part of a larger mechanism that strives to maintain a constant blood-glucose level. If the glucose level rises above a certain threshold, the pancreas will produce insulin, the hormone that helps the body lower blood-sugar concentration by transporting glucose into the cells, storing more glycogen in the liver, and converting glucose into fat. Insulin production is highest with sucrose or glucose and lowest with complex carbohydrates. For example, a meal of whole grains will produce a more sustained rise in blood sugar than a meal of cookies rich in simple sugars because the complex carbohydrates of whole grains will stimulate the least insulin production.[2]

"The difference between feeling up or down, sane or insane, calm or freaked out, inspired or depressed," William Dufty states in *Sugar Blues,* "depends in large measure upon what we put in our mouth."[3] Your energy level and ability to function will vary according to the source of your carbohydrates. Let's use an example.

For lunch you've had sweet pastries and the typical twelve-ounce soft drink that contains ten teaspoons of sugar—usually a combination of sucrose, glucose, and fructose. Shortly after eating, you experience a pleasant up as the glucose is absorbed into your blood. In trying to control this sudden rise in blood sugar, your pancreas releases a massive amount of insulin. Quite often, however, the insulin will lower the blood sugar below normal, and you will end up feeling down, down, down and desperately in need of more sugar so you can feel up, up, up again and start the sugar treadmill all over. Such blood-sugar imbalances have been linked to sudden and extreme shifts in mood and to mania, depression, anxiety, indecision and confusion.[4] If, instead of this sugar-laden lunch, you had had a cup of herbal tea and a sandwich of whole-wheat bread, bean sprouts, lettuce, tomatoes, and ground chick-pea patties, you would have avoided these mood swings.

William Dufty is eloquent about the increasing evidence of the dangers of sugar:

> The point is inescapable: as sugar consumption escalates, fatal diseases increase remorselessly. . . . Refined sugar is lethal when ingested by humans because it provides only that which nutritionists describe as empty or naked calories. In addition, sugar is worse than nothing because it drains and leeches the body of precious vitamins and minerals through the demand its digestion, detoxification and elimination make upon one's entire system. . . . Our body's tolerance and immunizing power become more limited, so we cannot respond properly to extreme attacks, whether they be cold, heat, mosquitos or microbes.[5]

Sucrose indeed impairs the ability of the immune system to fight bacteria. Because the immune system may not respond for up to four hours after the ingestion of sucrose, sucrose eaten at every meal may leave the body open to bacterial attack throughout most of the day.[6] Furthermore, one study on laboratory rats indicates that rats fed on sucrose are more likely to suffer from tumors brought about by carcinogenic substances than those fed on starch.[7] I myself have noticed an occasional soreness in my throat within a few hours after eating something with lots of sucrose such as dessert at a restaurant meal. If I have a sugar-rich food, like a milkshake, as my only meal, my throat often turns red later.

Under various guises, sucrose is added to practically every processed food under the sun and accompanies us from the cradle to the grave. It's in table salt, mayonnaise, salad dressing, tomato sauce, vegetarian beans, instant soup mixes, baby formulas, and

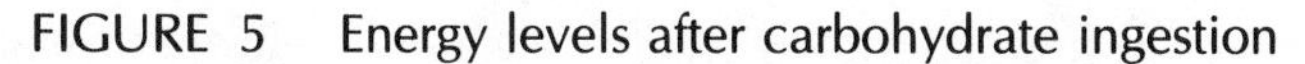

FIGURE 5 Energy levels after carbohydrate ingestion

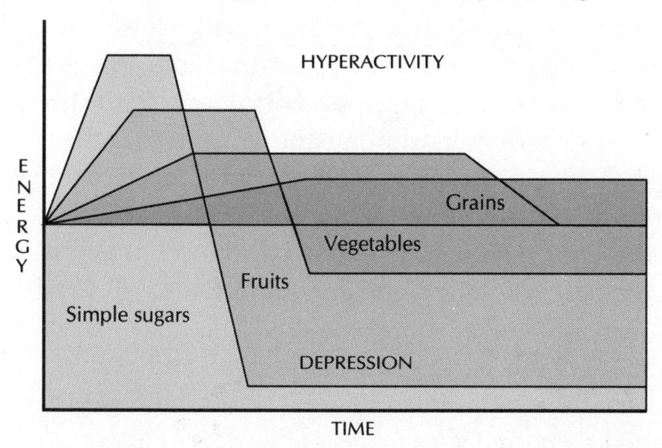

condiment mixes. Ketchup, for example, is about 29 percent sugar. In addition to the sugar naturally occurring in foods such as fruits and vegetables, the average American consumes about one-half cup of refined sugar every day. To avoid sucrose and all its aliases you will have to avoid practically all prepared or processed foods available on the supermarket shelf and gear yourself to the way people ate before twentieth-century "convenience."[8]

Many people regard honey,[c] molasses, and maple syrup as acceptable substitutes for table sugar. These sweeteners produce a glucose-insulin reaction almost as severe as that of sucrose; however, they are better than table sugar insofar as they are less refined and therefore retain some of the vitamins and minerals necessary for their breakdown. So-called natural cookies and cakes made with honey are, therefore, not much better than those made with regular table sugar.

Figure 5 plots the changes in energy (blood-sugar) levels that occur after the ingestion of different carbohydrates. Fruits provide a more sustained energy flow than simple sugars such as table or maple sugar, honey, and molasses because fruit fiber slows down the rate at which fruit sugars enter the blood. Vegetables constitute a further improvement. Grains, predominantly complex carbohydrates that are slowly digested and release steadily absorbed sugars, provide the most constant energy level of all carbohydrates.

We need to differentiate among the various starches. Refined starches, such as macaroni and white bread, have been stripped not only of vitamins and minerals but also of fiber. Without fiber, these starches will release glucose into the blood more quickly. On the other hand, a whole-grain diet high in fiber will produce sustained energy and fewer mood swings. This diet, supplemented with lots of vegetables and some beans, fish, and whole fruit, will supply most of the vitamins, minerals, and amino acids we need. Avoid refined carbohydrates.

For those whose health isn't at its optimum, consumption of sugar and refined carbohydrates might lead to other problems. It may aggravate infections by sugar-loving *Candida albicans,* a yeastlike fungus that causes thrush and can become an opportunistic pathogen in AIDS. Additionally, refined carbohydrates may aggravate impaired digestion. In some gastrointestinal disorders, the body stops producing one or more of the enzymes that aid in digesting sucrose, lactose, and maltose. Many people suffering from gluten-sensitive enteropathy, gastroenteritis, protein malnutrition, lymphatic blockage, and bacterial or parasitic diseases such as salmonellosis, shigellosis, and amebiasis are unable to digest lactose and, to a lesser extent, sucrose and maltose. In these cases, not only is the body unable to get energy from some of these double sugars, but the undigested sugars also draw a large volume of water into the intestines, causing bloating, cramps, and diarrhea.[9, 10]

If you have bowel problems, you should not consume dairy products, sucrose in any form, corn syrup, fruit juices, or more than an occasional whole fruit. You should probably also avoid potatoes and wheat and possibly rye, barley, and oats. In contrast to other starches, starches from wheat and potato products tend to produce more maltose, which is difficult to digest.[11] What's the use in eating any of these products—and sugar in particular—when they will provide little nutritional value and also may increase the incidence of diarrhea?

PROTEINS

Proteins are large and complex molecules that regulate most biological functions and are needed for building, repairing, and maintaining body tissue. Protein, in fact, is the main component of all living matter and is found in every body cell and all body fluids except urine and bile. The body, however, does not utilize proteins directly. It breaks them down into their individual constituents, the amino acids, and later reassembles them according to its needs.

A total of twenty amino acids make up all proteins. Those amino acids the body can produce itself are considered nonessential, whereas those the body cannot synthesize in sufficient quantity are deemed essential. Amino acids essential for adults are isoleucine, leucine, lysine, methionine, phenylalanine, threonine, tryptophan, and valine. In addition to these, histidine is also essential for infants.

Without these essential amino acids we die. But excessive protein in our diet can have disastrous results. Researchers have found that T lymphocytes do not function well when the blood contains high rather than moderate protein levels.[12]

Findings about our protein requirements run contrary to popular belief. Many people believe they need lots of protein in their diet, and that plant proteins are inferior to animal proteins and therefore need to be meticulously combined before the body can utilize them properly. This popular view holds that only animal proteins possess an amino acid ratio resembling that of the body's proteins.

Whole plant foods contain all the essential amino acids, but usually not in the proportions that our body needs for building protein. Plant foods should be combined so that foods that are rich in a particular amino acid complement those that are poor. We don't need to be rigorous about protein complementing, however, when we follow a varied, healthful diet. "Protein complementarity is not a myth," says Frances Moore Lappé in her revised *Diet for a Small Planet*. "It works. The myth is that complementing proteins is necessary for most people on a low or nonmeat diet. With a healthy varied diet, concern about protein complementarity is not necessary for most of us."[13] But we need to keep in mind that some of us will have to consume animal foods or complement plant protein sources carefully because we either need more protein or do not eat a varied diet.

How much protein do we require daily? The United States Senate Select Committee on Nutrition and Human Needs has recommended that an adult male with a 3,000-calorie diet should consume no more than 12 percent of those calories as protein—about 90 grams or 3.2 ounces of protein a day. This maximum is somewhat less than the usable protein in the customary eight-ounce American steak. On the other hand, the National Research Council has set a minimum recommended dietary allowance (RDA) at 4 to 5 percent of daily caloric intake, which translates to about 30 to 35 grams or 1.1 to 1.2 ounces of protein.[14] The World Health Organization also has established a minimum daily requirement of 5 percent. These lower limits set by the NRC and the WHO are well above the absolute minimum below which protein deficiency occurs. Studies have demonstrated that an adult male can maintain adequate health on about 20 to 24 grams, or about three-quarters of an ounce, of protein a day—the amount in four slices of whole wheat bread. The diets of most adults meet these minimums, provided they supply caloric needs through unprocessed starches.

To insure I get sufficient protein, nonetheless, I have complementary brown rice and beans daily, and, since I have found that some animal protein affords me greater energy, I eat seafood a few times during the week.

The Senate Select Committee was the only group to set a maximum for protein consumption and, in doing so, to recognize the dangers of too much protein. A high-protein diet means more work for the liver and kidneys. When too much protein is consumed, excess amino acids are not stored but are turned into glucose by the liver and used for energy by the body. The conversion of amino acids into glucose is less clean than the conversion of carbohydrates. It yields extremely toxic ammonia that the liver must quickly convert into the less toxic urea, expending energy in the process. Urea then enters the bloodstream and travels to the kidneys, where more energy must be spent for its excretion.

When the liver malfunctions, as it does in people with liver disease, it fails to convert all the ammonia into urea and instead may allow some to enter the bloodstream. Ammonia, even in small amounts, can cause brain damage and lead to coma or death. Viral infections such as cytomegalovirus infection (mononucleosis) and hepatitis attack the liver and reduce its ability to detoxify ammonia.

Too much ammonia in the intestines also can be deleterious. According to Willard Visek, professor of clinical sciences at the University of Illinois Medical School, "Ammonia behaves like chemicals that cause cancer or promote its growth. It kills cells . . . and it increases the mass of the lining of the intestines. What is intriguing is that, within the colon, the incidence of cancer parallels the concentration of ammonia."[15]

Excess protein itself might contribute to tumor growth. Diets deficient in protein have been shown to hinder the production of immunoglobulin G (IgG), a class of antibodies that warn T lymphocytes of the presence of microbes. But IgG cannot alert T lymphocytes to cancer cells. Too many IgG antibodies on a cancer cell will mask it from the T lymphocytes that would have otherwise killed it. The cancer cell will grow unchecked into a tumor. And because protein deficiency inhibits IgG synthesis, it may well be that the opposite—high protein consumption—could enhance IgG production and open the way for tumor growth.[16 17] Limiting protein consumption to the point of deficiency is harmful to anyone. On the other hand, those at high risk of developing cancer should avoid an excess of protein that could favor tumor growth.

A high-protein diet also might contribute to osteoporosis, the crippling loss of calcium from the bones. Some of the minerals in protein produce acids that the body must neutralize by drawing calcium from the bones. Too much protein may cause large quantities of calcium to enter the blood. The calcium is then excreted by the kidneys and lost to the body in the urine. Therefore, people who eat large amounts of protein may not have calcium in their bones even though their calcium consumption is high. Osteoporosis need not be an inevitable consequence of aging. Bone calcium loss starts around age fifty-five in Americans, but it has been found as early as age twenty in Eskimos, whose protein intake, not surprisingly, far surpasses ours.[18] High protein diets are also undesirable because they are usually high in fats. In the next chapter I will have more to say about the dangers of high-fat diets.

What are the best sources of protein? Practically every food provides some protein, but the amount supplied varies greatly. Apples, for instance, are one of the whole-food sources lowest in protein; only one percent of their calories comes from protein and the remainder predominantly from carbohydrates. Egg whites, on the other hand, are probably the highest source; 85 percent of their calories derive from protein.[19] Apples and egg whites, however, are on opposite ends of the protein spectrum and are not foods on which to build a stable diet. As I have said before, diets based on extremes are detrimental. Let's examine some other protein candidates to determine which ones belong to a more moderate, balanced, and healthful diet.

Table 8 lists the protein and fat content of several foods as a percentage of total calories. The table does not show the quality or usability of the protein. Most of the animal sources in the table are high in protein but also high in fat. Even so, the percentage of

TABLE 8 Protein, fat, and calories in selected foods

FOOD SOURCE	PROTEIN % *	FAT % †	CALORIES per gram	CALORIES per ounce
Barley	9	3	3.49	97.9
Beans, kidney	26	4	1.18	33.8
Beef, ground	34	65	2.90	82.9
Broccoli	45	9	.32	9.2
Brussels sprouts	44	8	.24	6.9
Carrots	10	4	.42	12.0
Cashews	12	73	5.61	160.4
Cauliflower	40	7	.27	7.7
Cheese, Swiss	30	68	3.70	105.8
Cherries	8	4	.63	18.0
Chicken, light and skinless	76	18	1.66	47.5
Corn, sweet	12	8	.84	24.0
Flounder	59	37	2.02	57.7
Lamb chops	22	76	2.52	72.1
Lentils	29	3	1.06	30.3
Lettuce	34	13	.14	4.0
Oatmeal	15	16	.55	15.7
Peas, green	30	4	.84	24.0
Rice, brown	8	5	1.19	34.0
Squash, summer	23	5	.19	5.4
Walnuts, black	13	85	6.28	179.6

*Protein and fat content expressed as a percentage of the total calories.
†Carbohydrates represent the caloric balance not shown.

Adapted from data in *Nutritive Value of American Foods in Common Units,* Agriculture Handbook No. 456, as presented by J. A. McDougall and M. A. McDougall in *The McDougall Plan.*

protein in broccoli, cauliflower, or Brussels sprouts is higher than that in ground beef. The low-calorie content of these vegetables, however, would require eating rather hefty portions if they were our sole source of protein. On the other hand, although one and one-third pounds of ground beef would give us most of the needed calories—about 1,800—they would deluge our bodies with fat in the process. Around 210 grams, or 7.4 ounces, of this beef would be usable protein. The rest, almost two-thirds, would be fat. The table does show that certain other foods contain at least as much protein as beef, thus dispelling the notion that the only way to get enough protein is to eat lots of meat. In fact, most of these foods would meet the 1.1-to-1.2–ounce protein RDA set by the National Research Council as long as they provided us with neither too few nor too many calories.

Barley, for instance, is representative of most grains. Just under two pounds would provide us with 3,000 calories and about 80 grams, or 2.8 ounces, of protein. Because 60 percent of this protein is usable, we would be consuming around 48 grams, or 1.7 ounces, more than the National Research Council's RDA and would still be eating a relatively low amount of fat. We can conclude that grains fill the body's caloric and protein needs while avoiding excess fat and thus come closer than any other food to being the core of a balanced, healthful diet. We shall talk about them again.

If you feel you cannot adequately judge your protein requirements and are concerned that you might be getting too little, you may want to follow Francis Moore Lappé's advice. Watch the condition of your nails, hair, and skin and how much time your nicks and scratches take to heal. Since all these require newly synthesized protein, they are a good gauge of whether or not you are getting enough protein. If you need greater reassurance, your physician can always test whether your body is getting the protein it needs.

FATS

Lipids—fats and fatlike substances—play an essential part in our diets. They are necessary for the transportation of fat-soluble vitamins, the absorption of calcium, and the insulation and padding of the body. They are the main constituent of all cell membranes. Because fats yield nine calories per gram when burned by the body (carbohydrates and proteins produce four), they act as the body's primary long-range reserve of energy.

Despite the importance of fats, our minimum daily requirements are small, and excessive amounts can prove dangerous. Only up to 5 percent of our dietary calories need to come from fatty acids,[d] a few of which are essential because the body cannot manufacture them from other fatty acids. One essential fatty acid is linoleic acid. A diet made up primarily of whole grains and vegetables will provide this polyunsaturated fatty acid in abundance. Some researchers also consider omega-3 and omega-6 fatty acids essential, because of their role in the production of the hormone-like prostaglandins that affect blood pressure, metabolism, smooth-muscle activity, and the fever mechanism of the body.[20]

Table 9 lists the fat and linoleic acid content of various foods. Although animal products have a high fat content, only a small percentage of that fat is the essential linoleic acid. Grains, on the other hand, are low in fat but possess a high percentage of linoleic acid. Most beans have the low fat, high linoleic-acid ratio of grains, except for soybean and its derivatives, which are high-fat foods. Nuts and seeds have not only the highest percentage of linoleic acid but also the highest fat content.

Cholesterol is another necessary, though not essential, lipid. It is present in all tissue and is the building block of certain hormones, bile salts, and a form of vitamin D. The body produces all the cholesterol it needs. Plants produce no cholesterol, so we are in

TABLE 9 Linoleic acid and fat in selected foods

FOOD	TOTAL FAT %	LINOLEIC ACID %	FOOD	TOTAL FAT %	LINOLEIC ACID %
Animal			**Beans**		
Beef (T-bone)	82	2	Chick peas	12	36
Eggs, whole	65	7	Soybeans	40	52
Milk	49	3	Soybean curd (tofu)	53	52
Grains			**Nuts and Seeds**		
Barley	3	50	Almonds	82	20
Corn	8	51	Cashews	73	7
Oatmeal	16	41	Peanuts	75	29
Rice, brown	5	35	Pumpkin seeds	76	41
Rye	7	62	Sunflower seeds	76	63
Miscellaneous					
Avocados	88	30	Margarine	100	28
Chocolates, sweet	56	2	Olives	98	8
Coconut, fresh	89-92	Trace			

Sources: *Fatty Acids in Food Fats.* Home Economics Research Report No. 7. U.S. Department of Agriculture and *Nutritive Value of American Foods in Common Units.* Agriculture Handbook No. 456. As presented by McDougall.

danger of consuming excess cholesterol only if we eat animal products. When, in addition, we consume insufficient plant fibers, the excess cholesterol of a high-fat animal diet will be more readily absorbed into the bloodstream and stored around the body, mainly in the blood vessels. Where and how cholesterol is stored depends on the relative amounts of other lipids in the body.

When cholesterol builds up on an artery wall, it eventually forms a growing plaque that hardens and narrows the artery, sometimes completely closing it. If this constriction occurs in a heart vessel, either from local build-up or from plaque that has broken loose elsewhere, the heart tissue fed by the blocked vessel might die, and if the affected area is large enough, so might the individual. If this vessel feeds the brain, a stroke or other brain damage could occur.

Excess cholesterol may contribute to a more rapid spread of HIV infection in AIDS and ARC. All cell membranes consist of cholesterol and the phospholipids phosphatidylcholine and phosphatidylethanolamine. The proportion of cholesterol to phosphatidylcholine determines the rigidity of the membrane and the exposure of the receptor molecules through which HIV infects the cell. The more the cholesterol, the more rigid the cell membrane and the more exposed to HIV its receptor molecules become. Conversely, the lesser the proportion of cholesterol to phosphatidylcholine, the more fluid the membrane and the more protected its receptor molecules.

A large portion of immunity is mediated through receptor molecules. When immune-cell membranes become too rigid, receptor molecules become frozen in place and fail to perform their immune-regulatory function. These frozen receptor molecules, now also excessively exposed to outside forces, wear down in the constant jostle against other immune cells. Immunity deteriorates. This cholesterol-induced membrane rigidity and loss of immune function happens not only with age but also during withdrawal from drugs.[21] This could be the mechanism through which excessive drinking and drug use may act as cofactors in AIDS.[e]

Although low cholesterol consumption alone is unlikely to alter cell membrane rigidity in people with AIDS or ARC, low cholesterol consumption and ingestion of a substance such as AL 721 will lower the proportion of cholesterol to phosphatidylcholine in cell membranes and may thus help contain the spread of HIV infection and restore immune function. A high-cholesterol diet, on the other hand, could neutralize the action of AL 721 or any phosphatidylcholine or lecithin supplements and contribute to the spread of HIV and the deterioration of immunity. For those with AIDS or ARC, keeping cholesterol consumption to a minimum is essential.

We get not only too much cholesterol but also plainly too much fat in our diets. The average American obtains over 40 percent of his or her calories from fats and fatlike substances. We simply love fats, and understandably so. Fats are rich and make our food taste better. They give us that stick-to-the-ribs feeling we get at the end of a satisfying meal. Their cost to our health, however, is devastating. A diet in which less than 25 per cent of our calories came from fats and oils would be more healthful.

Salad and cooking oils are an added, and often avoidable, source of fat in our diet. While in their nut, seed, or plant of origin, vegetable oils still contain vitamin E, which prevents their oxidation. Once processed, however, most oils lose their vitamin E, oxidize, and become rancid. When ingested, these rancid oils destroy many fat-soluble vitamins. Yet some oils might be beneficial when used moderately in salads and not in cooking. In implementing Dr. Russell Jaffe's AIDS protocol, Dr. Keith Barton recommends that a tablespoon of the following oils be taken, one oil per day in a four-day sequence: cod-liver oil, edible linseed, evening primrose oil, and raw sesame or grape seed oil.[22] These oils contain the omega-3 and omega-6 essential fatty acids that promote prostaglandin production. Since I eat animal products, fried foods, and oil in salads only occasionally, I consume small amounts of cod-liver and evening primrose oils and take one or two daily tablespoons of virgin, cold pressed olive oil. Olive oil is a good antioxidant (which may be why it helps relieve candida symptoms in some people),[23] helps lower cholesterol, is pleasant tasting, and will not go rancid outside the refrigerator. Instead of taking olive oil straight, you may want to add it to your salad.

In the frying of foods, unsaturated or polyunsaturated fats may cause more harm than saturated ones. Heating unsaturated or polyunsaturated oils to the high temperatures required for frying produces free radicals—certain atoms that are very chemically reactive and are thought to be carcinogenic. If you fry foods, you should use clarified butter or olive oil. Clarified butter is a high density saturated fat whose molecular structure remains stable and does not yield free radicals during frying. Monosaturated olive oil is noncarcinogenic for the same reasons.[24] Use these cooking oils judiciously; large quantities of them can increase vitamin E needs.

Margarine is produced by hydrogenating an oil or a mixture of oils. Hydrogenation uses nickel as a catalyst, and this nickel is not removed at the end of the process. Excess nickel has been shown to increase the amount of fats in the blood.[25] Hydrogenation also produces certain fatty acids that do not occur in nature[g] and are thought to be injurious. The McDougalls state that people who eat these manmade fatty acids are reported to have one of the highest rates of death from heart disease.

A high-fat diet may, of itself, increase your exposure to carcinogens. Substances such as herbicides, pesticides, nematocides, fungicides, and hormones are fat-soluble and concentrate in the fat of animals and plants. Prostate, breast, colon, and testicular cancers, as well as lymphomas, have been linked to high fat diets. The incidence of breast cancer among women increases dramatically in those countries with higher daily fat consumption.[26] J. Sattilaro, a Philadelphia physician who attests to a dramatic cancer recovery in *Recalled by Life,* states:

> The most widely held theory is that fat appears to promote cancer by influencing the metabolic processes of normal cells, making them more susceptible to the development of malignancy brought on by other agents. In other words, a high fat diet creates an internal environment that appears to make cells more vulnerable to

carcinogens, which might not be effective otherwise, and it has been suggested that fat acts like a solvent, which enhances the effects of certain carcinogens.[27]

Whichever way fat might promote the development of cancer, the body seems to connect fat with cancer in another way. During severe infections or a cancer outbreak, the macrophages of the immune system release cachectin, a hormonelike protein that forces cells to lose all stored lipids and blocks any further production of fat. The release of the protein causes continuous loss of weight, even if the individual is fed an adequate diet. But emaciation is not cachectin's only outcome. Researchers at Rockefeller University have identified cachectin as the elusive tumor necrosis factor. Cachectin, in other words, encourages the quick death of cancer tissue. Researchers believe that the substance depletes fat cells so it can use their energy to fight tumors.[28] Yet one wonders whether cachectin could also be the way the immune system recognizes a link between high fat levels and the onset of malignancy in a cell.

The immune system holds other aversions towards excess fat. A high fat diet has been shown to hasten the shrinking of the thymus, the organ that helps activate immune cells.[29] Researchers at the University of Cincinnati have linked high fat diets to reduced immune function. They have shown that certain blood fats, the low- and very low-density lipoproteins (LDLs and VLDLs),[h] substantially reduce the disease-fighting abilities of T and B cells by blocking the receptors through which these cells recognize foreign bacteria, viruses, and cancer cells. In addition, these fats prevent T cells from cloning and thus from relaying to other cells the message to to fight particular offenders. Large amounts of VLDLs and LDLs have been found to reduce immunological activity by as much as 70 percent.

These findings substantiate previous studies that found

TABLE 10
Fat and oil consumption

USE PREFERENTIALLY
Olive oil for frying and in salads
Clarified butter for frying
Sesame, linseed, corn oils (except for frying)

LIMIT
Animal fat in milk, eggs, and meat

AVOID
Lards
Hydrogenated oils
Polyunsaturated frying oils

impaired immune function in persons suffering from high-blood-cholesterol disease. Researchers say, however, that these fats do not necessarily compromise immune response in people with normal blood cholesterol. The part of the immune system not influenced by the fats should compensate for any suppressed immunity.[30] One might conclude nonetheless that persons with already impaired immune systems should avoid high amounts of low- and very low-density lipoproteins, which are prevalent especially in red meat, fowl, eggs, whole milk, and whole-milk products (see Table 10 for a listing of fats to use and to avoid).

FIBER

Americans have small stools and big hospitals. — DENNIS BURKITT, M.D.[31]

Fiber is composed of polysaccharides we cannot digest, such as cellulose, lignin, hemicellulose, pectins, gums, and mucilages.[i] Although it yields no nutrients, dietary fiber offers other benefits. It provides bulk, stimulates bowel movement, reduces food transit time through the colon, and slows the absorption rate of sugars into the bloodstream. More important, fiber lowers blood-cholesterol levels, encourages beneficial intestinal flora, and discourages harmful bacteria that might produce toxic wastes in the bowels.

The liver manufactures bile, a cholesterol-based substance discharged by the gall bladder to emulsify and help digest fats in the intestines. Once bile has performed its digestive function, it is normally reabsorbed into the blood to be collected and sent by the liver back to the gallbladder. If we eat a high-fiber diet, however, the fiber binds with the bile salts, thus preventing them from being reabsorbed and eliminating them from the body along with the feces. With the loss of the cholesterol-based bile, the liver has to scavenge cholesterol from all over the body to replenish the gall bladder's supply of bile. The interaction between fiber and bile thus helps reduce the amount of cholesterol present in the blood.

Fiber, by providing bulk and facilitating bowel movement, also reduces the transit time of food through the intestines. In countries such as India and Africa where high-fiber diets are prevalent, the typical transit time is about one day, whereas in the West it is usually a few days and sometimes even more than a week.[32] Reduced transit time means less exposure of the intestines to whatever toxins might be present in the food. Moreover, the added fiber dilutes the concentration of carcinogenic toxins, helping prevent their absorption by the intestines.

Where does dietary fiber come from? Certainly not from any animal sources, unless you were to eat fur, feathers, and claws. Fiber is most abundant on the exterior surfaces of whole grains, seeds, beans, vegetables, and fruit and is amply provided when we eat all of these unrefined, whole carbohydrate foods. A diet of complex carbohydrates can contain 60 or more grams of dietary fiber.

Most of us, however, consume a diet high in animal products and highly refined carbohydrates. Such a diet is very low in dietary fiber, supplying us with less than 10 grams per day. This low fiber intake, along with excessive fat and protein consumption, has been implicated in the increasing number of colon cancer cases.

One very common problem caused by a low-fiber diet is known as the irritable bowel syndrome, characterized by cramps and diarrhea, which sometimes alternate with constipation. Constipation can often lead to hemorrhoids. Other ailments linked to low fiber intake are diverticulosis,[j] gallbladder disease, gallstones, and even coronary artery disease.

Realizing they are not getting enough dietary fiber, many people have turned to bran supplements. Bran is the most concentrated form of fiber and is often, although incorrectly, thought to be the same as dietary fiber. Processed bran contains little of the fiber found in a varied diet of natural whole foods and does not adequately fulfill the body's needs the way vegetables, grains, beans, and fruit do. Bran supplements may in fact cause more problems by creating unnecessary phytic acid, which prevents the assimilation of calcium, and by blocking the absorption of nutrients in the colon. To cash in on this bran fad some food processors make "extra fiber" products by adding processed wood chips to the flour! Invariably this is the case when the label mentions "crude" rather than "dietary" fiber.[33]

The bran fiasco illustrates how crazy the food-processing situation has become. The industry starts with whole wheat, which was not dubbed the staff of life by accident, strips it of its protein, minerals, vitamins, and fiber, and ends up with a product that has eternal shelf life because it is eternally dead. Then they add another dead substance—wood—that is totally inappropriate for our needs unless we happen to have termite ancestry. The product is then advertised as containing "nutritious fiber." To add insult to injury, manufacturers are charging us more for a product that might be worse for us than Mom's worthless white bread. The industry seems to have gone mad, and so will we if we let ourselves be conned into accepting an illusion of bounty and wholesomeness while our bodies are being eaten up with cancer, intestinal disease, coronary failures, or possibly AIDS.

Eat only those whole foods suitable to whole humans!

VITAMINS

Vitamins are various unrelated, complex organic substances essential in small quantities for the normal functioning of the body. They are essential because the body does not produce them either at all or in sufficient quantities to meet its needs.

What our vitamin requirements are and whether they should be met through supplements are currently controversial issues. We are uncertain not only about the optimum amount of each vitamin we need but also about whether we've identified all vitamins. Vitamin research is quite new—most vitamins were discovered in the past sixty years and have been used in medicine only since the 1940s. Since our knowledge of how the known vitamins interact is imperfect, and because there might be many essential substances yet to be discovered in foods, we should strive for a balanced diet before relying on vitamin pills. As a case in point, one recent study suggests that the anticancer factor of some vegetables lies not in their vitamins but in some other unidentified substance.[34]

There are two broad classes of vitamins: water-soluble and fat-soluble. Most of the B vitamins and vitamin C are water-soluble. They exit the body quickly and need to be replenished daily. Vitamins A, D, E, and K are fat-soluble. They are stored in the body's fat and can be injurious if taken in large doses.

VITAMINS A AND D

Vitamin A is necessary to prevent night blindness, to build resistance to respiratory infections and shorten the course of a disease, and to promote growth and produce strong bones and healthy skin, hair, teeth, and gums. The U.S. recommended daily allowance of vitamin A is 5,000 IU.[k]

TABLE 1
Good sources of carotenoids*

Food	IU
Carrots, 2/3 cup	10,500 IU
Collard greens, 1/2 cup	5,400
Dandelion greens, 1/2 cup	11,700
Garden cress, 3 1/2 oz.	7,700
Kale, 3/4 cup	7,400
Mustard greens, 1/2 cup	5,800
Parsley, 3 1/2 oz.	8,500
Pumpkin, 2/5 cup	33,990
Squash, butternut, 1 cup	13,120
Squash, Hubbard, 1 cup	10,050
Sweet potato, 1 lg.	14,600

*all foods cooked

Source: Bowes and Church

Vitamin A *per se*—or, more correctly, its ready-made form, retinol—is found only in animals. Plants contain carotenoids, the precursors of the vitamin. The darker orange or green the vegetable, the higher its carotenoid content usually is. The body converts carotenoids such as beta carotene only when the need arises, so it is nearly impossible to overdose on vitamin A by eating vegetables rich in carotene or by taking beta carotene supplements. The worst that could happen would be getting a yellow or orange tinge to your skin. Such is not the case with vitamin A from supplements or animal and fish sources. Excessive vitamin A can cause headaches, hair loss, blurred vision, and liver damage. The carotenoids of plants may be more closely linked to a lower incidence of cancer than the retinol of animals.[35]

TABLE 12
Good sources of vitamin D

Eel, raw	5,000	IU
Herring, raw	900	
Salmon, raw	650	
Shrimp, cooked	105	

Vitamin D is actually a sterol, or hormonelike lipid, and because of its hormonelike structure can be immunosuppressive, much like the hydrocortisone discussed in chapter 1. Recent studies suggest that excessive vitamin D suppresses the production of interleukin-2, which is needed for the proliferation of the helper T cells that mobilize the immune system.[36] Vitamin D is necessary, in very small amounts, for the metabolism of vitamin A and for the utilization of calcium and phosphorus by the body.

Vitamin D can be produced by the body from a sterol found in the skin, if the skin is exposed outdoors to the ultraviolet rays of sunlight (ultraviolet rays do not penetrate window glass). But since vitamin D is stored in the body, it isn't necessary to go out in the sun every day. Exposing a few square inches of skin to the sun for a few minutes produces enough of the vitamin;[37] at the latitude of Washington, D.C., standing under the noon sun for five minutes in a bathing suit provides 200 to 300 IU.[38]

If you are strictly vegetarian and do not go out in the sun, you might not be getting the daily 200 IU of vitamin D recommended for adults. If this is the case, you need to include seafood in your diet or take a vitamin D supplement because grains and vegetables are poor sources of the vitamin. For example, one teaspoon per day of cod liver oil will suffice. An excess of the vitamin D, in addition to being immunosuppressive, can be toxic and might cause irreparable kidney, heart, and aortic damage.

THE B VITAMINS

Once thought to be a single vitamin, the B vitamins form a complex, or family, of vitamins. They include vitamin B_1 (thiamine), B_2 (riboflavin), B_3 (niacin), B_5 (pantothenic acid), B_6 (pyridoxine), B_{12} (cobalamine), and biotin and folic acid, also known as vitamins H and M. The B vitamins work in unison and should be obtained as a group; one without the others just won't do. They are necessary for digesting and utilizing carbohydrates, proteins, and fats; maintaining healthy skin, lips, tongue, eyes, blood, nerves, and digestive system; developing normal red blood cells and antibodies; and promoting appetite.[l] A diet rich in whole grains will provide most of the daily requirement of the B vitamins.[39]

Because it was once thought that vitamin B_{12} could be obtained only from animal sources, there is still some debate about whether a vegetarian diet provides enough of the vitamin. We now know that the only nonanimal source of vitamin B_{12} is bacteria such as those found in the root nodules of certain legumes.[m, 40] Foods rich in cobalamine-producing bacteria—sauerkraut, seaweed, tempeh, and miso (the last two are fermented soybean products)—will supply the vegetarian with an adequate amount of B_{12}. Moreover, since the body stores a three- to eight-year supply, we need not worry about eating cobalamine-rich food every day.[41]

Two clinical studies in the early 1970s initiated a debate about whether megadoses of vitamin C caused vitamin B_{12} deficiency. The studies suggested that doses over 500 mg per day lowered vitamin B_{12} levels in 2 to 3 per cent of those studied. Vitamin B_{12} deficiency results in fatigue, shortness of breath, and decreased resistance to infection. Many later studies, however, have found no correlation between increased dosages of vitamin C and lower levels of vitamin B_{12} and impute the earlier results to inefficient, nonstandardized methods of extracting and analyzing cobalamine.[42] Macrobiotic opinion maintains that members of the Solanaceae or nightshade family—tomatoes, potatoes, eggplants, and green and chili peppers—also will hinder the absorption of vitamin B_{12}. To my knowledge, no clinical studies substantiate this claim.

TABLE 13
Good sources of vitamin C*

Food	mg
Broccoli, 2/3 cup	90 mg
Brussels sprouts, 6–8 med.	87
Cauliflower, 7/8 cup	55
Collard greens, 1/2 cup	46
Lotus root, 2/3 segment	75
Mustard greens, 1/2 cup	78
Orange, fresh, 1 med.	80
Parsley, raw, 3 1/2 oz	172
Strawberries, fresh, 1 cup	85
Turnips, 2/3 cup	69
Watercress, raw, 3 1/2 oz	80

*cooked unless otherwise stated

VITAMIN C

Much has been written about vitamin C because it plays a large part in most biochemical processes. Part of the woof and warp of life, vitamin C is crucial for the formation of collagen, a fibrous protein that helps bind tissues together throughout the body and is the major structural element of bones and tendons. Thus, vitamin C aids in the healing of wounds, sores, burns, and bleeding gums, protects against bone fracture and disease, and prevents scurvy. Vitamin C also helps reduce blood cholesterol, lowers the occurrence of blood clots, and acts as a natural laxative.[43]

Vitamin C is also a powerful antioxidant that prevents the conversion of the nitrates present in many foods into nitrites and ultimately into nitrosamines, which are among the most potent cancer-causing substances known. In the same way, vitamin C captures free oxygen and prevents it from forming carcinogenic free radicals in combination with other substances. These oxygen–vitamin C complexes also help the body fight many viral and bacterial infections. Furthermore, several studies have shown that high doses of vitamin C increase the production of antibodies, the reproduction of T cells, and the synthesis of interferon, an antiviral substance.[44]

Animal sources do not supply vitamin C (unless, like the Eskimo, you eat whale blubber). Exposure to heat, air, light, and freezing temperatures destroys vitamin C. Frozen vegetables, for example, lose between 30 and 50 percent of the vitamin. A diet rich in vegetables and fruits adequately supplies the U.S. recommended daily allowance of 60 mg of vitamin C, yet many nutritionists, biochemists, and orthomolecular physicians doubt that this 60 mg RDA is adequate for humans.

Most animals are able to synthesize all the necessary vitamin C from other dietary substances, yet humans, along with apes, guinea pigs, and some birds, have lost this ability completely. We need to obtain all of our vitamin C from our diet. How much vitamin C do we need? Certainly not substantially less than any other animal, since we possess the same biochemical processes requiring vitamin C as other creatures. Some animals synthesize between 26 and 59 mg daily per kilogram of body weight. Assuming this rate of production is proper for humans, someone weighing around 154 pounds should consume at least between 1.8 and 4.1 *grams* of vitamin C per day, an amount 3,000 to 7,000 percent larger than the established RDA. Many other animals, including dogs and cats, produce about 10 grams of vitamin C for 154 pounds of weight. Our biochemical processes themselves tell us we shouldn't be that different from other creatures to need an amount two orders of magnitude smaller of such an essential substance. "The optimum daily intake of ascorbic acid for most adult human beings," says Nobel laureate Linus Pauling, the discoverer of vitamin C, "lies in the 2.3 gram to 10 gram range."[45]

You would have to eat quite a lot of parsley or oranges to get this amount of ascorbic acid. Vitamin C is one of the vitamins that should be taken as a supplement.[n] Indeed, vitamin C in much larger doses than the optimum mentioned by Pauling is being used therapeutically in AIDS and ARC as part of the Cathcart protocol printed in appendix C. Large doses of vitamin C, unlike those of vitamins A and D, are rarely toxic.[o] Unsubstantiated reports describe scurvylike symptoms when megadoses of vitamin C have been discontinued suddenly. Such symptoms may in effect indicate that you shouldn't have discontinued the vitamin in the first place, but if you feel you must do so, decrease vitamin C supplementation over a week or so to be on the safe side.

VITAMIN E

Vitamin E is the body's main antioxidant. It prolongs the useful lives of vitamin C and vitamin A by preventing oxidation, a natural process that nullifies the chemical properties of these vitamins. Because this antioxidative trait works on many other cellular substances, vitamin E retards cell aging in general. It also contributes to endurance by making the body use oxygen more efficiently and helping the capillaries to dilate. It hinders the formation of blood clots and prevents the formation of thick and deforming scar tissue on skin wounds. Like vitamin C, vitamin E inhibits the formation of carcinogenic nitrogen compounds and helps in the healing of burns.

The recommended daily allowance of vitamin E is 10 IU—in this case, 10 mg. A diet of whole grains, vegetables, beans, and seeds should provide this recommended allowance. Again, this RDA might prove insufficient for many of us. According to Pauling, vitamins A, B_{12}, and C and pantothenic and folic acid appear to fortify immunity when taken in larger amounts than those recommended.[46] Ten milligrams of vitamin E may be insufficient to prevent the oxidation of these larger vitamin quantities and perform its other functions in the body as well.

TABLE 14
Good sources of vitamin E

Apple, 1 med	1.8	IU
Beans, dry, 1/2 cup	1.6	
Broccoli, 1 cup	2.2	
Brussels sprouts, 3 lg.	2.3	
Corn, 1 ear	1.5	
Parsnip, 1/2 lg.	1.5	
Rice, brown, 1/3 cup	1.1	
Sunflower seeds, 2 tbs.	3.5	
Sweet potato, 1 med.	9.7	

Source: Bowes and Church

* * *

Under what circumstances is vitamin and mineral supplementation warranted? I wrestled with that question for over a year as I read and listened to differing opinions. The evidence from numerous laboratory studies and clinical histories led me to conclude that many of us need some vitamin supplementation to maintain minimum requirements and that most, if not all, of us need supplementation to achieve optimum health.

Unfortunately, vitamins can be very profitable to sell, and so supplements are being sold in exorbitant quantities, usually by people who know little about food and nutrition. These people talk as if vitamins were food and push the if-some-is-good-more-is-better philosophy of health. Just as detrimental, if not more, is the standard but unfounded macrobiotic tenet that holds vitamins are always harmful. These opposite views represent the excessive laissez faire of American materialism on the one hand and the rigid dogmatism of Orientalist thought on the other.

After attending a health seminar that pushed supplements, I took megadoses of vitamins and other supplements for a year. But these supplements appeared to have no correlation with the foods I ate or to my daily health. The seminar's vitamin pushers promoted the same pill mentality so common in our society today. Just as we expect pills to provide magical cures for all our ailments—whether medical, nutritional, or even spiritual—we believe vitamins will produce similar cures. The pecuniary interest those running the seminar had in my pill taking, however, eventually made me doubt their credibility. Spending $300 a month on vitamins cured me of my vitamin-popping craze, which I recognized as only the flip side of popping drugs.

Vitamin and mineral supplements are not food and do not compensate for a poor diet! The best vitamins and minerals are found in whole, healthful food, and one should not expect supplements to take the place of a better diet and a more healthful way of life.

Vitamin and mineral allowances drawn up by the Food and Nutrition Board's Committee on Dietary Allowance often miss the mark when vitamin supplementation does become necessary to ward off diseases other than those caused by vitamin deficiency. The committee had not only health but economics in mind when it developed its standards.

The idea of a list of necessary nutrients came about only as recently as the early years of World War II. At that time, the government had two concerns: providing soldiers with nutritionally adequate rations and assuring a minimum diet for large populations if ever the need arose for mass feeding programs. Research was geared to establish minimum daily amounts that would keep deficiency diseases at bay but not necessarily provide for optimum health. The result was the list of recommended daily allowances, in effect only a guide for planning and procuring food supplies for the nation during a war crisis.

The RDAs have been modified every five years since their establishment, but they address the same question—what amounts of X, Y, or Z nutrients will keep Joe and Jane Average from getting a vitamin-deficiency disease? Although a multitude of studies have identified many instances in which supplementation is beneficial, little research has been done to determine the optimum levels of vitamins that would rid us of the deficiency model of nutrition.

The Food and Nutrition Board's Committee on Dietary Allowance partly recognizes the shortcomings of the RDAs and emphasizes that they do not cover "special needs for such problems as premature birth, inherited metabolic disorders, infections, chronic diseases and the use of medications."[47]

The RDAs clearly are not enough for people with AIDS and ARC. Certain social and economic factors often prevent PWAs from obtaining regular sound meals that supply RDAs, thus compounding the need for supplementation. I believe that vitamin and mineral supplementation is necessary for most people with AIDS, although I am not qualified or allowed by California law to recommend a program of megavitamin supplementation. Such a program should be designed by a physician trained in orthomolecular medicine who knows your specific needs and health status. If you cannot get to an orthomolecular doctor,[p] at least read up on vitamins before you take any amounts larger than the RDAs.

Doctors Robert F. Cathcart III and Russell Jaffe are becoming well known in the fields of metabolic medicine and AIDS treatment. Both physicians have developed protocols that include massive doses of vitamin C. But since their proposed courses of treatment are still in the small-group testing stage, the exact role played by vitamin C and the other supplements in AIDS remissions will probably remain unknown for some time. Anecdotal evidence leads me to believe that the role might be an important one.

Food supplements may have negative effects that have nothing to do with the specific vitamin or mineral in the pill. Current federal regulations establishing vitamin and food-supplement purity are even less reassuring than those controlling drug and food additives. For example, a 1976 amendment to the Food, Drug, and Cosmetics Act prohibits the Food and Drug Administration from regulating vitamin and food-supplement potencies. Today's regulations allow for a 2 percent level of impurity in vitamins, in addition to the fillers, carriers, colors, and preservatives that may make up most of the pill or capsule. Allergenic substances such as the colorant FD & C Yellow No. 5 are often added. Because liberal doses of these toxic additives may be present yet none are regularly listed on the label, the health benefits of such contaminated supplements are somewhat dubious. Furthermore, many vitamins are made from yeast, sugar beets, and corn—substances that are typically allergenic to many people and counterproductive for those with candida.

False and exaggerated claims about vitamins can be made without any threat of prosecution. Worst of all, the government has not regulated the use of the term "natural," allowing it to be used deceitfully. Many vitamin companies want us to believe they manufacture their own natural vitamins when in fact they just package a substance produced by pharmaceutical companies like Hoffman–La Roche or Eastman Kodak. For example, some rose-hip vitamin C bottle labels suggest that the vitamin comes from natural rose hips. The manufacturing process, if it were described on the label, would indicate otherwise. Rose hips, which are not very good sources of vitamin C to begin with, are first ground into the bulk of the tablet; then laboratory-made ascorbic acid is added to provide the actual vitamin dose.[48] There is no need to label vitamin C as natural; ascorbic acid is ascorbic acid no matter its source.[q] Yet this kind of labeling practice seems to be the rule in the health-food vitamin industry. There are a few exceptions that are sometimes either high-priced or low in potency. Beware of what you buy.

Before deciding to use supplements, do some reading. *How to Live Longer and Feel Better* by Linus Pauling, *Earl Mindell's Vitamin Bible,* and *The Complete Book of Vitamins* published by the Rodale Press are good introductions to supplementation. Work with a doctor who appreciates whole foods and is trained in nutrition, metabolic disorders, and vitamin therapy. Always look to whole foods as your first and best source of vitamins and minerals.

MINERALS

Minerals are the elements that remain as ash when plant or animal tissue is burned. About 4 percent of our body weight is made up of mineral matter. Without the dozens of minerals in our bodies we would not live. Both mineral deficiencies and excesses have been associated with higher rates of cancer and other health problems.

Minerals need to be balanced within prescribed ranges for proper body function to occur. Since no mineral works alone, too much of one will upset the balance and function of the others. Extreme diets and improper supplementation can therefore overwhelm the body's delicate balance. The best assurance of a sufficient and safe supply of essential minerals is a diet consisting of a wide variety of unprocessed foods (food processing results in excessive mineral loss). By eating a balanced, whole-food diet you will be able to keep minerals in their proper ratio to one another without incurring possibly toxic excesses.

Some nutritional literature mentions that a vegetarian diet might be deficient in calcium, magnesium, iron, and zinc, the same minerals that, in addition to selenium, are most often recommended by supplement manufacturers.

If you listened to dairy commercials and read mineral supplement ads, you would think that dairy products are the only source of calcium, a mineral that supposedly none of us gets enough of in our diets. The fact is that, with few exceptions, the rest of the world consumes dairy foods in small quantities, if at all, and still has very little calcium deficiency even when calcium supplements are not used.

The problem in our diets is not too little calcium but usually too much phosphorus, and too many proteins and fatty acids. A fatty as well as a high-phosphorus diet, such as one of cow's milk, soft drinks, meat, and highly processed grains, promotes the formation of insoluble compounds that entrap calcium and prevent its absorption by the body. Oxalic and phytic acids present in some natural foods likewise can result in the formation of these insoluble calcium complexes. A high-protein diet also hinders the absorption of calcium.

The solution to the calcium problem lies not in eating more dairy products or in consuming calcium supplements but in cutting down on meats and fats; eliminating soft drinks; limiting foods high in oxalates, such as rhubarb, spinach, beets, coffee, and cocoa; maintaining an adequate source of vitamin D; and increasing the consumption of vegetable foods high in calcium. Leafy vegetables, broccoli, oranges, whole grains, legumes, green beans, sea vegetables, and fish (especially fish whose cooked bones can be eaten, like tuna or sardines) are good sources of calcium.

After calcium, magnesium is probably one of the minerals most prescribed as a supplement. There is definitely a need for more magnesium in our diets. In the past fifty years the amount of magnesium in the average diet has dropped by at least one-fifth. Much magnesium is lost in the process of refining flour. A diet rich in whole grains, fresh leafy vegetables, legumes, and sea vegetables will provide the body with adequate amounts of magnesium, without the need for added supplements. Prostate problems could be an indication of inadequate dietary magnesium.

While following a vegetarian diet, one should be aware that the body cannot utilize the iron in vegetable matter as well as that in meat and that processing further depletes the iron content of vegetables. Iron-deficiency anemia can result from too low an intake of iron, inefficiently absorbed iron, and excessive blood loss due to hemorrhage or parasitic infection. Milk has often been touted as a good source of iron. Studies of children, however, have shown cow's milk to cause intestinal hemorrhaging resulting in iron-deficiency anemia. Milk will also cause profuse diarrhea if parasitic infection is present.

People with AIDS often show low iron levels in the blood, and thus their physicians often recommend iron supplements. This could be a serious mistake, as excess iron can impair the ability of macrophages to fight pathogens and thus suppress residual immunity. Because many microorganisms need iron to reproduce, the body lowers blood iron levels through several mechanisms. Low blood iron levels during infection are akin to fevers. Both help the body fight disease. Any iron supplementation is counterproductive during infection.[49]

Only small amounts of the iron in our diet are absorbed by the body, but vitamin C will facilitate the process. So if you have a high vitamin C intake from supplements, you need not be concerned about getting enough iron. In fact, the body retains iron so well that it is possible to get too much, especially if you consume "enriched" ingredients like those present in most processed foods. This brings us back again to the fact that thoughtless supplementation, such as adding iron to refined grain products, upsets a natural balance and can be deleterious. Unprocessed foods like beans, peas, whole grains, nuts, and leafy vegetables are good sources of iron. Some signs of iron deficiency are chronic fatigue or malaise and frequent illness or infection.

Using iron pots for meals that take a long time to cook is a good way to insure against deficiency if your iron is inadequate. Be aware, however, that the exclusive use of iron pots can provide too much iron.

Zinc combats infection by increasing the stability of cell membranes, interfering with the reproduction of viruses, increasing the effectiveness of lymphocytes and stimulating the activity of phagocytes that ingest invading bacteria. Excessive levels of zinc, however, can depress all these activities as well as upset proper copper ratios, cause selenium deficiency, and possibly accelerate the development of some kinds of cancer.[50] Too much zinc in a diet often results in the same symptoms seen in zinc deficiency.

A vegetarian diet can be deficient in zinc unless it is rich in whole grains, leafy greens (especially Brussels sprouts), legumes, sea vegetables, and mushrooms. Symptoms of zinc deficiency consist of mental dullness, inability to concentrate, a notable loss of taste and smell (foods don't taste and flowers don't smell as good as they used to), the appearance of white flecks or spots on fingernails, a longer healing time for wounds and scratches, and loss of hair.

Our reaction to selenium is similar to our reaction to zinc: we need some to stay healthy, but too much can be toxic. If we eat food from various geographic areas, we need not be concerned about too much or too little selenium. The selenium content of soils varies so much from region to region that any excesses or scarcities average out over a wide geographical area. If you feel you need more selenium, however, whole grains, fish, garlic, mushrooms, onions, broccoli, carrots and radishes are good sources. The main symptom of selenium deficiency is premature loss of stamina.

As with vitamins, mineral supplementation sometimes becomes necessary, even with a good diet. Since small amounts of some minerals could be toxic, consultation with an orthomolecular specialist is of great importance.

SALT

The sea in which our remote ancestors evolved left its mark on us: the salts in our blood. At no time in our existence are we separated from salts. We need them. They are our lifeblood, and without them we die.

We should consume natural sea salts, not the refined sea salt usually found on the table. Sodium chloride is the only ingredient regular table salt has in common with natural sea salts. Since it is nearly pure sodium chloride, common table salt is an unbalanced product unsuitable for forming blood and other body fluids.

On the other hand, the salts of the ocean are, like the salts in the womb and body fluids, only about 90 percent sodium chloride. The other 10 percent consists of some eighty-odd mineral salts, including magnesium, calcium, sulfur, silicon, iodine, and bromine salts. These salts occur in sea water in nearly the same proportions as they do in the body and make natural sea salt a balanced product ideal for human consumption.

Ninety-seven percent of the mined, processed, and refined salt in the United States is used in industry. Since industry requires pure-grade sodium chloride, the refining process forcibly removes all trace minerals from sea salt, leaving a product eminently suited for industrial use. People consume the remaining 3 percent of all salt thus produced and get a worthless substance not suited to their needs.

The body needs salts in the same balanced proportions found in its fluids as well as in natural sea salt. Table salt provides the body only with sodium chloride and denies it other needed salts. The body, however, is often smarter than we are; it tells us what it needs. It sets up a craving for salts, expecting natural sea salt to provide the needed elements. But we grab the salt shaker and give the body more refined salt—more sodium chloride—which further aggravates the need for other salts. Thus, we enter an ever-widening spiral that results in excess sodium consumption and might even lead to salt poisoning.[r]

We often hear that a salt-free diet is ideal or that one should lower salt intake. If you consume meat, canned goods, and preprocessed foods and also eat at fast-food restaurants, this admonition might apply to you because you probably are getting too much sodium. Therefore, using additional salt in cooking or at the table would constitute an overkill. In fact, the average American who eats meat and processed foods consumes about two to five teaspoons of sodium daily, although the body needs only less than one-quarter teaspoon per day. Much of the excess, which we may consume unwittingly, comes from the sodium chloride added to processed foods such as canned soups and vegetables, breakfast cereals, and even fruit juices. If your diet consists predominantly of whole grains and vegetables, however, adding small amounts of high-quality salt can be beneficial.

Excessive sodium intake destroys the balance between sodium and potassium in the body and results in water retention, or edema, which in turn creates increased blood pressure and heart rate and contributes to circulatory and heart problems.

As I mentioned before, table salt is nearly—but not all—pure sodium chloride. Once its essential trace salts are removed, refined salt is treated with a group of additives. Ferrocyanide, yellow prussiate of soda, tricalcium phosphate, aluminocalcium silicate, and sodium tricalcium are used singly or in combination as anti-caking agents to prevent salt from mixing with water and hardening up in the box.[51] The salt is also iodized. Iodine oxidizes rapidly when exposed to light, so dextrose (sugar) has to be added as a stabilizer. The potassium iodide and dextrose combination turn the salt purple, so to bleach the salt to a more appetizing color sodium bicarbonate is added.

Salt has to be iodized because people with diets deficient in iodine produce insufficient thyroid hormone. This dietary deficiency results in part from the consumption of table salt whose iodine salt, along with everything else that isn't sodium chloride, has been removed in the refining process. So the iodine is added back in to remedy the thyroid imbalance. But since this amount is twenty times what occurs in nature, it sometimes causes other thyroid and glandular problems. What a vicious circle!

Natural, unadulterated sea salts are also beneficial in warding off infection and disease and are necessary for a healthy immune system.[52] Thus, if you would like your immune system to function better, I suggest you get rid of your salt shaker and all adulterated salt in your house and go buy yourself some natural sea salt.

Gray Celtic salt is the best natural sea salt available. It is collected on the coast of Brittany by sun drying sea water in clay basins. The Mexican salt collected by Noburo Muramoto also is of higher quality than what is sometimes labeled 100 percent natural sea salt. Various regulations in the United States require that salt sold in supermarkets for consumption must be at least 98 percent sodium chloride. Most salt advertised as "100 percent natural sea salt" in health food stores meets those requirements since it contains only 2 percent nonsodium salts rather than the 10 to 16 percent in real, natural sea salt.[53] If you have difficulty obtaining the sea salts I recommend, check with a local macrobiotic center or order from the Mountain Ark catalogue (see appendix H for addresses).

Once you have obtained your natural sea salt, it is important that you use it correctly. Salt should be used sparingly and added to food while cooking, not at the table. Cooking juices readily dissolve the salt crystals and thus allow the body to utilize salt better.

Adding salt to sautéing vegetables releases their water and reduces or eliminates the need for oil. Salt increases the body's ability to assimilate vegetables[54] and brings out the sweetness and natural flavors of foods. It also increases the flow of saliva and thus exposes food to more of the salivary amylase that begins starch digestion in the mouth.

It takes practice and patience to determine the proper amount of salt you need. Do not use so much that food tastes salty. A craving for sweets after you have given up animal products might indicate that you are still getting too much salt.

The only foods that should taste salty are the condiments you add to food after cooking. I use three of these on my grains: a condiment made from tamari-shoyu (water, soybeans, wheat, and sea salt), nori (a sea vegetable), and mirin (rice cooking wine); sesame salt, made from ten to twelve parts lightly toasted, whole, unhulled sesame seed and one part salt; and beefsteak-leaf condiment, made from beefsteak leaves pickled in brine, then dried, roasted at low temperature, and ground to a powdery or flaky texture.

WATER

Clean water is too often taken for granted. Just turn on the faucet and you think you have all you need. Unfortunately, high quality water is not readily available.

Our drinking water originates in wells, rivers, and lakes; its purity varies tremendously. You will never find truly pure water because water is a solvent that acts to a greater or lesser degree on all it comes in contact with. Currently, there are over 70,000 chemical compounds in our sewage and industrial wastes. Many of these are carcinogenic and leach into our water supplies, principally from landfills where these chemicals are routinely dumped. Thousands of tons of these pollutants have reached the ground water. There's no solution in sight to this problem. Once an aquifer becomes tainted, it is very difficult, if not impossible, to clean it up.[55]

I grew up in Nassau County, Long Island, and can remember hearing how fortunate we were to have such an abundant and pristine aquifer. Apparently, that is no longer the case. Volatile organic chemicals (VOCs) are commonly used as solvents or degreasers in many septic-tank cleaning products for home use. VOCs can contaminate rivers and lakes, but they present an even greater danger to ground-water sources. Water in an aquifer moves very slowly; unlike surface waters, it cannot disperse contaminants and so retains them for long periods. In 1979 Long Islanders used about 400,000 gallons of VOCs in their homes. An EPA study determined that these chemicals had polluted 13 percent of Nassau County's community water supply, thus forcing many private and public wells to close.[56]

Because most municipal water-treatment plants still use technology developed in the late nineteenth century, they are incapable of removing many of these harmful substances. Many remove only the suspended sediments from the water and then add chlorine in hope of killing microorganisms. Thus, although the water you drink every day might have been treated by the municipal plant, it is possible that it still contains sediments, microorganisms, and organic chemicals.

Ironically, the chlorine added to kill bacteria can combine with organic matter and other chemicals in the water to produce carcinogenic substances such as carbon tetrachloride, chloroform, and trihalomethanes. There are also indications that water chlorination might be partially responsible for the increase in heart attack rates and senility in the aged.[57] "If chlorine were now proposed for the first time to be used in water," states New Jersey biochemist Herbert Schwartz, "it would be banned by the Food and Drug Administration."[58]

More damage is done to water after it leaves the plant. As it journeys through the distribution system it picks up heavy metals, such as the lead used to solder copper pipes, and carcinogens, such as the asbestos from cement pipes. The EPA offers this advice about drinking water thus contaminated:

> Under certain conditions, such as when water remains in contact with metal for extended periods of time (overnight or longer) without flowing, sufficient metal can be dissolved by corrosive water to constitute a potential health risk. In general, first-drawn water should not be consumed, and hot water from the tap should not be used for cooking or beverages.[59]

As a temporary solution to metals in your drinking or cooking water, let the water run full force two or three minutes before you use it in the morning. This will help clear out the dissolved metals that might have accumulated in the pipes overnight.[s]

Every community water system that distributes to more than fifteen water meters or to at least twenty-five people is required by federal law to sample its water at least monthly for bacteria and yearly for various organic and inorganic substances. You can call your local water district's quality division to get a copy of these sampling tests and sanitary surveys. The EPA publishes standards by which to judge your local water (see appendix H for address). At my request the Water Quality Division of the San Francisco Water Department promptly sent me copies of their Mineral Analysis and Special Analysis. If your water department isn't as helpful, call your local newspaper or TV station. They might pick up on it and create some action.

For the month of December 1984, the San Francisco survey shows no detectable signs of insecticides, such as lindane, which is common in agricultural communities. Asbestos, however, was present throughout the system during the same period. The Crystal Springs reservoir had the greatest concentration: five times that of the San Andreas reservoir. It was also interesting to note that the Hetch Hetchy reservoir in Yosemite had a greater aluminum concentration in September 1984—the peak of the tourist season in the park—than on December of the same year.[60]

Until recently I used a popular San Francisco brand of bottled water. But then I called and asked for a copy of the company's most recent analysis. The laboratory report I received was totally inadequate. It contained no tests for aluminum, arsenic, cadmium, lead, mercury, asbestos, or pesticides. I was able to conclude that the chloride and nitrate contents of the bottled water were much lower than those of the San Andreas reservoir, which serves my area. It was nice to discover that the water contained no fluorides.[t] Diligence is required to obtain the facts about the water you drink daily; information might not be as readily available to you as it was to me.

In the short run, purchasing bottled water is simpler and cheaper than installing a filtration system. But once yearly bills for bottled water reach three digits—as they often do—you might be better off buying a filter. The cheapest but perhaps the least effective one is the activated charcoal filter; the smaller units usually do not contain enough carbon. If you do choose activated charcoal, try to avoid powdered activated carbon and instead buy a solid-block activated carbon filter.

The most effective system, and the one that needs the least maintenance, is the reverse osmosis filter. A pressure differential drives water through a membrane and thus removes all the impurities normally contained in water. The cost of this filter is high, though—up to $500. Another option is water distillation systems, which boil water and recondense the steam, thereby leaving the impurities in the boiler tank. Distilled water can have an odd taste unless the system reoxygenates it after distillation. Before buying any system, always carefully investigate the claims of the manufacturer.

Once you have procured a good, clean water supply, use it whenever you are thirsty. Drinking enough water every day helps eliminate toxins from the body. I disagree with those proponents of macrobiotics who claim that drinking only small amounts of liquids is best for your health. I myself find that whenever I quench my thirst with a full glass of water, I feel better instantly. Thirst-quenching properties aside, a high water intake reduces the burden on the kidneys because, according to clinical evidence, they do less work when excreting dilute rather than concentrated urine.[61] People with AIDS or ARC, who often have impaired kidney function, should thus drink plenty of water.

CHAPTER 7

The components of a good diet

GRAINS

Grains are the small, hard, edible seeds of cereal plants, such as wheat, rice, and barley. Since they contain a carbohydrate-to-protein ratio of approximately 7:1 and generally have no more than 8 percent fat, grains should make up the central core of one's diet. A whole grain cereal comes closer than any other plant source to providing adequate nutrition.

Figure 6 illustrates a typical whole grain. Both the aleuron layer and the germ contain the majority of the grain's protein, but the germ has the highest *usable* percentage. Protein content varies widely among grains. Rye, wheat, and oats have about 30 percent more protein than rice, corn, and barley. Rice, however, contains the highest percentage of *usable* protein by weight, equal to that of beef.[1]

Unfortunately, modern refining processes remove the better-quality proteins from grains, leaving only the endosperm, which is basically starch.[a] What little nutritive value is left begins to degrade upon contact with oxygen.[2] This is why grains should be freshly ground when flour is needed for cooking.

You should avoid flour products as much as possible, however,

FIGURE 6
A typical whole grain

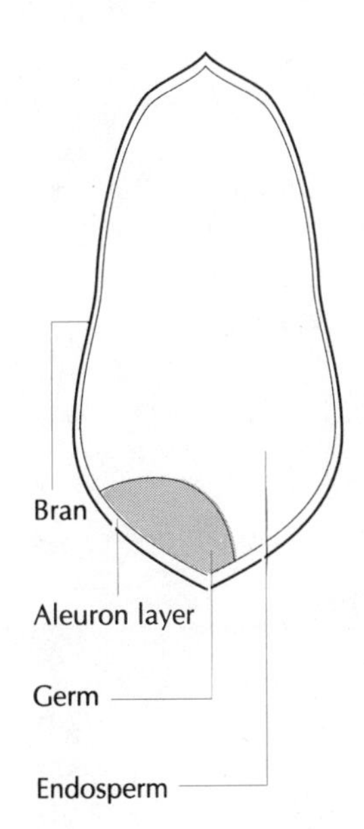

due to their inferior protein, mineral, vitamin, and fiber content. When possible, it is better to eat grains whole rather than as pancakes, muffins, bread, or the like. If you are ill, you should eat even a high-quality bread only a few times a week rather than daily because it may prevent the quick discharge of body wastes.[3]

If you include bread in your diet, eat only the highest quality. Look for a label that reads something like this: "Made from organically grown rye stone-ground fresh in our mills the day of baking. Water, rye starter, and sea salt; nothing else added." The word "organic" (the use of which is regulated in California) is important because nonorganic grain is often treated with cyanide gas to eliminate weevils and other vermin. "Stone-ground" means that the grinding stones have not removed the grain's germ and outer layers, as steel grinders would. "Day of baking" assures you that the stone-ground bran has not had a chance to become stale. (Refined flour does not become stale because everything that could spoil, such as protein and oils, is removed in processing. The price we pay for everlasting shelf life is flour that has no life).

"Naturally fermented" or "natural leavening" are other assurances of good quality. Avoid bread made with commercial yeast, which consumes most of the bread's nutrients. The wild yeasts harnessed by natural fermentation, however, are much less ravenous than their domesticated, commercial counterparts. They produce a bread that will not go stale and whose taste will improve with age. Additionally, bromides and ammonium persulfate are added to yeasted breads in order to accelerate leavening. Persulfate may be harmful; its use is forbidden in France, Italy, Belgium, and Hungary.[4]

Besides being healthful, whole grains are also tasty and filling. Brown rice made in a pressure cooker has a slightly sweet taste and an appealing texture. Oats cooked slowly for a couple of hours make an enjoyable, flavorful breakfast. Table 15 gives some

TABLE 15 Energy value of selected grains

	PROTEIN*	FAT*	CARBOHYDRATE*†	CALORIES/ GRAM
Barley, raw	9	3	90	3.49
Buckwheat flour, dark	14	7	87	3.33
Corn, sweet	12	8	94	.84
Oatmeal	15	16	71	.55
Rice, brown	8	5	86	1.19
Rye flour, light	11	2	87	3.57
Wheat flour, whole	16	5	85	3.33

*In percentages.
†Percentages do not always add up to 100.

Source: *Nutritive Value of American Foods in Common Units,* Agriculture Handbook No. 456, as drawn from *The McDougall Plan.*

nutritional information about a few cereal grains.

Before cooking or grinding grain, carefully remove any foreign particles, such as pebbles and seeds, that look as if they do not belong. Crotalaria seeds, which contain potent liver toxins, are found in wheat and corn fields in some areas of the United States and are often gathered with the crop by mechanical harvesters.[5] This is another reason to avoid refined grain products over which you have no control.

When you select rice, avoid polished, white rice. It has less fiber, protein, minerals, and vitamins than brown rice, and to prevent spoilage some of it is coated with glucose and talc possibly contaminated with asbestos. No matter how well the rice is washed, the asbestos remains, which may help explain the high incidence of stomach cancer in Japan, where white rice is a staple.[6]

Whole grains keep well for long periods of time provided they are stored securely in a cool place. The shelf life of cracked grains is appreciably shorter. Try to limit cracked grains in your diet. Avoid toasting bread, which might produce compounds with mutagenic or carcinogenic properties.[7] For proper digestion, chew grain products thoroughly, especially whole grains. Grains should be well mixed with saliva, which contains an enzyme that breaks down their carbohydrates.

The gluten in wheat, oats, barley, and rye seems to cause gluten-sensitive enteropathy in some people, bringing about weight loss, malaise, weakness, and diarrhea.[b] Elimination of wheat, oats, barley, and rye has brought about dramatic relief to many of those affected.[8] Wheat flour and barley malt are present in many prepared foods. If you experience the above symptoms, eliminate these foods as well and try eating rice, millet, and buckwheat instead. These are also safe grains if wheat, oats, barley, or rye seem to aggravate candida infection.

For thousands of years, whole-grain cereals have been humankind's primary food source and the mainstay of its great civilizations. Only after steel mills replaced the old buhrstones almost a century ago did industrialized societies switch from whole grains to refined flours that were better suited for new, fancier-looking yet nutritionally inferior baked goods. This diet change, along with increased consumption of meat, dairy products, and refined sugars, has been linked to the increase in degenerative diseases such as heart disease, colon cancer, and diabetes in Western nations. Such diseases are rare among less developed peoples.[9]

We should seriously consider returning to the diet of our ancestors, one in which the whole cereals constitute about half the total calories. The advances of modern medicine combined with more traditional food sources would allow us to benefit from the best of both worlds. But the return to a grain-centered diet, however, might not be welcomed by the powers that be. According to William Dufty, "A vogue for natural grains could raise havoc with the vitamin pushers, the sugar pushers and the pharmaceutical companies and their partners in the disease establishment."[10]

Table 16 presents some acceptable and unacceptable grains and grain products.

TABLE 16 Grains

USE AS A STAPLE	
Barley, regular and pearl	Quinoa (from South America)
Buckwheat	Rice, short and medium brown
Corn	Rye
Millet	Wheat
Oats	

EAT OCCASIONALLY	AVOID
Anything with yeast (avoid completely if you have candida)	Any grain products containing preservatives, coloring agents, flavor enhancers or any such additives
Bulgur	Anything bleached
Corn grits, corn meal, and rye flakes	Breads, noodles, and other products made from refined flours
Couscous	
Naturally leavened whole-wheat or rye bread	
Rice cakes	
Seitan (wheat gluten prepared from whole wheat flour)	
Steel-cut oats and rolled oats	
Sweet brown rice and mochi (pounded sweet brown rice)	
Unleavened bread*	
Whole-wheat noodles	
Wheat germ (its oils go rancid very quickly)	

*Except for religious observance, avoid completely if you do not take mineral supplements. The phytic acid in unleavened bread could interfere with mineral absorption.

VEGETABLES

Vegetables are the edible leaves, stems, roots, and flowers of plants. They are good sources of fiber, vitamins, minerals, protein, and carbohydrates and give variety to our diets with their many colors, textures, and flavors.

Whole vegetables can be eaten in unlimited quantities and should be eaten every day. Because vegetables are high in vitamins A and C and low in fats, the caloric proportion of vegetables in our diets should be second only to that of grains. Most vegetables should be lightly cooked. Occasionally raw or pickled vegetables may be consumed. If a person is critically ill, all vegetables should be cooked.

If you have a problem with candida, some vegetable juices, stripped of the fiber that protects against the absorption of too much sugar, could be a problem when consumed in large amounts. Carrot juice, one of the most common vegetable juices, is

TABLE 17 Vegetables

USE AS A STAPLE			
Bok choy	Cauliflower	Mustard greens	Shiitake mushrooms
Broccoli	Collards	Onion	Scallions
Brussels sprouts	Daikon	Parsnips	Turnips
Burdock	Dandelion	Parsley	Squash, acorn
Butternut squash	Kale	Pickles	Squash, yellow
Cabbage	Leeks	Pumpkin	Watercress
Carrots	Lotus root	Sauerkraut	
EAT OCCASIONALLY			
Alfalfa sprouts[1,2]	Eggplant	Okra	Swiss chard[4]
Artichokes[3]	Endive	Potatoes[3]	Tomatoes[5]
Asparagus[1]	Escarole	Plantain	Tanniers
Bamboo shoots	Fava beans	Red radish	Taro
Bean sprouts[2]	Fennel	Rhubarb[4]	Wax beans
Beets[4]	Garlic	Snap beans	Yams
Bell pepper	Jerusalem artichoke	Snow peas	Zucchini
Celery	Kohlrabi	Sorrel[4]	
Chives	Lettuce	Spinach[1,4]	
Cucumber	Mushrooms[2]	Sweet potatoes	

1 Because their saponins may destroy some red blood cells, avoid if you have anemia.
2 Except for shiitake mushrooms and freshly sprouted seeds and beans, avoid because of mold problems if you have candida.
3 All but the certified organic are usually high in pesticides.
4 Because their oxalic acid blocks calcium absorption, avoid if you do not take mineral supplements.
5 May aggravate joint swelling and pain in people with rheumatoid arthritis.

very sweet, and its sugar can aggravate yeast symptoms. If you don't have a problem with sugar content, however, you can consume vegetable juices as often as you like as long as the juice is very fresh. Cancer researcher Virginia Livingston-Wheeler recommends drinking carrot juice daily because a particular type of vitamin A analogue found in carrots may help prevent cancer.[11]

Choose a wide variety of vegetables that are fresh, organic, and locally grown (I do admit that living in California makes this easier). Unfortunately, many of us grew up where only a few vegetables were available during cold weather, and we neither acquired a taste for various vegetables as children nor became inquisitive about new vegetables as adults. Next time you go shopping, buy a vegetable you've never had before and try incorporating it into your diet.

Include vegetables that are deep yellow, orange, or green; they are rich in beta carotene, a precursor of vitamin A. Vegetables that should be eaten routinely are Brussels sprouts, cabbage, cauliflower, broccoli, turnips, parsnips, and mustard greens (see table 17). These vegetables are all members of the cruciferous family and contain substances [c] that enhance the activity of the intestinal enzymes that block the action of carcinogens present in food.[12]

BEANS

Beans, the edible seeds of various leguminous plants, are rich sources of vitamins, minerals, fiber, protein, and amino acids—particularly lysine, in which cereal grains tend to be low. Indeed because of the high protein and amino acid content of beans, certain bean and cereal combinations, such as any kidneylike bean[d] and rice, equal or surpass meat in protein quantity and quality. Lysine makes beans an important addition to the diet of people

TABLE 18 Beans

USE AS A STAPLE	
Adzuki beans	Lentils
Chick peas or garbanzos	Soybeans, black
EAT OCCASIONALLY	
Blackeyed peas	Navy beans
Black turtle beans	Pinto beans
Carob[1]	Soybeans
Great northern beans	Tamari
Kidney beans	Tempeh
Lima beans[2]	Tofu
Miso	
AVOID	
Fava or broad beans[3]	Peanuts[4]

1 a stimulant.
2 contains minute amounts of cyanide.
3 may raise blood pressure.
4 may be contaminated with aflatoxins unless otherwise certified.

with herpes. Lysine blocks the action of the amino acid arginine, necessary for the replication of the herpes virus.

The most essential bean product in my diet is miso, a rich-tasting, fermented soybean purée. It is an excellent source of vitamin B_{12}, minerals, and protein, and it also contains zybicolin, a substance said to help eliminate heavy molecules—metals, pollutants, and radioactive poisons—from the body.[13] Miso is fermented by bacteria rather than by yeasts or molds and so should not present any yeast problem to people with candida. The bacteria in miso may actually help re-establish the beneficial intestinal flora that control the growth of candida.

Since beans are also high in saponins—soaplike substances that can destroy red blood cells—and sometimes in fat, eat beans only about once a day or every other day, depending on your health. Choose beans that are low in both fats and saponins such as chick peas (garbanzos), adzuki beans, and lentils. Raw beans contain phytic acid, which interferes with the body's absorption of calcium, zinc, and iron. Furthermore, the combination of proteins, starches, and sugars in beans frequently creates intestinal disturbance, making their digestion difficult for the sedentary person.[14] Adding a strip of the sea vegetable kombu during cooking can make beans more digestible. Soaking them overnight in water diminishes their gasifying properties. If even after following these measures, you find getting used to beans difficult, eat only a small quantity for a while and then build up slowly until you can tolerate beans well. You may also want to eat fish regularly during this build-up period if you feel you're not getting enough protein.

Soybeans (the beans, not their products), besides being high in fat, saponins, and phytic acid, also increase the body's requirement for iodine. If you eat soybeans, include sea salt and sea vegetables in your diet.

These negative points about beans are not meant to scare you. Beans and soybeans are excellent, inexpensive, and versatile sources of protein. Restricting our diet to the same foods day in and day out, however, can create problems by magnifying the negative effects of these foods. Remember to emphasize not only quality but also variety in your diet.

SEA VEGETABLES

What are sea vegetables? If I said seaweed, you might think, "Ah, that smelly stuff that litters the seashore." Seaweed certainly doesn't smell appealing, and the idea of eating the stuff might be downright sickening. I've had such feelings myself. Unfortunately, we usually see only the unpleasant side of sea vegetables. If you ran into a long-dead chicken, cow, or pig on the road, the stench would make rotten sea vegetables smell like perfume in comparison, yet you most likely eat chicken, beef, or pork.

Like flesh, sea vegetables have a more pleasant side; you have been eating them all your life, probably without knowing it. Extracts of sea vegetables are found in many prepared foods such as puddings, jellies, ice cream and salad dressings. Any food requiring stabilizers or thickeners is likely to contain agar, algin, or carrageenan—all sea-vegetable extracts.

If you have eaten sushi at a Japanese restaurant, then you know the sea vegetable nori, the green wrapping around the rice. Nori is more than just a clever Japanese wrapping for rice; there's more to it than its beautiful luminescent dark green. Ounce for ounce, nori has four times the calcium and protein and eight times the vitamin B_{12} found in milk, with only one-sixth the fat.

Sea vegetables, in fact, might be the most nutritious food on earth. Their nutritional value has long been recognized in the Orient. Indeed, they are so popular in Japan that natural crops are insufficient and artificial aquaculture has become necessary to meet the demand.

The healing properties of sea vegetables also have been known in the East for centuries. One of these is their ability to alkalinize the blood if it is too acid and reduce excess fat and mucus. The alginic acid found in the sea vegetables kombu and wakame transforms toxic metals in the intestines into easily eliminated salts. In 1964 researchers at McGill University in Montreal demonstrated that sea vegetables could remove radioactive strontium 90 from the body.[15]

Opinion varies as to the human ability to digest carbohydrates in seaweed. Experimental data is inconclusive and differs according to seaweed species and the individuals who consume them; nevertheless, carbohydrates in all sea vegetables except nori appear to be indigestible. Eleanor and John Lewaller present a differing opinion in their book *Sea Vegetable Gourmet Cookbook and Forager's Guide* (a good source of sea-vegetable recipes):

> The carbohydrates (sugars and starches) in all sea vegetables were thought, until recently, to be indigestible by the human body. Now the prevailing opinion is that one's body acquires the ability to assimilate sea-vegetable carbohydrates after one eats sea vegetables regularly for a week or so.[16]

Everyone agrees, however, that sea vegetables are highly nutritious. They contain little fat and are loaded with minerals, vitamins, and proteins. Table 19 details the protein, fat, and carbohydrate composition of sea vegetables.

TABLE 19 Energy value of sea vegetables*

SEAWEEDS		WATER	RAW PROTEIN	FAT	CARBO-HYDRATE	FIBER AND ASH
Hijiki	*(Hizikia fusiforme)*	16.8	5.6	0.8	29.8	47.0
Wakame	*(Undaria pinnatifida)*	6.0	12.7	1.5	47.8	22.0
Kombu	(*Laminaria* sp.)	18.0	6.7	1.6	49.1	24.6
Arame	*(Eisenia bicyclis)*	19.3	7.5	.6	49.1	24.6
Nori	*(Porphyra tenera)*					
lower		13.4	29.0	0.6	39.1	17.9
middle		11.1	34.2	0.7	40.5	13.5
upper		11.4	35.6	0.7	39.6	12.7
Sea lettuce	(*Ulva* sp.)	15.2	23.8	0.6	42.1	18.3

*as a percentage of total weight

Source: Seibin and Teruko Arasaki, *Vegetables from the Sea*, Japan Publications, Tokyo, 1983.

Sea vegetables are rich in protein. Nori is usually sold in thin rectangular sheets and contains almost twice the protein of most meats, without the accompanying fat. The average fat content of sea vegetables is no more than 1.5 percent, whereas in meat it is often more than 30 percent.[17] The amino acid composition of sea-vegetable protein is of very high quality, higher than that of land plants. It closely resembles the composition of ovalbumin, the egg-white protein used as the standard for protein quality. You should limit your sea vegetable intake, however, if you have herpes. Sea vegetables are high in arginine, an amino acid that promotes the replication of the herpes virus.

Sea vegetables are also high in vitamin content. Nori has a vitamin A content at least ten times greater than that of spinach and a hundred times greater than that of tomatoes. Nori's most outstanding attribute, however, is its high vitamin B_{12} content. Most standard clinical nutrition textbooks claim that a purely vegetarian diet is deficient in vitamin B_{12} and recommend B_{12} supplements. Land vegetables, seeds, and nuts contain minute quantities of vitamin B_{12}, but seaweed can be included in the vegetarian's diet to augment the B_{12} supplied by miso and other fermented foods.

Sea vegetables convert inorganic minerals in sea water into organic mineral salts and therefore contain more minerals—7 to 38 percent of their dry weight—than any other food source. They supply sufficient quantities of all the minerals required by humans, including sodium, calcium, magnesium, potassium, iodine, iron, and zinc, as well as trace minerals. Hijiki has 14 times the calcium in cow's milk, 8 times the iron in spinach, and 120 times the iodine in shellfish. Therefore, contrary to popular myth, strict vegetarians who take no supplements can get plenty of iodine, calcium, and iron if they consume sea vegetables.[18]

Sea vegetables are storehouses of proteins, vitamins, and minerals, but if they taste terrible and look gruesome, who wants to eat them? Let me dispel a myth: sea vegetables are very tasty. Macrobiotic cooking makes ample use of sea vegetables.

FRUITS

Fruits are the edible pulpy tissues surrounding the seeds of plants or trees. They are usually rich in vitamins, minerals, and fiber and serve as good intestinal cleansers. Fruits, however, contain mostly simple and compound sugars that are quickly absorbed by the blood and may bring about the problems associated with high blood-sugar levels. For this reason, fruits should be consumed whole—not as juice—and in moderate quantities. The fiber in whole fruits, as opposed to fruit juices, slows the rate at which the sugar is absorbed by the blood and helps to moderate blood-sugar and insulin levels.

Because of their high sugar content, fruit juices will exacerbate candida symptoms and should be avoided at all costs. A small amount of whole fruit may be okay, however. Fruit sugar content varies widely according to the kind of fruit, the season, and the growing conditions, so there's really no such thing as a list of safe

TABLE 20 Fruits

EAT OCCASIONALLY			LIMIT
Apples	Pears	Oranges, lemons, limes, and grapefruit [1]	Avocado[2]
Blueberries	Plums		Banana[2]
Cantaloupe	Prunes		Figs
Cherries	Raisins		Grapes
Currants	Raspberries		Mango[2]
Papaya	Strawberries		Pineapple[2]
Peaches	Watermelon		

1 Only if they can grow in your area.
2 If you live in the tropics, these may be consumed occasionally.

fruits. I myself eat fruit infrequently—maybe one serving of tart green apples, pears, or berries twice a week. You will have to figure out by trial and error which fruits do not present a problem and how often you can eat them.

If you choose to include fruit in your diet, you may be best off eating those fruits that grow in your geographical region and are currently in season. A possible exception is papaya. Readily available in the tropics, it is believed to be beneficial to the digestive system; in temperate climates, eating papaya once or twice a week could be okay.

NUTS AND SEEDS

Nuts and seeds are good sources of protein, but their oil content is so high that they should be eaten only occasionally and in small quantities. Sunflower seeds, which are 17 percent protein and 76 percent oil, and sesame seeds, which are 13 percent protein and 83 percent oil, make excellent condiments.

Nuts should be purchased in their shells, which protect the nut meat from the air and delay rancidity. Because of the problem of rancidity, nuts do not store as well as grains and should be kept no longer than a few months. Nuts and seeds are best eaten raw.

TABLE 21 Nuts and seeds

EAT OCCASIONALLY		AVOID	
Almonds	Pecans	Brazil nuts[1]	Peanuts[2]
Cashews	Pumpkin seeds	Chocolate[3]	Pistachios[4]
Chestnuts	Sesame seeds		
Hazel	Sunflower seeds		
Macadamia	Walnuts		

1 Sometimes contain aflatoxins.
2 Most likely contain aflatoxins.
3 A stimulant.
4 Mold problems.

If you roast nuts, don't use oil, and consume them immediately because roasting hastens rancidity.

Nuts and seeds are best avoided if you are critically ill. Furthermore, nuts are high in arginine, the amino acid that favors the replication of the herpes virus.[19] Avoid them if you have herpes or cold-sore problems.

THE GARLIC BREAKFAST

Hippocrates, the father of medicine, recommended garlic for its medicinal effects. Whenever I feel a cold coming on, I include raw garlic in my breakfast. Taking garlic for a day or two is usually sufficient to make me feel better.

Garlic has been used with great success to treat nasal and bronchial congestion, dysentery, cholera, parasites, and blood disorders such as high blood cholesterol, triglycerides, and arteriosclerosis. Louis Pasteur talked about the antibacterial properties of garlic. Albert Schweitzer is said to have used garlic in treating amebic dysentery in Africa, and research has recently confirmed folk-medicine claims about the effectiveness of garlic as an antiseptic and powerful antibiotic. "Moreover," states Eric Block in the March 1985 edition of *Scientific American*, "garlic juice exhibits a broad spectrum of activity against 200 pathogenic fungi and many strains of yeast, including some that cause vaginitis."[20]

In other words, garlic is mighty powerful stuff. It can suppress a strep throat and Salmonella and is particularly effective against all but two of twenty-six strains of *Candida albicans*.[21] There is even some preliminary research that suggests garlic may increase immunity to cancer due to its high selenium and germanium content.[22]

There are several ways to take garlic. While chewing fennel seed to prevent garlic breath, I finely chop six to eight cloves of garlic, then quickly swallow about one teaspoon of the minced garlic followed by some water. I continue this process until I have downed all the garlic. Pretty soon my stomach starts feeling fiery, but eating a piece of bread usually settles it immediately. Use only one clove the first time you try this garlic breakfast, and slowly work your way up over a few weeks. Parsley with the meal helps cut the garlic's odor.[e]

A friend of mine has a system for taking garlic that is a lot easier on your stomach but takes more time. He chops the garlic very fine and puts it into gelatin capsules. Then he fills another capsule with pulverized fennel seeds and swallows the garlic- and fennel-filled capsules.

For further information on garlic, read *The Miracle of Garlic* by Paavo Airola and *The Book of Garlic* by Lloyd J. Harris.

CHAPTER 8

The pitfalls of ingestion

TOXINS

Diet and nutrition are not synonymous. Diet is simply the total of what we ingest, whether it is peanut butter, cheeseburgers, vegetables, coloring agents, or pesticides. Nutrition implies consuming foods the body can utilize effectively for energy, growth, repair, and health. In this chapter we will look at toxic, nonnutritive substances that are often part of what we eat. The subject matter has been broken into four topics suggested by Corine H. Robinson and Marylin R. Lauler in *Normal and Therapeutic Nutrition:* food contamination by bacteria, parasites, molds, and fungi; toxins inherent in food; sensitivity to foods; and food contamination by toxic chemicals like pesticides and additives.[1] Food sensitivities will be discussed in a separate chapter.

BACTERIA, PARASITES, AND FUNGI

Bacteria such as the salmonellae that cause gastroenteritis, the staphylococci that produce boils and blood infections, and the shigellae that cause dysentery are the primary causes of many food-borne bacterial illnesses in the United States. If you are in good health and get food poisoning from these bacteria, your illness, though uncomfortable, will probably be brief. But if you have an impaired immune system, one of these ordinarily minor infections could kill you.

Salmonellosis and other diseases such as typhoid and scarlet fevers, tuberculosis, strep throat, botulism, amebic dysentery, and infectious hepatitis may result either from intimate contact with a sick person or from eating one of the following: an infected animal or plant; food contaminated by insects, flies, roaches, or rodents; food that has been in contact with sewage or polluted water (as shellfish often are); or food contaminated by someone who has ignored personal hygiene or acceptable food-handling practices.[a] While investigating this last contamination source, I learned from the Department of Health of the city of San Francisco that restaurants in the city are routinely inspected four times a year and even more frequently if there are complaints. The California Restaurant Act also requires physicians who are treating infectious diseases to ask their patients if they handle food at a public establishment. If so, the physician must advise the Bureau of Disease Control which informs the Health Department, which in turn makes sure the patient is no longer handling food.

Food handlers, however, are not required to undergo any routine medical tests. An employee infected by *Entamoeba histolytica*, staphylococci, or salmonella might contaminate what you eat because he or she is ignoring good hygiene while preparing your food. Restaurant inspectors have broad powers to keep a restaurant employee from handling food if they notice open sores, persistent coughing, or other indications of disease, but it is difficult to tell whether a food handler has an infection when the disease presents no outward manifestations.

Although not every restaurant is a potential source of contamination, eating out or purchasing prepared meals will increase your chances of encountering food that is not carefully prepared. You will thus court the risk of opportunistic infection. Because my health is now good enough that I need not avoid eating out, I will do so occasionally, usually at a vegetarian, seafood, Japanese or Chinese restaurant. Were I in the bad shape I was two years ago, I would restrict myself and prepare more meals in my own kitchen. You should decide what is appropriate for you.

If you eat out a lot, I suggest taking a healthy dose of raw garlic at least once a week. Garlic contains a potent substance that inhibits the growth of many bacteria that cause dysentery.[2]

Of all the fungal toxins found in food, only aflatoxins and trichothecene toxins need concern Americans. Aflatoxins are produced by a mold, *Aspergillus flavus*,[b] that infests many plant foods, especially peanuts, Brazil nuts, cottonseed, and improperly harvested grains such as corn. Peanuts with toxin levels above FDA standards cannot be used to manufacture peanut butter, but there is no way to eliminate aflatoxins completely from peanut products.[c, 3]

Aflatoxins can cause liver damage and may contribute to liver cancer. Animal experiments suggest that aflatoxins are also immune suppressors. Exposure to them is likely to worsen any existing infection or predisposition to infectious disease.[4] In fact, *Aspergillus flavus* has been observed as an opportunistic infection in some AIDS patients.[5] Because of these things, I stopped eating peanuts a year ago.

According to nutritionist Paul Newberne, trichothecene toxins in foods and crops are said to be "more widespread and significant than . . . aflatoxins."[6] The trichothecene toxins produced by molds of the genus Fusaria have been found in a high percentage of all dry corn in the United States. Studies indicate that some of these toxins are the cause of alimentary toxic aleukia (ATA), a food-poisoning reaction characterized by progressive loss of lymphocytes and granulocytes, extensive pin-sized hemorrhages throughout the body, tissue necrosis, and a swelling of the larynx that often results in strangulation and death. Although not all trichothecene toxins produce ATA, their ubiquitousness in the food supply is a cause for concern. Many people seem to be allergic to corn products. Perhaps such an allergic reaction is not so much a sensitivity to corn itself as to its trichothecene toxins. You can continue to enjoy corn on the cob and loose grain, however, provided the kernels are not shriveled or damaged and thus possibly infested by mold and contaminated by tricothecenes. But you might want to avoid corn syrup, cornstarch, and other prepared corn products in which these toxins could be present.

One more word about molds. Some molds are extremely toxic, so throw away *all* moldy food. Don't risk eating it!

TOXINS INHERENT IN FOOD

Plants produce a myriad of chemicals, some of which are as toxic and injurious to your health as contamination by bacteria, molds, or parasites.

One of the most common plant toxins in the United States is the solanine found in the Solanaceae plant family, which includes nightshade or belladonna, tobacco, eggplant, tomatoes, potatoes, and bell and chili peppers. Solanine is especially prevalent in potato leaves and stems but occurs in low concentrations in the tuber. The eyes of the tuber are high in solanine, however, so they should be removed before cooking. Light concentrates the toxin; when potatoes grow close to the ground's surface or are stored in a bright place, their skins become greenish, indicating a high solanine content. Store potatoes in a dark place, and discard any that have sprouted or turned green or that show major blemishes from mechanical injury. Eating potatoes whose green areas have not been completely removed may cause pain, vomiting, jaundice, diarrhea, and prostration. After you've peeled your unblemished, nongreen potato, cook it quickly. (Because of the standard excessive application of highly toxic chemicals to the potato crop by farmers,[d] I avoid potatoes altogether unless they are certified organic.)

Phytic acid, another toxin, is a phosphorus compound found in the outer husks of all grains. It readily binds with calcium, zinc, and iron, making them insoluble and therefore unavailable to the body. If you eat products with added bran or add bran to your food, you may be consuming a high concentration of this toxin. Soaking, sprouting, or cooking grains helps break down phytic acid. Leavening bread is also an effective way of eliminating phytates. As the bread rises, fermentation releases an enzyme that destroys the toxins. As explained in chapter 7, you should buy only naturally fermented or naturally leavened breads, however, and avoid unleavened breads or those leavened with commercial yeast.

Saponin toxins are common in beans (particularly soy), spinach, asparagus, horse chestnuts, and sugar beets. They are also used as stabilizers in confections, beer, and soft drinks, so these products should be avoided.[7] Large doses of saponins characteristically destroy red blood cells and interfere with the body's use of vitamin E.[8] Although I don't mind cutting out alfalfa, spinach, horse chestnuts, and asparagus, soybeans are an important part of my diet. I believe their advantages outweigh their disadvantages (see "Beans" in chapter 7), but I suggest that you use any bean product only as a supplemental or secondary food that constitutes no more than 10 to 15 percent of your diet. Soy products should compose no more than 3 to 5 percent.

Another bean to avoid is the fava, also known as the broad bean. Eating this bean, *either raw or cooked*, might contribute to the destruction of red blood cells, leading to anemia. Lima beans, too, can be toxic; they contain a substance that may turn into hydrocyanic acid and cause cyanide poisoning. Eating lima beans once in a while is okay, but it is best to leave them alone altogether.

Oxalic acid, a poisonous compound used as a metal cleanser and laundry bleach occurs in spinach, purslane, swiss chard, beet tops, sorrel, and rhubarb in concentrations of over 10 percent. Rhubarb—and sometimes sorrel—can be especially toxic when ingested, causing gastroenteritis, diarrhea, vomiting, and occasionally convulsions and coma. The other vegetables might not be as overtly toxic, but your body will still have to neutralize their oxalic acid, and this process puts an extra burden on your immune system. If you take large doses of vitamin C, it is important to keep consumption of foods high in oxalic acid down because ascorbic acid metabolism adds to the oxalic acid levels in your body.[9] Furthermore, even very low concentrations of oxalic acid from food are said to neutralize the salivary amylase that begins starch digestion in the mouth.[10]

FOOD ADDITIVES

The best source I have found on food additives is Beatrice Trum Hunter's *Fact Book on Food Additives and Your Health*. The book is a real eye opener; unfortunately it is out of print at this time, so I will summarize the author's major points:

1. Each and every year most of us consume over four pounds of chemical preservatives, stabilizers, coloring agents, flavor enhancers, and other additives.
2. These chemicals may produce changes in the food itself or combine with the natural constituents of the food to form new toxic compounds, and the toxicity of the chemicals can increase considerably through interaction with one another.
3. Over 3,000 chemicals are deliberately added to our foods.[e]
4. Over 1,000 of these chemicals have never been tested

for their likelihood of causing cancer, genetic damage, or birth defects.

5. Under the aegis of the Food and Drug Administration, manufacturers of these untested chemicals have the exclusive right to determine the safety of a food additive.
6. Food manufacturers and processors, the end users of these chemicals, do not have to inform the FDA of their use.

About twenty pages in the *Fact Book* are devoted to various types of toxic additives and their functions. One popular additive is the bleaching agent used to whiten flour (dough made from unbleached flour turns unappetizingly gray if stored uncooked for any length of time). Other common additives are food colors derived from coal tar, emulsifiers made from plastics, and flavor enhancers such as MSG. The danger in food additives lies in how they interact with each other. Just one food additive alone might prove harmless, but the wrong combination could be fatal! And given the 63,000 chemicals commonly used in food today, the odds for an unlucky combination are fairly high.

Most of these substances are added to food not because they offer nutritional value but because they make the food look, taste, or feel better. It's all for cosmetic illusion. Some common food additives are discussed in greater detail in appendix D.

If food additives are slowly poisoning us, what then are the effects of pesticides specifically designed to destroy life? Current pesticides make no distinction between insect and human life. The deaths of 2,500 people in Bhopal, India, in 1984 attest to this fact.

Every year, farmers apply over 2.3 billion pounds of insecticides, nematocides, herbicides, and fungicides to the plants and soil from which we draw our nutrients. It is not uncommon for chemical residues to remain on and *inside* foods at the time of purchase or for such residues to contaminate our water supplies.[g, 11] Despite laws to the contrary, untested pesticides are still in use.

> In 1972, Congress rewrote the 1947 Federal Insecticide, Fungicide and Rodenticide Act to require that all pesticides be tested for their effect on health before being sold. While the act exempted 600 of the ingredients in use at the time, it required that they be proved safe by 1976. After an extension, the deadline was changed to 1978. To date [1985], only about 100 of the 600 ingredients have been reviewed by the EPA, and only four have been completely tested for their health effects.[12]

Aside from being toxic, many pesticides are immune suppressants even in the smallest quantities. Aldecarb,[h] the Union Carbide chemical that devastated Bhopal, is one of these.[13]

Try to purchase food that is organically grown without the application of deadly chemicals.[i] Also avoid fish, such as tuna, that are the last predators in a long predator-prey chain and whose tissues therefore contain a high concentration of chemical residues. Animal fat readily retains toxic chemicals, so animal products such as meat and milk generally contain higher levels of these dangerous substances than do vegetable sources.[14]

FOOD ALLERGIES AND SENSITIVITIES

There's little value in a well-planned diet if some of its elements, even though whole, unprocessed, and chemical-free, prompt the body to reject food, thereby causing malnutrition.

This can be the case with food allergies and sensitivities. Allergies engage the immune system and divert it from healing and warding off disease. In people with AIDS or ARC, food and chemical sensitivities are common and sometimes aggravate certain conditions such as Kaposi's lesions and lymphadenopathy.[15]

What causes allergies? Why do certain people show an unusual reaction to a substance that, in similar amounts, would not affect others?

An allergy is basically an immune response that causes tissue damage. When a food fragment or foreign chemical enters the body, the immune system acts upon and neutralizes it as it would any other antigen. In a hypersensitive person, however, the antigen—now called an allergen—hooks onto special cells before the normal immune response goes into action. These cells, called mast cells in the tissues and basophils in the blood, bristle with a particular antibody, immunoglobulin E (IgE), which binds very strongly to the allergen. After the allergen and the cell-bound antibody grip on to each other, the cell explodes, releasing chemicals that produce the allergic symptoms.

The food and chemical sensitivities found in AIDS patients are mediated not by IgE but by the lack of certain enzymes, usually the digestive ones. In these enzymatic deficiency allergies (EDAs), the enzyme needed to break a particular protein into its component amino acids is lacking. The food fragments containing this protein are therefore not broken up and may adhere to the intestinal wall, damaging its mucous lining and other tissues. This process creates intolerance to a particular food.

The origin of many food and chemical sensitivities remains controversial. Conventional immunology cannot explain them. In fact, some immunologists scoff at the word *allergy* when applied to food or chemical sensitivities that are not mediated by the IgE–mast cell mechanism. On the other hand, clinical ecology, an interdisciplinary offshoot of environmental medicine,[j] explains these sensitivities differently. It proposes that a sensitivity is not of itself a disease but rather the symptom of an underlying disorder resulting from the accumulated exposure to low doses of stressors —chemicals, pollutants, common foods, airborne particles, even emotional stress—on the rise in our environment. *Clinical Ecology* by physician Iris R. Bell is an excellent and very readable book on the subject.

One probable cause of food sensitivity, especially among people with AIDS, is chronic infection by *Candida albicans*, which will be discussed at greater length in chapter 12. This fungus is usually under check in most people, but under certain conditions it will infect the mouth—producing the white patches known as thrush—or the vagina. When the immune system isn't fully operational, candidiasis can spread to the bowel. Candida's rootlike growths will penetrate the intestinal mucosa and allow entry of incompletely digested proteins and unneutralized toxins into the blood vessels, which in turn may produce allergies or sensitivities.[16] These allergies usually clear up after treatment of the infection.

It is also believed that the AIDS virus itself might increase sensitivity to certain chemicals and foods, although it is not yet known why. Severely ill clinical ecology patients, however, show several of the immune abnormalities also present in people with AIDS: low absolute T cell counts, increased production of autoantibodies (antibodies directed against the body), and most significant, high levels of immune complexes[k] or antibody-antibody agglomerations.[17, 18] Food and chemical sensitivities, therefore, might be as-of-yet-unrecognized signs of immune abnormality—not necessarily IgE-mediated—caused by environmental or biological factors. In any case, both food allergies and sensitivities engage residual immunity when the neutrophils set out to repair tissue damage, neutralize toxins, and clean up debris in the affected areas. Food and chemical intolerances in people with AIDS should therefore be given special consideration.

The absence of normal bacteria or the presence of abnormal ones in the bowel, a condition known as dysbiosis, might also cause sensitivities. Normal bacteria help the intestinal lining absorb substances at a normal rate. When there are not enough normal bacteria or too many abnormal ones, the lining becomes more like a colander with large holes than the fine sieve it usually is. The results are like those of candidiasis: toxins and partially digested foods enter the body and cause an allergic reaction. Common causes of dysbiosis are weakening illnesses, antibiotic therapy, and diets rich in refined foods. Cultures of live beneficial bacteria, such as those in acidophilus and miso, along with a whole-food diet may help alleviate this condition.[19]

We eat too much of the same foods, day in and day out. The 1977–78 Nationwide Food Consumption Survey revealed the lack of variety in our diets. Potatoes, tomatoes, lettuce, beans, peas, and corn accounted for 73 percent of all vegetables in the average U.S. diet. Wheat, milk, eggs, corn, and cane sugar were consumed daily.[20] Not surprisingly, these common foods are the ones most likely to trigger allergies.[21] The more frequently one eats a food, the more likely it is that one may develop a sensitivity to it. And strange as it may sound, the reaction against one food might lead to dependency or addiction and turn overconsumption into a closed loop out of which it is difficult to escape.

The allergy-addiction response seems to operate independently of substance. It comes as a result of food, alcohol, or drugs. After an unpleasant initial reaction to a food, repeated exposure seems to desensitize a person. At this stage, repeated exposure overstimulates, producing a much-sought-after sensation of well-being —a pick-me-up. But the sensitivity remains hidden. Repeated exposure quietly wreaks havoc on the body (on the liver and the brain with alcohol and drugs, on insulin-glucagon production with sugar). A person may consume the same amount of alcohol or an offending food for years without experiencing symptoms. The disease progresses, however, and finally all of its symptoms blossom. In an attempt to counteract these, the person increases consumption of the same substance. The symptoms worsen, and more and more of the substance is needed; the increase in consumption causes greater and greater deterioration. With alcohol and drugs, the allergy-addiction cycle can happen faster than with food.

Of course, food offers one alternative that alcohol or other substances don't. You can always switch to a food that doesn't trigger the allergy-addiction cycle, unless you're a compulsive eater who has to reduce all food consumption. Despite the efforts of many alcoholics to change brands of liquor, you cannot really change to a safe kind of alcohol. For the compulsive user, all alcohol and drugs are equally damaging.

Even when allergy or sensitivity symptoms appear, it is often difficult to recognize them. The obvious symptoms are headache, stuffy nose, watery and puffy eyes, pressure on the chest, and a white coat on the tongue. Other symptoms, however, might mimic those of other diseases—muscle pain, intermittent and unexplained joint aches, abdominal cramps, diarrhea, constipation, swelling of the hands or ankles, persistent fatigue, nervousness, irritability, foggy-headedness, depression, and excessive sweating unrelated to exercise (some of these can also be candida symptoms).[22]

Since symptoms can be nonspecific or disjointed, food sensitivities are often dismissed as psychosomatic or as caused by stress. When symptoms blend with those of other diseases such as candida infection or AIDS, food allergies might go undiagnosed. Food sensitivity is often the last factor a doctor will consider, if he or she considers it at all. Appendix E discusses several tests used to discover food and chemical allergies and sensitivities.

FLESH, FOWL, AND FISH

Animal flesh—whether from land or sea—is not necessary for your nutritional well-being. In fact, its inclusion in your diet could be lethal in some cases. If you do feel the necessity for animal protein, however, you should try to confine your intake of it to fish, lamb, or *organically* raised chicken.[l]

Beef is high in fat and has been related to cholesterol problems. About 50 percent of beef's calories come from fat. As a result, many people have switched to chicken in the belief that they're doing something better for their health. Chicken meat, unfortunately, may be as bad for you as beef, not because of its fat and cholesterol content—poultry is somewhat lower in cholesterol and a good deal lower in fat than other animal foods—but because antibiotics such as penicillin and tetracycline are routinely fed to chickens and other farm animals to stimulate growth and improve feed efficiency. These antibiotics, however, are given in dosages insufficient to kill all the bacteria that might plague the chicken, thereby often allowing the development of strains of microorganisms resistant to medication.[m] When we eat contaminated meat, this resistance might be passed along to the bacteria in our intestines—bacteria interchange genetic material frequently—and from our intestinal bacteria to other, more harmful bacteria that might infect us. Antibiotics might then be ineffective during illness caused by such resistant pathogens. In *Nutrition for a Better Life* Nan Bronfen states: "In tests, 30 percent of cooked sausage contained antibiotic-resistant *E. coli*[n] which are a common cause of infection. *E. coli* are capable of transferring antibiotic resistance to *Salmonella* bacteria, the organism responsible for food poisoning."[23]

In addition, commercially grown chickens are usually crammed into cages that don't even allow the birds to flap their wings. Crowded conditions make the animals so hostile that they routinely have to be debeaked to prevent them from pecking each other to death. To make things worse, their quarters are lit twenty-two hours a day because chickens won't eat in the dark. Such cruel treatment subjects these chickens to great stress, increasing their incidence of infection (thus necessitating more antibiotics) and tainting the quality of their meat with toxins. Perhaps their secret revenge for the suffering we impose on them is to give us the increased health risks of antibiotic-resistant bacterial infections and food poisoning.[24]

Meat, poultry, fish, eggs, and dairy products are the most common source of salmonella, the usual cause of bacterial food poisoning in the United States.[25] There are over 20,000 confirmed cases every year, although the actual number is probably over 100,000. Salmonellosis is likely to be benign in most adults, but sometimes it might have serious complications leading to peritonitis, endocarditis, osteomyelitis, urinary tract infection and meningitis.[26] Moreover, in the elderly and the very young as well as those weakened by illness, even an apparently mild infection such as salmonellosis can often lead to serious complications or even death.[27]

There have been increasing reports of recurrent salmonella infection in AIDS patients. Infection has not confined itself to the gastrointestinal tract; in some cases, salmonella has invaded the bloodstream, attacked the inside lining of the heart, and formed lethal abscesses in the brain. Gastrointestinal and blood infections by salmonella have responded to antibiotics up to now, but doctors fear that the prolonged hospital stays of many AIDS patients may allow the pathogens to acquire resistance to treatment from resistant bacteria in the wards.[28]

The best way to avoid salmonella and resistant *E. coli* is to limit consumption of meat, poultry, fish, eggs, and dairy products and to eat a vegetarian diet. The McDougalls explain: "Fresh plant foods, which are very different from us in their biochemical makeup, do not contain microorganisms harmful to humans unless they are contaminated with products or excretions from diseased animals or people."[29]

A butcher's block, kitchen counter, or kitchen utensil can be the source of contamination from any other food with which it comes in contact. For example, a restaurant employee cuts up salmonella-contaminated chicken on a wooden cutting board. The chicken is cooked and its bacteria are killed, but the board on which it was cut is only quickly rinsed and then used to cut the salad vegetables. You are then served the decontaminated, cooked chicken along with the salad, which is now contaminated by the chicken salmonella from the board. One cannot be sure that all restaurant workers handle food in a way that avoids such contamination. If you eat out, you should therefore consider limiting yourself to vegetarian restaurants, which prepare no meat in their kitchens. And if you live with meat eaters, use separate cutting boards and knives. Keep the kitchen immaculate and wash everything carefully.

You'll probably find it easier not to eat at anyone else's home unless he or she understands your dietary restrictions. This is extremely tough on friends who are unenlightened about diet. In all societies, eating is a means of initiating and maintaining relationships. Well-intentioned friends, often unaware of the danger certain foods could represent to your condition, will try to convince you to eat whatever they serve. Try a polite refusal first, something to the effect that the food doesn't agree with you. If they then insist with a line like "Have just one; it won't kill you," try a straightforward no and tell them why it might indeed kill you. Most people will rarely nag you again.

Meat can also be a source of carcinogenic substances, both natural and manmade. Malonaldehyde is a powerful natural carcinogen that appears as a breakdown product when an animal is slaughtered; it is especially prevalent in beef.[30] Fourteen percent of the meat and chicken sampled by the U.S. Department of Agriculture between 1974 and 1976 showed signs of illegal and potentially harmful drugs, pesticides, or environmental contaminants. Even if the meat you bought were free of such substances, it could still become carcinogenic in your kitchen. Cooking meat over high heat, especially over a charcoal fire, will bring about chemical changes that produce carcinogens. "A one-pound steak broiled over charcoal," say the McDougalls, "can contain as much benzopyrene as 600 cigarettes. Benzopyrene is a powerful carcinogen used since the 1940's to cause lymphomas, thymomas [thymus cancers], stomach cancer and leukemia in laboratory animals.[31]

Worst of all, meat is hard to digest. The body must expend a great deal of energy to metabolize it—energy that is then no longer available for fending off disease or for healing. If this section has not convinced you of the ill effects of meat, then at least try to avoid liver and processed meats such as wieners, sausages, and bologna.

People who insist on including animal protein in their diet but who are nevertheless ill should try limiting themselves to deep-sea

TABLE 22 Seafood

EAT OCCASIONALLY		AVOID	
Anchovies	Perch	Bluefish[3]	Lobster[3]
Cod	Salmon[2]	Carp[4]	Oysters[4]
Flounder	Shrimp	Catfish[4]	Scallops[4]
Haddock	Smelt	Caviar[4]	Swordfish[3]
Halibut	Sole	Clams[4]	Trout[4]
Herring, fresh	Striped Bass	Herring, packed in oil[2]	Tuna[3]
Mackarel[1]			

1 High in omega-3 and omega-6 lipoproteins.
2 High fat content.
3 High on the food chain—concentrated pesticides and toxins.
4 Subject to various pollutants.

fish a few times a week. As one regains health, chicken, lamb and even beef may be appropriate occasionally provided they are organically raised and range-fed. The key word is *occasionally.* Perhaps because of their metabolic requirements, some people seem to do better on some animal protein, but never in the colossal amounts common to the American diet. With a diet rich in vegetables, grains and beans, however, you probably will not need any red meat to get adequate protein. If you do eat meat, poultry, or fish, consider it tainted with infectious agents until properly cooked (that should answer any questions about sushi).

DAIRY

Milk is our first food as children and thus symbolizes the security of infancy. Based on that pleasant association and on other, less-than-accurate insinuations, the dairy industry is able to sell its products. Dairy industry advertisements suggests that women who don't get enough milk products in their diet run a high risk of developing osteoporosis. In reality, one of the contributing factors to the rising incidence of osteoporosis in the United States may be the high amount of phosphorus in diets rich in dairy products and other animal protein. The body counteracts high phosphorus concentrations in the blood by leaching calcium from bone and expelling it in the urine.[32]

After weaning, most people in the world subsist on diets that contain no milk products, but calcium deficiency is relatively unknown among them. In the United States we believe that cow's milk is suitable not only for calves but also for human babies and adults. This is not the case. A calf needs to increase in size very quickly; the rich milk of its mother permits a fast increase in weight. A human baby, on the other hand, needs to develop primarily its nervous system; only human milk can support this process adequately.[33]

Cow's milk contains three times the casein—the protein in cheese—and three times the total protein in human milk (but only one-half the carbohydrate). Casein is used to make paints, glues, and plastics. Too much cow's milk in the diet is said to create viscous mucus secretions that easily dry out and adhere to the cilia lining the respiratory tract, impairing their function and thus allowing pathogens, such as the ones that cause colds, to invade more easily.[34]

Cow's milk is also a ready source of lactose. Lactose, however, cannot be absorbed by the body unless it is broken down by the enzyme lactase. In the United States alone, about 10 percent of the whites, 70 percent of the blacks, 75 percent of the Mexicans, 60 to 80 percent of the Jews, and 90 percent of the Asians lack this enzyme and therefore cannot tolerate lactose in their diet. Lactose intolerance is characterized by stomach cramps, intestinal gas, and diarrhea.[o, 35]

Parasitic infections such as salmonellosis, shigellosis, amebiasis, and typhoid fever can injure the intestinal lining to the point that it loses its ability to produce lactase. This pathogen-caused lactose intolerance adds to the severity of the diarrhea that accompanies such infections.[36] AIDS patients suffering from these diseases should avoid dairy products at all costs. Lactose also supports the growth of candida.[37] For those with lactase deficiency, yogurt causes less of a problem than milk because it contains some lactase produced by the culture and because some of its lactose has been predigested by fermentation. Yogurt, however, contains no nutrients other than those present in the milk from which it comes.[p] Also, like regular milk, yogurt and acidophilus milk may cause a thicker mucus.

Milk and yogurt may contain bacteria, antibiotics, hormones such as estrogen, and carcinogens such as aflatoxins, nitrates, nitrites, pesticides, and radioactive elements. The antibiotics present in milk can kill many of the intestinal bacteria that keep candida in check.[38] Hormones like estrogen are steroid compounds that can be immunosuppressive.

According to *The McDougall Plan,* dairy foods also might be associated with Hodgkin's disease, a cancer of the lymphatic tissue. "Continuous over-stimulation of the immune system by dairy proteins," the McDougalls say, "may eventually lead to the breakdown of the immune system into this form of cancer."[39] Possibly linked to this phenomenon is a virus that produces leukemia in laboratory animals[q] and is found in a substantial percentage of dairy cows.[40]

Yogurt and certain cheeses—Brie, Camembert, Cheddar, Emmentaler, Gruyère, and Stilton—also contain large amounts of tyramine, an amino acid produced by bacterial fermentation. Tyramine interacts with certain drugs used as antidepressants or in chemotherapy[r] and may precipitate a hypertensive crisis characterized by high blood pressure, severe headaches, palpitations, and in a few cases death. Other foods that may interact similarly with these drugs are ale and beer, avocados, bananas, caffeine, Chianti wine, chicken and beef liver, chocolate, cola drinks, fava or broad beans, herring, soy sauce, tea, vanilla, and yeast.[41, 42]

One last danger in dairy products is caused not by the food itself but by the vitamin D_2 that is added to cow's milk to combat vitamin D deficiency in cities where there's too little winter sunlight for the body to produce this vitamin. In contrast to vitamin D_3, the true form, vitamin D_2 can rob the body of magnesium and has been linked by Nobel researcher Hans Selye to calcification problems and kidney stones.[43,44]

Most books classify eggs as a dairy food, which they really are not, although they can cause similar problems and allergic reactions. Some of the constituents of egg albumin can inhibit the digestive enzyme trypsin;[s] another egg-albumin constituent, the protein avidin, binds to the important B vitamin biotin, preventing its use by the body. Egg yolks are notorious for their high cholesterol,[45, 46] which neutralizes the anti-HIV activity of active lipids such as phosphatidylcholine and phosphatidylethanolamine. The phosphatidylcholine in egg yolk seems to work against HIV only when a process similar to that used for making AL 721 removes the cholesterol.

Eggs may also contain estrogen, antibiotics, and pesticides, so if you do eat eggs, make sure they come from hens that are not given hormones or antibiotics and are range fed—that is, allowed to hunt and peck freely for the nutritious worm.

One final note about dairy and eggs. Dairy- and egg-derived semisolid foods such as custards, cream fillings, sauces and dressings, and mayonnaise in all its permutations can pose a very real danger of food poisoning from staphylococci by providing an ideal growth medium for these airborne bacteria. The bacteria multiply rapidly when these foods are left unrefrigerated for a few hours, so a person can come down with acute gastroenteritis after eating some potato salad left on the kitchen counter through a hot summer afternoon. Food poisoning from *Staphylococcus* is abrupt and severe and can last from one to three days in a relatively healthy individual.[47] In a person with a suppressed immune system, symptoms can be much worse.

HERBS AND SPICES

Herbs and spices have been used through the ages in teas and as therapeutic agents and flavor enhancers. There's been a recent upsurge in their use in the United States, particularly in the herbal teas that are currently replacing coffee and black tea.

Herbs are used in healing and have many therapeutic effects. Do not forget, however, that herbs contain drugs, albeit in impure form, and should be used with discretion to avoid negative effects.

For example, sassafras—once widely used—contains safrole, an oil now known to cause liver cancer in laboratory animals.[48]

Other common herbs that could be deleterious if used continuously are alfalfa, comfrey, lady's mantle, yellow dock, shave grass, peppermint, and chamomile. If you are allergic to ragweed, asters, or chrysanthemums, you should avoid chamomile, since it might cause a severe allergic reaction.[49] An occasional cup of these herbal teas will not be harmful, although long-term consumption could.

Many spices are best avoided because their volatile oils might irritate the kidneys.[50] These oils are often natural insecticides produced by plants to ward off insects and are not necessarily fit for human consumption. Some spices, such as cloves and black pepper, however, contain natural antibacterial and antifungal substances. Nonirritating spices that could be used occasionally are dill, paprika, turmeric, capsicum, and caraway, fennel, and celery seeds. For more information on spices, I recommend *The Complete Book of Spices: Their Medical, Nutritional and Cooking Uses* by John Heinerman.

Some holistic physicians have been recommending various herbs in their protocols for strengthening the immune system of their AIDS patients. Although many of these herbs have been used extensively in folk medicine, conventional medicine has done little laboratory work to investigate their properties.

Infusions of ginseng root have been used traditionally in the Orient as a cure-all and supplement for good health. Ginseng is considered a tonic, that is, a medicine that invigorates by increasing or restoring body tone. The Jaffe protocol recommends it as an "adaptogen," an herb that increases the body's ability to adapt to stress.[51] Ginseng contains certain physiologically active compounds that can be beneficial[t] yet can also produce serious side effects when taken in large or prolonged doses. Nervousness, insomnia, blood pressure changes, and, in older women, sore breasts and vaginal bleeding have been reported after excessive use. But small amounts of the root are probably harmless. Beware of the ginseng you buy. One-fourth of the fifty-four ginseng supplements available in the United States are said to contain no ginseng at all and over half to contain so little as to be of no practical value.[52]

Echinacea augustifolia, long promoted by native Americans for the treatment of infections, and ginger, traditionally used to relieve colic and to ease cold symptoms, are also recommended as adaptogens in the Jaffe protocol. In his version of this protocol, physician Keith Barton says that *Echinacea* might be a general immune stimulant. Allegedly its properties have been investigated in Germany, but I have seen no results in writing. The data on both *Echinacea* and ginger seem to come from the clinical experience of the practitioners who use them. One such person is Misha Cohen, doctor of Oriental medicine and head of the Quan Yin Acupuncture and Herb Center of San Francisco. In appendix F she writes about her experience with various herbs as complements to the treatment of AIDS and ARC.

If you plan on using any herbs as medication, I suggest that you first consult with a knowledgeable physician or an acupuncturist-herbologist and read up on the possible side effects of the herbs. *The Guide to Medicinal Plants* by Paul Schauenberg and Ferdinand Paris is a useful book that covers over four hundred plants with therapeutical properties.

PREPARED AND PROCESSED FOODS

Nature has been the leader of the food industry for eons, and her products remain unsurpassed. They support life. None of the industry's newcomers has done a better job. Most of them, in fact, have done no job at all as far as our health is concerned. Therefore, my advice is to avoid *all* processed foods.[u]

You are mistaken if you believe you can eliminate harmful or empty foods by reading labels. First of all, the harmful ingredients might not have dangerous-sounding chemical names. Take, for instance, the benign-sounding cottonseed oil and partially hydrogenated oils listed on a can of cream of celery soup. Cotton is one of the U.S. crops most heavily treated with pesticides, and its seed readily concentrates these poisons. Partially hydrogenated oils probably contain traces of the nickel used to catalyze the hydrogenation process. Metallic nickel has been linked to certain kind of cancer, especially those of the lungs and the nasal passages.[53] In addition, hydrogenation converts an unsaturated oil into a saturated fat—saturation, after all, means that a fat has more hydrogen. Cottonseed and partially or totally hydrogenated oils are best avoided.

Many harmful substances are not even mentioned on the label. There are several hundred substances on what is known as the GRAS (generally recognized as safe) list that can be added to food without any mention on the label. Many of these GRAS additives have never been tested for safety. Most were in use prior to the Food Additives Amendment of 1958, and a "grandfather clause" exempted them from the regulations of this bill. Among the GRAS additives you will find acidulants, alkalis, anticaking agents, antimolding and antistaling agents, antioxidants, buffers, emulsifiers, artificial colors, and bleaches, some of which are discussed in either the "Toxins" section of this chapter or appendix E.

Do not trust the term *natural*. It tells you nothing about the product and is often used deceitfully. Neither the Food and Drug Administration, which regulates labels, nor the Federal Trade Commission, which regulates advertising, have defined the use of this adjective. Until they do so, the word *natural* can be applied to any product that originally comes from nature, and since most things in the universe fall into this category, foods containing lead, white table sugar, MSG and coal-tar coloring can and will be advertised as natural. The terms *naturally fermented* or *naturally leavened* are an exception because they describe the lack of an ingredient—commercial yeast. A statement that a product doesn't contain a certain ingredient could be subject to labeling and advertising regulations.

Industrial food processing not only adds substances that are unhealthful but removes those needed for health. One example is the loss of vitamins and minerals when whole grains are turned into flour for bread and breakfast cereals. After the food processors have taken almost all the good and desirable substances out of the grains, they make a big show of putting a small portion of the nutrients they removed back in—thus, their product is fortified in an X number of ways whereas nature's product was originally fortified in innumerable ways.[v] Unfortunately, the vitamins that enrich processed products do not include pyridoxine or B_6, folic acid, and pantothenic acid, three vitamins that are essential for a healthily functioning immune system. Whenever one of these is absent, the body has difficulty in manufacturing antibodies.[54]

In addition to removing vitamins and minerals, food processing reverses the sodium-potassium ratio in foods, contributing to the high sodium content of our diet. Foods in nature are usually low in sodium, which the body conserves and therefore does not require continuously, but they are high in potassium, which the body loses easily and needs to replenish constantly. Corn flour, for example, contains 1 part of sodium for every 120 parts of potassium. When the flour is made into corn flakes this ratio changes to 1,160 parts of sodium to 120 parts of potassium.[55]

Refining and processing also remove fiber from food. A low-fiber diet increases food transit time through the intestinal tract; as a result, toxins spend a longer time in contact with intestinal mucosa, and animal products putrefy in the intestines. This puts added strain on a body if it is already overtaxed by stress and improper eating habits. Diseases associated with processed food consumption are increasing. The list includes tooth decay, heart disease, ulcers, hemorrhoids, cancer, gallstones, obesity, and diabetes. Time and again, a marked increase in physical and mental disorders has been observed whenever "primitive peoples" such as Eskimos, Yemenite Jews, Polynesians, and Zulus become "civilized" and adopt a diet of refined carbohydrates.[56] Furthermore, adding bran to food can compound health risks. Avoiding the health hazards of low-fiber diets is simple enough: fiber should not be removed from food in the first place.

Most food processing is geared toward cosmetic appearance rather than nutrition. What matters is how the food looks and keeps on the shelf, not how it enhances your health and well being. A winner in this contemporary tradition is the most recent food-processing technique, irradiation. Proponents of this latter-day marvel tell us that irradiated food will keep longer, eliminating the need for many harmful preservatives. They assure us that low- to medium-dosage irradiation[w] kills insects, controls sprouting, and reduces bacteria and that nutrient loss will be no greater than what is lost by canning. But here is where the beast shows its teeth. Loss of nutrients has long been considered a major problem in canned foods. Likewise, studies show that reduction of vitamins A, B_1, B_6, B_{12}, C, and E is often drastic after irradiation. In addition, the dosages approved for food irradiation will not kill the bacteria that cause botulism but will kill their natural enemies, thereby not only allowing but actually increasing the possibility of contracting this fatal disease from irradiated food. Food irradiation will put to good use all that worthless nuclear waste we're having so much difficulty getting rid of and will keep our food looking good for years without refrigeration. Luckily, the FDA still considers irradiation a

TABLE 23 Processed foods

EAT OCCASIONALLY	
Apple butter	Sesame seed oil
Corn oil	Sunflower oil
Grain syrups	Vinegar
Olive oil	Whole-grain, unleavened breads
Safflower oil	Whole grain products
Sesame seed butter	
EAT RARELY	**AVOID**
Canned, frozen, and packaged foods	Honey
	Maple sugar and molasses
NEVER EAT	
Additives, all foods with	Peanut products
Corn syrup	Saccharine and other artificial sweeteners
Cottonseed oil	Sugar, white and brown
Oils, commercially processed	

food additive, and irradiated food has to be labeled accordingly.[x] Be on the alert for it!

Even nonirradiated food on the shelf can present some hazards. Infinitesimal amounts of the vinyl chloride, acrylonitrile, and other plastics used in packaging will occasionally get into food. Vinyl chloride is commonly recognized as a potent human carcinogen, and acrylonitrile has caused tumors in laboratory animals.[58]

The food-processing industry provides us with a product that's good to look at and sometimes good to taste but that really is not all that good to eat. The industry's cosmetic solutions to problems of spoilage, waste, and appeal indeed might force many of us to get the greatest cosmetic job of them all: the mortician's.

FAST FOODS

Even though fast-food establishments call themselves restaurants, their methods and products have more in common with those of commercial food processors. Fast foods are processed foods and should be avoided for many of the same reasons. They are high in fat, which provides 53 percent of the calories in a Big Mac, 59 percent in Arby's sausage-and-egg croissant, and 72 percent in Hardee's shrimp salad. For the frequent fast-food patron, limiting fats is very difficult indeed. To those whose immune system can be further impaired even by a moderate fat intake, fast-food establishments should be anathema.

Fast foods are also too high in sodium. We only need about 1,100 mg of sodium per day. McDonald's sausage biscuit contains 1,380 mg; Wendy's taco salad, 1,100 mg; Jack-In-The-Box chicken supreme sandwich, 1,582 mg; and Arby's fried chicken-breast sandwich, 1,323 mg. It is the combination of high fat and high sodium that has earned one of the most popular fast food hamburgers the nickname "Coronary Unit Special."

But even if you could manage to avoid all the high-fat and high-sodium items sold in a fast-food establishment, you still wouldn't be safe. The most alarming aspect of fast foods is that they are loaded with additives. Although some of these additives constitute a threat to your health, many fast-food companies refuse to list the ingredients in their products, using the argument that they would be divulging trade secrets. If regular restaurants are exempt from such a requirement, they maintain, fast-food restaurants also should be. But regular restaurants are exempt for reasons that do not apply to fast-food establishments. In a regular restaurant there is no package that can bear a label listing ingredients. The menu, and therefore the ingredients themselves, can change daily.

Fast-food outlets, on the other hand, are not really regular restaurants; they are small, decentralized food manufacturing facilities. In all their franchise establishments, the same ingredients are used and the same standard items are produced. The menu is limited and doesn't change much. Most fast food is packaged in containers that could easily show a list of ingredients and nutrients.[y]

Of all the major fast-food chains, only Arby's fully answered a recent questionnaire sent by the editors of the Nutrition Action Healthletter[z] requesting ingredient information. Burger Chef, Long John Silver's, and Wendy's ignored the questionnaire altogether. Burger King, Church's Fried Chicken, Hardee's, Jack-In-The-Box, Kentucky Fried Chicken, McDonald's, Pizza Hut, and Roy Rogers maintained that either such information was not available or that it was confidential and could not be divulged.[59] What great proprietary secrets could be exposed by revealing the ingredients in french fries, hamburgers, and shakes? One cannot help but wonder what these companies are really hiding. Could it be something like the sulfiting agents many of these establishments use as preservatives in their fresh salads, dried fruits, uncooked vegetables, avocado dips, wines, beer, and shrimp?

These agents have caused severe reactions—weakness, cyanosis, chest constriction, shock, coma, and even death—in sensitive individuals.[60] Widespread use of these compounds brought severe criticism from the chairman of the House Energy and Commerce committee, Democratic Congressman John Dingell of Michigan, for the FDA's failure to alert the public. Although the FDA had been urged as early as October 1982 to ban or limit the use of sulfites in food, the agency has yet to take any action. Sulfiting agents, the only additives that in the past twenty years actually have been shown to kill people , remain at large.[61]

ADVERTISING AND THE POLITICS OF FOOD

In our economy, how much the consumer needs or desires a product determines, in theory, how well the product will sell and how much money it could make for its manufacturer. So we might conclude that if a product sells well, it fulfills a vital need and therefore is valuable. Wrong. By appealing to the emotions of consumers, advertisers create an imagined need for a product with dubious benefits. In fact, the more ads you see for a product, the less benefits you are likely to derive from it. Truth is never an obstacle in advertising.

The food industry resorts to extensive—and often deceptive—advertising. Soft-drink companies alone spent about $82.4 million in the first quarter of 1985 just on television advertising.[62] According to the McDougalls,"the food industry and associated allies are spending billions of dollars a year to teach us incorrect, profit-oriented concepts of nutrition that have caused illness and suffering for parents and their children worldwide for the past several generations."[63] What we enjoy eating and believe is good for us is often the product of indoctrination, not of correct nutritional information.

Advertisers use several strategies to create appeal for their products. They portray ingestible products—sometimes even real food—in a highly attractive way or in situations that suggest social status, group acceptance, and fun. Coca-Cola executives have learned through careful research that American youth is searching for what is "real." The company pushes the illusion that "Coke is the Real Thing!" in one of the most striking ad campaigns ever. The *real* real thing is never shown: the rotting teeth many of these beautiful kids will soon acquire, just as their parents did one generation ago, courtesy of Coke.

Children are a prime target of advertising, and advertisers play on peer pressure and adult authority to convince them of what their parents should buy. Children identify with role models such as sportsmen, spacemen, he-men, entertainers, cartoon characters, father figures, mother figures, and even the kid next door. They believe the often incorrect information about food these role models offer them. Breakfast foods, the so-called cereals that are 35 to 40 percent sugar, are notorious for being sold in this fashion.[64]

If role models and peer pressure don't work, maybe good old scare tactics will. Or at least that's what the dairy industry seems to think. Their well-planned advertising efforts have convinced many dietitians, doctors, and parents that milk is nature's most perfect food and that a diet lacking generous portions of dairy products will inevitably result in calcium deficiency and poor health. People who do not consume milk and its products worry about calcium deficiency, an illness virtually unknown in the world even though most humans stop consuming all milk products after being weaned. Furthermore, the dairy industry fails to consider that cow milk and infant formula preparations might be one of the causes of the sudden death syndrome that accounts for approximately 20 percent of all deaths in American infants in the first two months of life.

Even after consumers have become aware of the shortcomings of a food product, food companies often do not abandon their efforts at dubious advertising; they just move on to where the pastures are greener. Such is the case with infant formula manufacturers. Infant formulas, when they replace mother's milk rich, in antibodies and other immune promoters, are a risk to the health of babies. Formula feeding has been linked to an increase in infant mortality caused by gastroenteritis and respiratory ailments. When many fearful mothers in the industrialized world returned to breast feeding, infant formula companies launched a very effective campaign to convince mothers in Third World countries to bottle-feed their babies. By 1981, an estimated one million deaths of children under one year of age in developing nations resulted from the diarrhea and malnutrition caused by infant formula prepared with contaminated water.

When the World Health Organization asked infant-formula companies to curtail their excessive advertising practices, only one nation failed to join the other 117 member nations in their request. In voting no, the United States was responding to lobbying pressure from the formula industry.[65] Because I am a financial planner, my interests lie in strong free enterprise and a healthy business environment. I do not for a moment think that big business exists to make a buck by exploiting the masses. But should corporate profits be placed above the health and welfare of people, especially children? The infant-formula controversy shows us that our government often thinks so.

Politics affects much in our lives, and food is no exception. Due partly to our status as the world's largest purveyor of dairy products and to the political clout of dairy states, the federal government has occasionally suppressed information about the possible ill effects of milk and its derivatives. When the Department of Agriculture planned to print a relatively noncontroversial pamphlet—*Food/2*—that recommended the reduction of dietary fats and cholesterol, food lobbyists, including the dairy industry, had little trouble getting the department to abandon publication.[66] The tobacco industry's abuse of political power is probably one of the most obscene cases. The federal government subsidizes tobacco cultivation even though the Surgeon General of the United States cannot find stronger warnings about the dangers of cigarette smoking. For governments worldwide, there are substantial financial incentives against curtailing the growth of the tobacco industry. Since cigarettes and tobacco products are taxable, they provide U.S. federal and state governments with about $6 billion a year.

And in the eyes of the British government smoking is a boon: it reduces life span and therefore cuts down on the cost of old-age benefits.[67] The health and well-being of citizens are not necessarily a government's first concerns.

It was no surprise when in 1985 the government official entrusted with much of our health and well-being, Department of Health and Human Services Secretary Margaret Heckler, was accused by Congress of violating public trust and the law. In 1960 Congress banned all dyes in foods, drugs, and cosmetics that tests showed to cause cancer in humans *or animals.* Congress decided in favor of such a strict prohibition because it thought that dyes, having no medicinal or nutritional use beside their purely aesthetic value, weren't worth even the smallest risk of cancer. Although by the end of 1984 ten coal-tar-based dyes shown to cause cancer were still in the market, six of them seemed to be on their way out. FDA experts had proposed prohibiting all six, and three successive FDA commissioners had advised banning one or more in the group.

Yet in early 1985 Secretary Heckler and the FDA gave in to what some FDA officials and consumer groups called "industry pressures." Secretary Heckler announced that she would allow all six dyes to remain on the market, maybe indefinitely. She argued that Congress hadn't meant to ban dyes shown by tests to be of little risk to humans during normal use, even if they had caused cancer in animals. Heckler wished the law to be interpreted so as to give her department the power to choose which dyes were to be proscribed, a power not written into the law by Congress twenty-five years earlier. Congress said no and censured her, but that did not absolve it of its own responsibility in the controversy. The least Congress could have done was to require labeling for all items containing these dyes so consumers themselves could decide about the risks.[68]

True to form, in that same year the Secretary downplayed the severity of the AIDS epidemic and announced that breakthroughs against the disease were at hand and a successful vaccine was imminent. Whatever AIDS breakthroughs have occurred up to now are certainly not a result of Heckler's lame attempts to support research funding. (Heckler is now *former* Secretary.) Moreover, some of the physicians fighting AIDS in recent years have complained—in private, understandably—that although FDA regulations might prevent some of the inevitable quackery brought on by an epidemic, in the case of AIDS, an illness where most conventional therapies fail, the regulations have also dissuaded many honest physicians from pursuing alternative avenues of treatment. One is forced once again to wonder whose interests the FDA protects—those of the multinationals that seek to monopolize profits from AIDS drugs or those of the public seeking relief and release from the disease.

CHAPTER 9

Making the change

Usually we are not aware of harmful eating habits. Like any other habits or attitudes, lifelong eating habits and attitudes toward food are difficult to change. But learning to eat differently becomes easier if you understand your attitude toward food, allow yourself a supportive environment, learn how to cook while discovering sources of unadulterated whole foods, and, above all, persevere.[a]

First of all, food should provide us with energy and help us maintain a healthy body. It should also look good to the eye, taste good, and give us pleasure. Yet we often use food to ease anxiety and mental pain or as a substitute for unfulfilled emotional needs such as companionship, love, and even sex. When seeking such oral gratification, we tend to eat foods that are harmful, usually sweets and oily or highly processed foods. Once we learn to fulfill our emotional needs in other ways, however, food can assume its proper place in our lives, and we will hardly have time to think about the unwholesome, unhealthy foods we once craved.

I would be the last to suggest that eating changes are easy to make. The way we eat is usually so far from the way we should be eating that just the thought of such a vast change fills us with despair.

The first step in change is to weigh things and decide whether you want to change or not. Is feeling better worth changing what you eat? It is natural to avoid such yes-or-no questions. Face your reluctance and try to make a clear-cut decision. If you make the decision to change, commit yourself to it. In your mind's eye, picture yourself as a strong, loving, worthy, and healthy person who has achieved your goals.

Commitment does not imply rigidity. Don't try to be a stickler for compliance, or you may end up copping out because you can't make it all the time. Rigidity implies dogma, and dogma closes our lives to new information that provides potential for growth and transformation. Remember that the smallest beneficial change takes you one step closer to wellness. Life is a process of learning and changing through such small steps.

All this sounds fine, but what do you do when you crave a particular food and can think of nothing else? If you've eaten a piece of cake in five minutes, then all you've had is five minutes of enjoyment. Imagine how long the enjoyment of that food will last. Food gives you pleasure only while you eat. As soon as it's eaten, it no longer does so, although it will cause harm to your body. Force yourself to abstain for five minutes or whatever short time you actually would have enjoyed a food, and soon you will realize that avoidance need not be an awesome chore. You need to be disciplined only a few minutes at a time.

If you give in temporarily, don't put yourself through a guilt trip, and don't punish yourself by saying you can't do it and give up completely. Anxiety and guilt benefit no one. Never question the value of your commitment when it's being tested. Tradeoffs might be necessary. If you absolutely have to eat something, then go ahead. Rather than battle natural urges, think about why you crave a particular food and eat a small amount of it occasionally until the craving subsides.

Another strategy when strict adherence becomes too difficult is to establish "Junk Food Day." Stick to your commitment for six full days and then eat whatever you want on the seventh. It will be reassuring to know you have to be strict only for six days; the seventh day rewards you for your good behavior. Most likely, however, after a few weeks you will find that you don't feel as well on "Junk Food Day"or the day after; this will reinforce good eating habits and diminish your craving for junk food.

Don't try to change everything else in your life at the same time you change your eating patterns. During the first months, recognize that you are trying to break a deeply embedded habit. Be easy on yourself. Baby yourself with other pleasures. Once you start feeling comfortable with your new diet, you can then apply yourself to breaking other habits.

A habit is learned, so it can be unlearned. With gradual change, moving in the right direction is more important than the actual details of the daily struggle. Change should start slowly and build up speed as comfort increases. But it should not be so slow that we remain stuck in old patterns.

In the beginning, try substitution. Sweets are usually the most difficult foods to give up. If you have an ice cream habit, for example, buy brands made with honey or maple sugar rather than cane sugar; then switch after a few weeks to brands that use rice syrup or barley malt. You should find it easier to cut down on ice cream as you change over to a better quality of sugar. Eating red meat may increase your sugar craving, so cut back on it if you are trying to consume less sugar.

Taper off foods gradually. Do not feel daunted by the idea of eliminating certain categories of food from your diet. Once you develop an appreciation for new and better foods, you will find it easier to give up those that are not health-enhancing.

The gradual approach doesn't work for everyone. Making a

slow, smooth transition may not be feasible if you don't have the time; you may need to adopt a strict diet immediately. Other people, especially those whose habit has become a compulsion, find the cold turkey route works better. Old ways and established tastes may linger unless a clean break is made. Whether to slowly slide into or white-knuckle a new diet is a matter you will have to decide for yourself.

It is easier to avoid a food when you don't have it around. If you live by yourself, collect all foods in your home that might threaten your commitment, throw or give them away and start from scratch. Thus, you will make it easier on yourself when the foods you crave are not in the kitchen but a trip to the store away. The corner grocery store rarely offers a cornucopia of healthful foods. Therefore, always keep plenty of food handy so you don't have to run out to buy products that conflict with your commitment. Plan a weekly menu and do not rush your shopping. When I take a trip to a place where I'm not sure proper food or any food will be available, I usually bring my own.

Eliminating harmful foods means changing our lives, and such a realignment of priorities may be upsetting or threatening. Food is not only a matter of nutrition but also one of social custom and tradition. As you exercise your decision to change your diet, you may feel strong social pressures to conform to the dietary status quo. Do not expect everyone to understand. If people question your diet (usually because they know nothing about food), your explanations may be a waste of time. People may think you are weird. Let them.

You also may find you no longer can eat with some of your friends or colleagues because they see no reason to sacrifice and restrict their choice of foods. You will probably feel pulled between the need for friends and the need for health. In some instances, you will have to avoid people altogether if food is the focal point of the occasion. One solution to this dilemma is to make new friends who eat a similar diet. Getting together with them will eliminate the feeling that you are developing your new eating habits alone. Don't alienate yourself. Reach out and get all the support you need. It's much easier to change with the support of others whom you in turn can support. Regular social contact can provide a multitude of benefits.

Learning or relearning how to cook will also make your change easier. Learning how to cook macrobiotically, for example, not only is fun but might even provide you with a new source of friends and social activities. While I do not agree with all macrobiotic philosophy—partly because I sense some dogma in it—I find much of the information helpful. Until you have seen macrobiotic foods prepared and have tasted them, you may not fully appreciate the diet nor have a standard against which to measure your cooking.

I strongly recommend you learn to cook from a qualified macrobiotic instructor. For a copy of the Worldwide Macrobiotic Directory, a list of centers and instructors, send $2 to the *East-West Journal* at the address listed under "Macrobiotics, General" in appendix H.

A short fast is often touted as an effective way to start a new diet. A four- to five-day fast is said to give your body time for withdrawal from certain addictive foods, and besides, a few days with little food will make anything taste good. But fasting is not to be embarked upon lightly, since the toxins the body produces during a fast may cause acute withdrawal symptoms. A fast may also exacerbate the symptoms of a pre-existing condition. You should avoid fasting if you are very ill or bedridden.[b]

Some toxic effects, withdrawal, and worsening of pre-existing symptoms can happen during the change to a simpler diet. Do not panic. These seemingly adverse reactions are part of the healing process, signs that our body systems are regenerating and throwing off the accumulations of a lifetime. If the symptoms seem excessive or too uncomfortable, you can ease the discharging process by modifying your new diet to include foods such as animal products and sugar in small amounts. Avoid the use of over-the-counter medications to relieve symptoms because these products may only add more toxins for the body to eliminate, thereby compounding the problem.

As you get over the difficulties of withdrawal and healing reactions, the transition will become more and more easy. Simple foods will seem strange at first, but before long you will develop a preference for them.

WHERE TO GO

You have probably realized by now that you won't be able to buy most of your food at the typical supermarket. Ideally, it would be best to grow your own food, but this might not be possible for various reasons. Search for alternative markets that sell organic foods.

Start with health-food stores. If most of the store is stacked with vitamins and other food supplements, I would look elsewhere. You want a store that sells whole foods. In San Francisco we are lucky to have several of these stores, such as Rainbow and Real Foods. If you cannot find a nearby store that can supply your needs, you can purchase many nonperishables by mail order. See "Mail- Order Whole-Food Companies" in appendix H for selected addresses. In addition, the Worldwide Macrobiotic Directory offers additional information about whole-food stores in your area and mail-order distributors.

* * *

A further note on organic foods: Even though the word organic is defined by law only in three states, California, Oregon, and Maine, there is a good chance you are getting what you expect—a product grown without the use of synthetic pesticides, insecticides, and fertilizers—when you buy something labeled organic. According to an expert buyer for the New England Food Cooperative Organization, 90 to 95 percent of all these claims turn out to be legitimate when verified. Legitimate organic growers and packers offer a product that is more healthful than the usual crop, and they are highly preoccupied with care and quality.[1]

Unfortunately, there are warnings that people with AIDS should stay away from organic foods because they may have been fertilized with human or animal waste that contains disease-causing bacteria. Nothing could be further from the truth. U.S. environmental pollution laws prohibit the use of raw human sewage (night soil) in agriculture. Sludge from sewage is produced using several methods that kill pathogenic bacteria and is then subjected to high heat that renders it safe for commercial and agricultural use. Animal manures yield better results when cured than when fresh.[2]

Moreover, the goal of organic farming is to build the richness of the soil so as to preclude commercial fertilizers and harmful pesticides. Organic fertilizers, manure being only one of many, are usually applied well before planting and not right before harvest time as commercial ones are. The beneficial bacteria in the soil thus have enough time to take care of any harmful bacteria that might have slipped through in the curing process. I would worry more about the pesticide-laden produce in the supermarket than about the organic lettuce you buy.

CHAPTER 10

Living with food

MACROBIOTICS

The word *macrobiotics* comes from the Greek *makrobiosis*, or "longevity," *makros*, meaning "long," and *biosis*, "a way of life." Accordingly, macrobiotics is not just another diet but a way of life that seeks to promote longevity through a philosophy of balancing foods according to our environment and bodily condition. Macrobiotics holds that balanced nutrition brings health to the body and hence to the mind, assuaging mental extremes such as fear, hate, and envy.

Although echoes of this philosophy are heard as far back as Hippocrates ("Let thy food be thy medicine"), macrobiotics focuses more on Far Eastern (specifically Japanese) thought. This Oriental background can become a stumbling block to the macrobiotic newcomer in the Western world. While many macrobiotic practices are supported by dietary findings, a few seem to be based only on Oriental yin-yang philosophy. Thus, to understand these practices we need to understand yin and yang thoroughly, which means trying to think in a very different way from that to which we are accustomed in the West. Since most of us never achieve this new way of looking at things, we either abandon macrobiotics altogether or accept it without understanding, turning it into one more of the dogmatic Orientalist cults that exist only in the West.

Out of this blind Orientalism, much standard macrobiotic fare in the U.S. ignores the macrobiotic principles of geographic appropriateness of food and, whether in California or Massachusetts, offers basically a traditional Japanese peasant meal. For many of us, this kind of diet can be too high in whole grains and too low in fats and animal protein. Rather than adopting a diet foreign to our environments and needs, we have to re-evaluate our food and create a balanced way of eating in tune with ourselves and our surroundings.

Moreover, in the cultist approach to macrobiotics, food can become *too* important and drive us away from the balance of health sought by macrobiotic philosophy. How can you achieve health by worrying constantly about tomatoes or potatoes? Although food is the one key to health that we can most readily use, it isn't the only key to healing the sick in body and spirit. The role of proper foods, lovingly prepared and lovingly eaten, is to give added life to our bodies so that our minds may have the extra time to unlock other doors to health. Macrobiotics lies in this way of thinking and not in any one kind of food.

The macrobiotic diet is not specific; it will vary according to the individual. In striving to restore or maintain balance, macrobiotics takes into account geography, climate, age, lifestyles (sedentary or active), and personal needs. It seeks to restore the proper relationship between the individual and the environment that provides sustenance. "Everything in this planet is macrobiotic," says San Francisco macrobiotic cook and Kushi Institute graduate Susan Broad Stokes. "It's how you combine it, when you take it and how much. Quantity can change the quality of everything. Variety is very important."[1] More specifically, a macrobiotic diet for the tropics or the temperate zones is usually pesco-vegetarian. It includes plant foods, occasional fish, and limited poultry but excludes milk, eggs, and meat. Not all pesco-vegetarian diets are necessarily macrobiotic, however, since they might include processed and chemicalized foods shunned by macrobiotics.

Macrobiotics allows us a look at what our preindustrial ancestors ate for thousands of years. What was this diet like? Human anatomy provides several clues. Each of us has thirty-two teeth: twenty molars and premolars, eight incisors, and four canines. The molars and premolars are best suited for grinding hard foods such as grains and seeds, the incisors for cutting or biting softer foods like vegetables and fruits, and the canine teeth for tearing flesh. The grinding-cutting-tearing ratio of 5:2:1 suggests an evolutionary trend toward a diet of five parts grain to two parts vegetables to one part flesh.

Other components of the digestive system offer further insight. For instance, human saliva contains the enzyme amylase, which digests complex carbohydrates exclusively. But the saliva of carnivorous animals lacks this enzyme. Additionally, our intestines are long like those of herbivores, allowing for the lengthy digestion period needed for plant foods. The short intestines of carnivores, on the other hand, rapidly digest flesh and excrete the waste, reducing or eliminating putrefaction in the intestines. (By the same token, the possibility of putrefaction is enhanced by our much longer digestive tracts.) Finally, the human liver does not possess the capacity of the carnivore liver to eliminate large amounts of cholesterol. Because of this inability, excess cholesterol from animal products (the only source of cholesterol) will deposit in the arteries, causing several cholesterol-related diseases. These facts, though not conclusive, point toward early human adaptation to a primarily vegetarian diet. Anthropological evidence both from present-day hunter-gatherer societies and preserved sites of early human habitation indicates that most humans, although omnivores, favor a diet consisting primarily of plant foods and the occasional animal protein. Macrobiotics offers precisely such a diet.

Many people mistakenly believe that vegetarian or quasi-vegetarian diets are deficient in protein, vitamin B_{12}, and several minerals. On the contrary, a properly formulated vegetarian diet offers all necessary nutrients. Properly planned and prepared macrobiotic foods are even better. The macrobiotic diet has been judged nutritionally adequate by a U.S. House subcommittee chaired by Congressman Claude Pepper. Macrobiotics has advocates even in the medical profession. For over two years the Lemuel Shattuck Hospital in Boston has offered macrobiotic meals to its doctors and staff.[2]

The goals of macrobiotics are the same as those established in 1977 by the Senate Select Committee on Nutrition and Human Needs: to increase consumption of complex carbohydrates and to reduce refined or processed sugar intake as well as overall fat, saturated fat, and cholesterol consumption. A macrobiotic diet can accomplish all of these goals in a pleasant, tasty, and, above all, emotionally satisfying way.

COOKING

Macrobiotic cooking is a judicious balancing of selected nutrients to produce nourishment as well as pleasure; it is the loving art of creating life. Blandness, however, is not one of its requisites. Macrobiotic food need not be tasteless and monastic but rather should delight your eyes and satisfy your taste buds.

Like all cooking, macrobiotic cooking is very simple once basic techniques are mastered. Developing these requires time, discipline, social support, and, most important, proper instruction. Cooking classes at a local macrobiotic center are essential for learning how the foods should look, taste, and be prepared. Once you have mastered basic techniques, you can develop variations to suit your cooking style. Macrobiotic techniques can be adapted to any cooking style, from plain American home cooking to nouvelle cuisine.

As a general rule, ingredients should come from your surrounding area and be suited to your environment. For example, an Eskimo eats plenty of animal flesh to provide fat for warmth, whereas a person living in the tropics eats plenty of fruits and vegetables to provide water lost in perspiration. Those of us in the temperate zones need an in-between diet centered on grains for calories and vegetables for water and bulk.

If you are not used to cooking, working with fresh, unprocessed ingredients will at first seem too time consuming. The first few wholesome dinners I served seemed to take hours to prepare. I was overwhelmed by the required orchestration. But once I learned how to see, smell, and feel the ingredients making their way to my dinner plate, all effort became natural and easy. And the reward of a healthful diet was worth the adjustment.

There are other rewards as well. Cooking is a discipline, and when properly practiced it can help relieve the stresses and ill feelings of daily life. Strive toward peace and serenity while cooking your meals. The best cooks agree that the most important cooking ingredient is love.

Preparing your ingredients in advance is essential. Always clean them carefully. Wash vegetables briefly but thoroughly; letting them soak might leach away water-soluble B vitamins and vitamin C.[a] Before you wash grains, remove stones and foreign particles.

Use the least energy necessary for cooking. Avoid cooking over high heat except to bring things initially to a boil. High-temperature cooking can make proteins indigestible; low-heat cooking, on the other hand, increases the digestibility of all foods. Cooking methods you should use regularly are boiling, steaming, sautéing and stir-frying in water, and pressure cooking. Try sautéing or stir-frying in oil and baking occasionally. Stir-frying in oil coats food particles and slows the body's absorption rate, thus increasing tolerance in those people with food sensitivities.[3] Always avoid deep-frying and broiling because they can create carcinogens.

I recommend you buy a pressure cooker, something like the Italian hinge-on-the-lid kind, the Æternum, which seems to be safer, easier to use, and more durable than others. I use my pressure cooker mostly for cooking organic brown rice and garbanzos.

Sautéing in a small amount of water is my favorite way to cook. One of the first dishes I learned at my local macrobiotic center was carrots with leeks and tamari. Wash two medium carrots and one leek and slice them into diagonal pieces no more than a quarter inch thick. Fill a stainless steel pan or a cast-iron skillet one-fourth full of water and place on high heat. When the water boils, add the carrots, lower the heat, cover, and let simmer for ten minutes. Stir the carrots, add the leeks, and let simmer another five minutes. Add one tablespoon of tamari, stir again, and simmer another four minutes. Serve warm. It serves two.

Don't worry if you put in too much or too little water, use too high or too low a flame, or add too much or too little tamari. With time, even those for whom cooking has been a mystery can master certain techniques. Cookbooks are very useful. I especially recommend *The Book of Whole Meals* by Annemarie Colbin, *Introducing Macrobiotic Cooking* by Wendy Esko, and *The Whole World Cookbook* by the editors of the *East-West Journal*. Let me add that if even I have learned to cook for myself, then almost anyone else can as well.

THE RAW VERSUS THE COOKED

A common question is how should one eat food—raw or cooked? I believe in a judicious mixture of both. Meat and animal products should be thoroughly cooked. Grains should be sprouted or cooked. Vegetables should be eaten raw or lightly cooked. Carrots (perhaps as juice), onions, and mature greens are particularly beneficial when eaten raw.

Sometimes cooked food is better. Many foods contain anti-nutrients such as oxalic and phytic acids, substances that interfere with the proper functioning of vitamins and minerals and protein digestion. Cooking usually destroys these substances.

In addition, cooking increases the digestibility of some proteins and increases their biological value. Cooking ruptures the walls of starch cells, allowing digestive enzymes ready access while making vitamins and minerals available to your body. In other words, cooked food is easier to digest.

The most important reason food should be cooked is to kill any parasites or fungi. The yeastlike fungus *Candida albicans* and the protozoan parasite *Toxoplasma gondii,* the cause of common opportunistic AIDS infection, are food-borne pathogens.

Cooking food briefly on a low flame is preferable. Low heat makes protein more digestible by breaking the links that hold it together. Excessive heat, on the other hand, creates additional linkages that our enzymes cannot break down, thus making some amino acids unavailable to our bodies. Certain common breakfast cereals processed at high temperatures are subject to such losses. Excessive heat also promotes the formation of carcinogenic substances.

It is advantageous to eat some foods raw. All seeds and nuts and the mature greens of fresh vegetables contain abscisic acid. This acid, also called dormin when it acts as a plant hormone, may inhibit tumor growth. Unfortunately, abscisic acid is destroyed at 275° F, but pears, apples, strawberries, fruit blossoms, mature leafy vegetables, tomatoes, onions, spinach, and root vegetables all provide rich raw sources of it.[4]

EATING

Before discussing when, where, and how to eat, it is important to address when not to. You shouldn't eat when rushed, overheated, fatigued, worried, angry, fearful, in pain, or not hungry, or just before heavy physical work. Food consumed at these times will not receive the body's undivided attention and could indeed produce negative results.

Avoid eating when angered or stressed. After sitting down to your meal, collect yourself and put your mind at ease. Be silent, take a few breaths, allow the tensions of the day to vanish. If you wish, give thanks for the sustenance of your food. This is also a good time to congratulate yourself for the efforts that brought food to your table.

The beginning of a meal is a good time to drink a moderate amount of liquids. Drinking during or after a meal tends to dilute the digestive fluids. Avoid ice-cold liquids that can halt the digestive process. Eat your food slowly and chew it well.

Chewing serves several functions. Mechanically, it breaks up food and enables saliva to begin starch digestion. Psychologically, it is relaxing and provides a healthy outlet for aggression. According to some psychologists, chewing channels aggression into its proper biological place (the mouth is the primary tool of aggression in most animals, humans included) and integrates the emotion into one's personality rather than sublimating, exaggerating, or suppressing it.[5]

There should be no distractions during your meal. Avoid TV or emotionally charged conversations that prevent you from being aware of what and how you eat. I usually eat dinner while gazing out my dining room window at the San Francisco skyline illuminated against the background of the distant Berkeley and Oakland hills. I feel naturally connected to and at peace with everything and everyone. Despite what many San Franciscans will tell you, however, you don't have to move to this beautiful city to enjoy a tranquil meal. Your own city, the countryside, a small garden, a tree, a fireplace, anything that's restful to you will do. Most important is your own placid state of mind.

Just one meal all day long won't do either. Eat two to four properly spaced meals a day, as many as you can comfortably fit in. Spacing your meals allows the digestive system a rest. If you must eat between meals, snack on foods that will not interfere with your next meal, such as sunflower seeds or, if you have no candida problems, carrot juice, apples, or pears. Do not eat within two hours of bedtime so your body can use its resting period to work on healing rather than digesting. Leave the table satisfied but not full. We often eat too much food to satiate feelings of emptiness and loneliness. Let other sources fill your emotional needs.

In developing new ways, do not turn eating into a religion. Always allow yourself the ability to change, love, and grow.

COMBINING FOODS

The human digestive tract was not designed to accommodate complex meals. Efficient digestion occurs only when we eat simply and moderately. Inefficient digestion does not allow your body to take full advantage of a meal and, besides causing flatulence, abdominal pains, and even food sensitivities, causes inadequate nutrition. Proper food combinations and timing of meals are therefore especially important if you are sick. Compatible food combinations and well-timed meals will allow your digestive tract to perform maximally and deliver the true bounty of food to your body. But don't ever force yourself to eat. If you are in pain or are not hungry, it's better not to eat at all.

A well-balanced meal does not necessarily consist of a combination

TABLE 24 Improper food combinations

ACID AND STARCH

Acids destroy the salivary enzyme that digests starch.

PROTEIN AND STARCH

Starches undergo fermentation in the stomach while awaiting the digestion of the protein.

PROTEIN AND PROTEIN

It is best to consume only one type of protein at a meal. This does not exclude eating two or more kinds of nuts or seeds at a meal.

ACID AND PROTEIN

Acids inhibit gastric juice production. (Exception: Protein foods such as nuts and seeds can be eaten with acid foods.)

FAT AND PROTEINS

Fats inhibit the flow of gastric juices. Fat in-take should be limited.

SUGAR AND PROTEIN

Like starches, sugars are held up and ferment in the stomach while proteins are being digested.

SUGAR AND STARCH

Starches could stay longer in the stomach than sugars, allowing the latter to ferment.

Source: Herbert M. Shelton. *Food Combining Made Easy.* Willow Publishing, San Antonio, Texas, 1982.

TABLE 25 Low- or non-starch vegetables

(Can be eaten with either starches or proteins)

Alfalfa sprouts
Asparagus
Beans, green
Bok choy
Broccoli
Brussels sprouts
Cabbage
Cauliflower
Celery
Chinese cabbage
Collards
Corn, sweet
Cucumber
Eggplant
Endive
Escarole
Garlic
Kale
Kohlrabi
Lettuce
Mushrooms
Okra
Onion
Parsley
Peas, green
Pepper, sweet
Radish
Sorrel
Spinach
Squash, summer
Swiss chard
Turnips

Source: Herbert M. Shelton, *Food Combining Made Easy.*

of the four food groups in the dietician's litany. A meal of steak, french fries, lettuce, fruit, and ice cream for lunch or dinner most likely will assure you an unpleasant afternoon or evening. Let me explain. Steak, a protein food, needs about four hours in the highly acid medium of your stomach to be properly digested. Sugars (white sugar, sweet fruits, syrups, etc.), on the other hand, undergo digestion in the intestines rather than in the stomach. The sugar in your meal will sit with the steak in the stomach for several hours and ferment. Result: gas and heartburn. When eaten alone, sugars are moved relatively quickly to the intestines to be digested.

But most whole foods, you may be thinking, are a combination of proteins, sugars or starches, and fat. Grains are one such example. The body possesses the ability, however, to adapt its secretions to particular foods. It's only when we eat two or more dissimilar foods that the body's various digestive juices get confused and cannot function as well. Keep meals simple. Give yourself plenty of time between meals. Meals spaced too closely will have the same effect as improper food combinations. Allow at least four hours after a high protein meal, two hours after one of carbohydrate, and one hour after one of fruit.

The energy spent digesting daily meals is equivalent to at least four hours of work. Eating simple meals will lessen the burden of digestion and give us more energy for warding off disease and repairing its ravages.

For more information on combining food, I recommend *Food Combining Made Easy* by Herbert M. Shelton. Dennis Nelson's *Food Combining Simplified* can also be helpful.

CHAPTER 11

My diet

The overall goal of my diet is simple: to avoid or limit those foods that may tax my immune system and thus worsen the quality of my life. I have found that to accomplish these goals I don't need to constantly remember the dangers or benefits of every single food I eat, but only to keep in mind certain broad categories of foods that may be injurious.

These are the main things I watch for:

- Simple sugars in fruits and many refined products can lower the effectiveness of lymphocytes against pathogens.
- The fats in meats and animal products may promote the spread of HIV infection and worsen underlying immunodeficiency. Cholesterol in particular can make cell membranes more rigid and, therefore, more susceptible to HIV attack. Monounsaturated fats and high-density lipoproteins such as those found in olive oil and deep-sea fish may help keep cholesterol levels down.
- Certain vegetables and foods contain natural toxins or carcinogenic substances that tax the immune system.

- Most meats and animal products contain hormones, antibiotics, and pesticides that may likewise suppress immunity.
- A few foods can harbor disease-causing fungi or bacteria that may present a grave risk to anyone whose immunity is compromised.
- If candida is present, one also should avoid all those foods that could provide ideal growing conditions for this yeastlike fungus (these are summarized in chapter 12, "Detoxifying the Body: Offenders").

Let me illustrate these various dietary points by describing my diet, which I must emphasize suits only my needs and should not be imitated. There is no single diet that is right for everyone because each of us is biologically unique. As you get more in touch with your body, you will find out what your specific needs are and should adjust your diet accordingly. If you are gravely ill, you should follow a diet more restricted than mine; if you are healthy, on the other hand, you will have greater freedom than I do.

Over a few months my total diet is made up of about 35 percent whole grains, 30 percent vegetables, 10 percent beans, 10 percent fish and seafood, 5 percent refined carbohydrates, 4 percent sea vegetables, and 2 percent each of fruits, nuts and seeds, and meat and animal products.

The most important foods in my diet are cooked whole grains—mostly rice and oats. Rice provides calories and bulk, and oats supply the water-soluble fiber that helps lower blood cholesterol. To provide variety, I try to rotate these grains with millet, wheat berries, rye, barley, buckwheat, and quinoa, a quick-cooking South American grain. Besides those vegetables that are currently in season, I eat lots of winter squash, carrots, onions, and broccoli. My veggies are usually unprocessed except for the carrot juice I drink almost every day. No one food contains all necessary nutrients in adequate amounts, so it is important to eat a variety.

Meat is infrequent in my diet. If I eat in homes where my well-intentioned but uninformed hosts serve meat, I usually eat it. Some foods are acceptable if prepared with love. Mind you, I do not often get myself into this type of situation. At home I have organic chicken three or four times a month and organic beef once.

Animal products such as eggs and dairy products are unusual in my diet. I sometimes eat one or two eggs a month. I love pizza, however, and in eating it I allow cheese in my diet two or three times a month. I consume almost no milk or yogurt, but may allow myself an occasional butter croissant or buttered bagel. I limit my consumption of these animal products for health reasons, not out of religious conviction.

My refined carbohydrate intake is mainly bread and noodles. About once a month I will have a fruit pie or cookies sweetened with fruit juices. Sometimes after eating these sweets I feel the effect of the unusual amount of sugar, but they are a special treat I still give myself occasionally. Many macrobiotic advocates think we shouldn't eat bread. But I find properly prepared whole-grain bread to be an important source of complex carbohydrates and fiber in my diet and have some almost every day as part of a meal. (Even some of the naturally leavened breads, however, can exacerbate candida symptoms in a few people. Limit your bread consumption if you find this to be the case. Avoid all yeasted breads if you have candida.)

Refined sugars (sucrose), as well as honey and maple sugar, are rare in my diet. So are preservatives, coloring agents, and other food additives. I consume less than two dozen canned products a year and rarely prepare any frozen vegetables, which may have lost essential nutrients and flavor during the freezing process. I go through several jars of both apple butter and sesame salt condiment yearly. Besides loving pizza, I am extremely fond of chips and crunchy things, so I have a few corn chips or rice crackers three or four times a week. I am fully aware, however, that I may react negatively to fried foods such as the corn chips, and I eat them this frequently only when my health is good.

Because of its sugar content, fruit isn't big in my diet. I have about two fruit servings a week. I enjoy bananas and have one or two every month, and I use apple butter once in a while on bread.

A random daily menu might include the following:

BREAKFAST

Whole oats
Miso soup

LUNCH

Fish (a B12 source)
Broccoli, quickly boiled
(Breakfast or lunch is my high protein meal because protein digestion too late in the day can use up the energy the body needs for its nightly healing chores).

DINNER

Sautéed carrots and leeks
Kale, quickly boiled
Pressure-cooked brown rice

Appendix G provides a sample cleansing diet prepared by physiotherapist and macrobiotic consultant Ellen Lipsius of Toronto, Canada. This diet may serve as a preliminary guideline from which to develop a more elaborate, general diet.

Whenever I feel well, I go out to dinner two or three times a week at a local vegetarian Chinese restaurant with friends who support my self-imposed dietary restrictions. The restaurant tends to use too much oil—cottonseed, at that—but the food is excellent and otherwise follows much of my dietary regime. Although too much oil sometimes seems to lower my resistance, this seldom happens when I listen to what my body tells me. I know what I can get away with when I'm in good health.

An open macrobiotic diet that truly establishes a food balance suited to my individual needs has helped me achieve my dietary goals. Since I have followed this diet, I've had fewer colds, stomach problems, and upper respiratory and throat complaints and less fear of illness and of life in general. My health is now good enough that I can cope with excess oil, pizza, chips, cookies, and yeast bread. When I feel my health slumping, I avoid the treats and the restaurants.

But in following my diet I have to constantly remind myself that I avoid or limit certain foods to improve the quality of my life. Any diet that imposes limits greater than the benefits it provides defeats my purpose. I cannot organize the rest of my life around daikon radishes, Brussels sprouts, or tofu. I cannot allow the guilt of eating a tomato or a buttered bagel to govern me. Too strict and too long a diet may erode the quality of my life. I have seen many macrobiotic eaters turn food into an obsession, as if each morsel were some sort of miracle drug on which their lives depended. These people have failed to realize that healing comes from within. Their attitude defeats macrobiotics, whose purpose is not to cure but to re-establish a physical and mental balance in which the equilibrium of health can take place.

Getting in touch with your body allows you to determine what is best for you. Once you are tuned in to your body, you can choose foods while remaining fully aware of your part in the consequences. Self-awareness is often the biggest stumbling block on the road to recovery. It is indeed difficult to accept that the reins might, after all, be in one's own hands.

Part three: Healing the body

CHAPTER 12

Detoxifying the body: offenders

Nourishment comes not only from our food but also from how we digest and assimilate it. Improper diet, a sedentary lifestyle, polluted air, and everyday stress favor the production and accumulation of toxins in our bodies. Most of us end up with an internal toxic waste dump that interferes with metabolism. The immune system has to expend energy to clean up these unnecessary wastes. That energy, already at a premium because a poisoned body cannot draw full nourishment from food, would be better spent against disease. Detoxification can make your passage to better health a quicker and less traumatic experience.

The first step toward detoxification is to cleanse our bodies of accumulated food wastes, environmental toxins, and dangerous intestinal parasites. For many of us, the place to start is the gastrointestinal tract. An improperly functioning bowel prevents the efficient assimilation of food. Once the bowel is cleansed, however, less energy is spent on digestion, more energy is extracted from the same amount of food, and thus more energy is available for fighting disease and for healing. How much cleansing is needed depends on the state of your bowels and the nature of your bowel movements.

Natural as it may be, defecation is not a pretty subject. There is no way, however, to avoid it on the road to a healthier life.

Do you have one or two daily bowel movements? Do you void all your feces easily within seconds after sitting on the toilet? Are your feces firm as they pass out, and do they then crumble somewhat in the water? Do you rarely have intestinal cramps or diarrhea? Do you have infrequent and odorless intestinal gas? Are your feces clear of blood and mucus?

If you answered yes to all these questions, then there's a good chance your gastrointestinal tract is in good shape. If you answered no to some or all, then there's probably something amiss either in your food or somewhere between your mouth and rectum.

One common cause of bowel disturbances is intestinal parasites. Native mostly to the tropics, these pests have spread through the gay population by sexual transmission.

Through eons of evolution, parasites have become experts at foiling the efforts of the human immune system and may be a cofactor in the development of AIDS. Perhaps it is no coincidence that parasitic infection is so common in world communities where AIDS has spread into all segments of the population—central and eastern Africa, Haiti, and Belle Glade, Florida.[a,1] For people with AIDS, intestinal parasites may either cause fatal opportunistic infections or open the way to other pathogens that may do so. Therefore, prompt and safe treatment of these parasites could enhance prognosis.[2]

In addition to dealing with intestinal parasites and bowel cleansing, this section discusses other parasites that play a role in AIDS and explains the complications of candida and certain viral infections. It ends with a discussion of several general body detoxification methods, including exercise, saunas, and hot baths.

PARASITES

Intestinal parasites and yeastlike molds challenge our immune systems day in and day out. A healthy immune system usually meets this challenge, but when immunity is compromised, as in AIDS, the immune system is further weakened by parasitic attack. Indeed, some of these parasites, acting as cofactors, may open the door to the HIV infection that brings about AIDS.

Recent studies at the University of California School of Medicine in San Francisco strongly suggest that the healthy immune systems of most people can handle an HIV attack. Researchers believe there must be a factor or factors already suppressing immunity for HIV infection to occur.[3] Because of their immunosuppressive invasion tactics, the intestinal parasites so widely found among gay men are possible candidates, although it may be that other factors—alcohol or drug abuse, for example—permit HIV infection to proceed and also allow parasites to take a greater toll. Whether parasites come before or after HIV infection, however, they make the job of the virus easier. HIV spreads among helper T cells that are actively fighting disease. Parasites may produce a sizable number of activated helpers T cells that provide fertile ground for the growth of the virus. In addition, parasites may breach the intestinal wall, making it easier for other AIDS opportunistic pathogens to get into the blood.[4] Most parasitic infections should be diagnosed and treated.

The incidence of parasites among gay men in metropolitan areas has increased to epidemic proportions—nearly tenfold since the mid-1970s, just two or three years before the AIDS onslaught.[b] Several studies suggest that around 60 percent of urban homosexual men harbor one or more parasites, most commonly the protozoans *Entamoeba histolytica* and *Giardia lamblia*.[5]

ENTAMOEBA HYSTOLITYCA AND *GIARDIA LAMBLIA*

Entamoeba histolytica brings on serious illness in a small percentage of people; between 85 and 95 percent of those infected will show no symptoms. In those who are symptomatic, intestinal amebiasis is the more common manifestation. Its symptoms include dysentery, characterized by blood or mucus in the stool; colitis, characterized by abdominal pain and flatulence; and lack of appetite, loss of weight, and chronic fatigue. *Giardia lamblia* can produce asymptomatic infection, which disappears spontaneously in most individuals. Spontaneous disappearance, however, seems to depend on T-cell activity; it does not occur in "nude" mice, a special strain of mice that possess no thymus gland to activate T cells, or in children, in whom the thymus is not yet working at full capacity. Symptoms of giardiasis are diarrhea, intestinal gas, lack of appetite, queasy stomach, abdominal cramps, and steatorrhea (light-colored, foul-smelling stool that contains excessive amounts of fats). The infection might cause a malabsorption syndrome that, even after treatment, may result in a persistent intolerance to lactose.[6]

One of the first epidemiological studies of AIDS, conducted by New York and Columbia universities, found a greater incidence not only of sexually transmitted diseases but also of *E. histolytica* and *G. lamblia* among those who developed Kaposi's sarcoma. Seventy percent of those with KS—as opposed to 42 percent of the controls—showed signs of amebiasis;[7] thus, parasitic infection was among the top three risk factors before HIV was discovered. And although recent studies report the strain of *E. histolytica* in many healthy homosexual men to be nonpathogenic—that is, causing no invasive amebiasis or gastrointestinal symptoms[8]—there are other reasons for concern about these protozoa.

Studies show that *E. histolytica* produces one of a class of substances, called lectins, that render the immune systems of laboratory animals unable to fight viruses, fungi, bacteria, and parasites and to destroy cancer cells. One particular lectin, ConA, brings about an increase in the number of suppressor T cells akin to that in the low helper/suppressor T ratio of people with ARC and those with KS who develop no other opportunistic infections.[9] Moreover, the amebic lectin may stimulate helper T cells infected with HIV to undergo mitosis (divide). Mitogenic stimulation of HIV-infected cells causes quicker replication of the virus and leads to quicker cell death. Therefore, by eliminating a major source of mitogenic stimulation, parasite treatment may help prevent further deterioration of immune function in people with AIDS or ARC.[10]

In 1983 Cornell University researcher Jeffrey Laurence isolated from the blood of AIDS patients an immunosuppressive factor whose potency did not diminish even when diluted a thousand times. The factor resembled a "lectin-induced macrophage inhibitor" and was also present in men with the persistent, generalized lymphadenopathy (swollen lymph glands) often seen in ARC. In test tube trials by Dr. Laurence, antioxidants such as vitamins C and E and the amino acid alanine were the only substances that blocked the suppressor factor and allowed immune cells to respond normally.[11]

Diagnostic tests for intestinal parasites are time-consuming and require expert examination under a microscope. A parasitologist from the Tufts University School of Medicine declares that "having watched a seasoned protozoologist examine a properly collected warm stool sample for an hour before finding the elusive *E. histolytica* permanently weakened [my] confidence in the average hospital laboratory to be similarly successful."[12] Understandably, stool specimens are not the most popular items in many laboratories, and are often shunted to the most junior and least experienced technician.

If a parasite is found, it is often misidentified because of confusion with a nonpathogenic species. *Entamoeba coli,* an intestinal protozoan that does not cause disease, can be confused with pathogenic *Entamoeba histolytica.* A person often ends up either being treated needlessly for a nonpathogenic parasite or *not* being treated at all for a pathogenic one. Even respected authorities disagree on whether or not certain species are parasitic. For instance, *E. hartmanni,* a cousin of *E. histolytica,* is believed to be a pathogen by some but not all clinicians.

New experimental techniques involving culturing of suspect amoebas in a special medium and subjecting them to a process called isoenzyme electrophoresis can distinguish between pathogens and nonpathogens. These tests, however, are available to only a few clinicians, and the controversy of whether or not to treat remains at issue.[13]

Freshness of stool samples is crucial for the detection of many protozoans. Even if a combination of techniques are used, a single stool examination will detect only 25 to 50 percent of all *E. histolytica* infections. Up to six examinations are sometimes necessary to achieve a 90 percent certainty. Many parasitologists recommend stools obtained by purging—that is, by using laxatives—when searching for the elusive *E. histolytica.* Because *E. histolytica* dies rapidly when exposed to air, unpreserved liquid or soft samples become worthless unless examined within half an hour of production. Fully formed stool can wait three to four hours but should be refrigerated nonetheless.[14] You should ask the laboratory to provide you with a suitable preservative if you can not bring the samples in within the above time limits.

Some specialists recommend the use of a disposable proctoscope to view the bowel wall and scrape specimens directly from an infected area. "A stool specimen," says AIDS researcher Kevin M. Cahill, "is only a vehicle passing by; amebic organisms do not live in fecal matter, they live in the bowel wall."[15]

Several substances interfere with diagnosis or treatment of parasites. Antibiotics taken up to a month before obtaining a stool sample decrease the chances of protozoan detection. The barium sulfate used for intestinal x-rays interferes with microscopy if taken up to one week prior to sampling. So do compounds containing kaolin (a fine white aluminum silicate clay used in antidiarrheals such as Kaopectate), bismuth salts (one of the active ingredients in Pepto-Bismol), milk of magnesia, antacids, oil laxatives, and sulfonamides (some of the sulfa drugs used to treat PCP, for example). Specimens should be obtained, if possible, before any of these substances are used. Enemas are not advised. Urine in the specimen also prevents detection.[16]

Intestinal amebiasis can be completely cured. Perhaps the most widely used drug against amebic and giardic infections is metronidazole (Flagyl). It is the drug of default when amebiasis has propagated from the intestines to other parts of the body, but it has serious side effects. In a small percentage of people, metronidazole can cause seizures, serious numbness of the extremities, and a reduction of white blood cells. It can promote the growth of candida and produce headaches, loss of appetite, vomiting, diarrhea, constipation, and abdominal cramps.

If parasitic infection is only intestinal, other, less toxic drugs can be used. Paromomycin (Humatin), a broad-spectrum antibiotic, is often used in combination with tetracycline. Paromomycin, however, can promote overgrowth of certain organisms such as fungi and cause toxic damage to the kidneys when seriously ulcerated bowels allow its passage into the blood. Tetracycline can reduce the number of neutrophil and eosinophil white blood cells that are still functional in people with AIDS.

Another drug used against intestinal amebiasis is diiodohydroxyquin, or iodoquinol (Diodoquin, Yodoxin). Iodoquinol can cause serious nerve damage, especially in the optic nerve, and numbness in the extremities.[17] Parasites often develop a resistance that calls for alternating several of these drugs.

One last interesting note on parasites. The usual *turista,* or traveler's diarrhea, is caused not by any of the aforementioned pathogens but by a normally friendly bacterium, *Escherichia coli.* This bacterium is part of the intestinal flora that live in symbiotic relationship with your body. It takes some time for your body and *E. coli* to get used to each other and live in peace. Several regions in the world harbor distinctly different *E. coli* populations; these strains take some getting used to. Pepto-Bismol helps the process along. The problem in travelling to certain countries—Mexico, India, and parts of Africa and the Orient, for example—is not getting *turista,* however, but rather contracting serious amebic or bacterial dysentery from contaminated food. Keep this in mind if you travel.

PNEUMOCYSTIS, TOXOPLASMA, CRYPTOSPORIDIUM, AND *CRYPTOCOCCUS*

Immune suppression may result from an interaction between parasites such as *Entamoeba histolytica* and other factors such as alcohol, drugs, poor nutrition, and acute stress, opening the way for HIV and subsequent opportunistic organisms. Protozoa like *Pneumocystis carinii, Toxoplasma gondii,* and Cryptosporidia and fungi like *Cryptococcus neoformans* are parasites that proliferate only in immunocompromised hosts. All of us familiar with AIDS have heard of *Pneumocystis carinii,* the airborne organism that produces the pneumonia that is the greatest killer in AIDS. But only a few of us are aware of *Toxoplasma gondii,* a protozoan found in many vertebrate hosts, especially domestic cats and other felines.[c] *T. gondii* can also be found in improperly cooked meat—often in fast-food places.

Toxoplasmosis is usually benign. In fact, most adults and children show only generalized symptoms, if any at all. When symptoms do occur, they may resemble those of infectious mononucleosis: chills, fever, headache, muscle pain, inflammation of the lymph nodes, and extreme fatigue.[18] In AIDS, toxoplasmosis can spread through the body and severely affect the lymph nodes, brain, and eyes; it is one of the most common causes of encephalitis—inflammation of the brain—and can be fatal. If discovered promptly, the infection can be treated with a combination of a sulfa and an antimalarial drug, but such treatment usually needs to be continued indefinitely since it doesn't actually kill the parasite.

Cryptosporidia protozoans cause an AIDS opportunistic infection for which there is no current treatment. Found in humans, puppies, kittens, and many farm animals, these parasites are sometimes responsible for brief and benign diarrheal episodes in veterinarians and other animal handlers but has not been otherwise associated with human disease until recently. In immunocompromised people, cryptosporidiasis causes severe, chronic diarrhea that leads to malabsorption and emaciation. Eventually, even intravenous feeding will not provide adequate nutrition or maintain fluid balance. In addition, Cryptosporidia—as well as *Toxoplasma*— can cause pneumonia. Several drugs are said to hold promise against these deadly parasites.

Cryptococcus neoformans is a ubiquitous yeastlike fungus that flourishes in pigeon droppings, roosts, and nests. A rare disease in the U.S. before AIDS, cryptococcal fungemia causes tumorlike lesions in the lungs and can spread to the spinal cord and brain, where it results in meningitis or encephalitis. Cryptococcosis is treated in normal patients through an extended course of toxic drugs that commonly cause permanent brain damage. In AIDS, such treatments have not been effective to date.[19, 20, 21, 22]

Parasitic infections account for most AIDS deaths. This fact surprised many American physicians who, until AIDS came along, thought that parasitic infections were exotic diseases found only in countries where poverty and unsanitary conditions abound. "The majority of American medical schools," says Dr. Cahill, "offer no instruction in clinical parasitology. Few physicians in the United States have had any experience in the diagnosis and management of these ailments."[23] If you have AIDS or ARC, make sure your primary-care physician has more than textbook knowledge about parasites.

CANDIDA

Candida albicans, formerly called *Monilia,* is a yeastlike fungus that lives in the human alimentary tract or the vagina. Candida (pronounced with the stress on the first syllable) usually does not produce chronic infection in normal individuals but causes one of the most common opportunistic infections in people with AIDS.

More than 20 percent of AIDS cases reported by 1983 to the Center for Disease Control (CDC) showed signs of candida infection, most commonly in the mouth and esophagus.[24] A breakdown of the equilibrium that normally exists between the fungus and the immune system, candidiasis, or thrush—cheesy white patches in the mucous membranes of the mouth—is sometimes seen in adults after treatment with broad-spectrum antibiotics and in young children.

The mere appearance of thrush in an at-risk individual who is under no medication does not constitute a sign of AIDS. The CDC considers candidiasis indicative of AIDS only when it shows up in the esophagus, and then only if other AIDS criteria are met, such as positive antibody tests or viral cultures for HIV, a low number of helper T cells, and a low ratio of helper T to suppressor T cells.[25] Nonetheless, thrush in an at-risk individual may be a danger signal indicating an immune deficiency that, though not necessarily conducive to AIDS, should be monitored.

Unchecked, candida becomes a parasite,[d] and as such its relationship to AIDS is complex. Besides being an opportunistic organism that flourishes in a weakened immune system, candida might also be a cofactor in weakening immunity further. Similar to some other infections, candidiasis by itself can impair immune function as AIDS does—reducing the number of T cells and the helper/suppressor T ratio and also producing food and chemical sensitivities.[26]

Under certain conditions, candida can produce rootlike structures called hyphae that penetrate the mucosa of the intestinal tract and break down its boundary with the circulatory system. Thus, the harmful result of candidiasis is like that of other parasitic infections: a breakdown of the intestinal wall that allows incompletely digested food and toxic substances to enter the blood and exert a powerful assault on the immune system.[27] White blood cells then attack the half-digested foods and toxic substances and sustain damage in the attempt, releasing immunoglobulins and more toxins into the blood.[28] This mechanism may explain the interrelationship parasitic infections such as candida have with immunological dysfunction and food and chemical sensitivities.

Candida is a normal inhabitant of the intestinal tract and is kept in check by both a healthy intestinal flora and a functioning immune system. When these controls are missing, candida can flourish. A diet consisting of lots of sugar and refined carbohydrates reduces beneficial flora and white-cell function and nourishes candida, thus promoting its growth. Broad-spectrum antibiotics, in addition to killing friendly intestinal bacteria, reduce the number of lymphocytes that keep candida's rootlike structures in check. Cortisone-type drugs, birth control pills, chemotherapy, acute distress, and several illnesses have similar negative effects.

It is important to distinguish between superficial and systemic candidiasis. Candida infection is called superficial when it occurs on the skin, nails, mouth, tongue, and esophagus. Experimental data suggest that such infection is kept at bay mainly by macrophages and helper T lymphocytes. Systemic candidiasis occurs when the infection disseminates into deep-seated tissues such as the kidneys, lungs, and heart. The main controls against disseminated candida seem to be the neutrophils that account for residual immunity in people with AIDS. It is not surprising, then, that although superficial candidiasis is common in AIDS, systemic candida infection is not, unless it is brought about by the administration of immunosuppressive drugs and therapy or of antibiotics via a catheter inserted in a blood vessel. Systemic candidiasis is likely to be fatal in people with AIDS.[29]

Candidiasis is easy to diagnose when thrush coats the tongue and spots the gums and mouth or when the fungus covers nails and skin. But candidiasis can also present nonphysical symptoms that might be ascribed to "nerves": insomnia or excessive sleepiness; loss of memory, concentration, and self-confidence; and uncontrollable crying, irritability, anxiety, and lethargy. Other symptoms are so generalized they might be attributed to other illnesses. These include dry, scaly skin with or without acne, a metallic taste in the mouth, dizziness, blurred vision, night blindness, headaches; all the familiar manifestations of allergy, such as nasal and sinus inflammation, sneezing, stuffiness, and postnasal drip; increasing sensitivity to certain foods and chemicals; and heartburn, intestinal growling and bloatedness, painful constipation, urgent and frequent urination, urethritis, jock itch, rectal itching, and mucus or blood in the stool. A frequent symptom of candida is an overbearing craving for sugar, carbohydrate-rich foods, or alcohol.

With such a litany of symptoms, the lack of a simple diagnostic test for chronic candida infection does not seem surprising. Unfortunately, no smear or culture test can differentiate between the benign and pathogenic phases of the fungus. Such a distinction does not show under the microscope, because diagnosis depends on the extent to which the organism spreads throughout the body and not on its appearance. Diagnosis of chronic candidiasis can often be accomplished, however, after an invasive procedure such as a biopsy or an examination with an endoscope.

Treatment should follow diagnosis or strong suspicion of chronic candida infection by your physician. There is a greater chance of minimizing or even eliminating the chances of full-blown AIDS if candida infection is treated promptly. If candidiasis is left unchecked and AIDS ensues, the infection might prove intractable or, at best, very difficult to treat. Therefore, the goal of treatment should be to reduce the amount of fungus to the lowest possible level and to enhance the factors that check its proliferation in the intestines.

Treatment of chronic candidiasis should consist of seven steps: following certain dietary restrictions and recommendations, avoiding antibiotics, avoiding cortisonelike and immunosuppressive drugs, avoiding distress, taking anticandida medications, being vaccinated or desensitized against the fungus, and making certain environmental changes. These measures reduce the overall load on the immune system and thus help recovery. It is very important to take all these measures under the direction and supervision of a physician who uses a holistic approach rather than merely drugs in treating candida.

The first step toward recovery is to eliminate certain foods from your diet. Start with sugar. Candida has a voracious appetite for simple sugars such as beet, cane, and maple sugars, corn syrup, fructose, and honey, all of which promote candida growth. As agents of fermentation, yeasts and yeastlike fungi cannot survive on proteins and fat, but they do thrive on refined carbohydrates. Limiting consumption of simple sugars and refined carbohydrates thus deprives candida of its preferential food and slows the rate at which it multiplies.

Avoid eating fruits if you have chronic candida infection. According to experts, fruits and sugars promote yeast growth; vegetables and whole grains do not. Because vegetables and whole grains are slowly digested, they don't seem to release enough simple and double sugars at one time to allow candida to ferment. For some people, however, gluten-rich whole grains, such as barley, oats, rye, and wheat, may trigger candida growth. In such cases physicians recommend low-carbohydrate diets to fight candida. But be careful not to give up complex carbohydrates completely. At least 200 to 400 of your daily calories should come from carbohydrates, to offset the undesirable effects of protein and fat utilization. A diet rich in complex carbohydrates is generally beneficial. You must therefore find out, often by trial and error, how much good complex carbohydrate you can tolerate. As your condition improves, you should gradually reintroduce complex carbohydrates into your diet.

A useful technique is to try three levels of carbohydrate avoidance until you hit on the one that benefits you. The first level is to avoid foods containing beet, cane, maple, and corn sugars, honey, fructose, and other refined carbohydrates. In level two, stick to the restrictions of level one but, in addition, eliminate fruits and milk[e] and limit whole grains and vegetables such as potatoes, yams, and corn that are high in carbohydrates. If this isn't enough, proceed to the third level, which consists in avoiding, beyond the restrictions of levels one and two, all gluten-containing grains, nuts, and sweet vegetables.

Many yeasts and molds possess cross-antigenicity with candida —that is, their antigens may cause the same symptoms of candida in those whose immune systems are sensitized to the pathogen.[30] You will probably also need to avoid foods and beverages that contain a high amount of yeast or mold and perhaps even those whose preparation involved these organisms. Many canned and frozen foods, for instance, contain citric acid manufactured from cornstarch or beet sugar by a mold. Table 26 lists foods that favor the growth of candida.

TABLE 26 Foods that promote candida

DEFINITE ELIMINATIONS	

Alcoholic beverages
Breads containing yeast
Cakes
Candies
Carob
Cheese, eggs, beef, and chicken, nonorganic
Coffee and tea
Condiments, sauces and foods with vinegar:
  ketchup
  mayonnaise
  mustard
Corn syrup
Fruits, dried and candied
Fruit juices, especially canned and frozen
Green olives
Honey
	Ice cream
	Malt, all foods containing
	Maple sugar
	Meats, processed and smoked
	Melons, especially cantaloupe
	Milk
	Sugar, all foods containing
	Packaged and processed foods
	Peanuts
	Pickles
	Pistachios
	Soft drinks
	Vitamins containing yeast
	White flour
	Yeasts

PROBABLE ELIMINATIONS	
Citric acid, all canned or frozen foods with Fruits Leftovers Mushrooms and edible fungi	Sauerkraut Sprouts Vegetables, starchy, like potatoes and yams
POSSIBLE ELIMINATIONS	

Grains containing gluten:
  barley
  oats
  rye
  wheat
	Shiitake mushrooms
	Tamari
	Vinegar

One should add to the diet several foods that could help control candida, the best of which are onions and garlic. As mentioned in the garlic section, several studies show garlic to have antifungal properties. In *The Yeast Connection*, physician William G. Crook mentions studies that have found garlic to possess an *in vitro* potency against *Candida albicans*, but he points out that large-scale controlled trials of garlic have yet to be conducted under the auspices of the FDA.[31]

Oleic acid, a fatty acid, is important in your diet. It prevents candida from changing into its invasive form. For this reason, several holistic physicians recommend virgin or cold-processed edible linseed, evening primrose, sesame, grape seed, and olive oils, to be taken as supplements.[32] These oils should be consumed uncooked, and care should be taken to avoid fried food, dairy, eggs, and meat, which would then add too much fat to the diet.

Taheebo, also known as *pau d'arco, lapacho, or iperoxo,* is an herbal tea derived from the inner bark of two South American trees, the *lapacho colorado* and *lapacho morado* (red lapacho and purple lapacho). The tea contains antifungal substances that are said to benefit both those who have been on antifungal medications previously and those who have not. People who drink it usually have four cups a day. Although both Argentina and Brazil currently export the tea, you should buy only the Argentinian brand, for there is a good chance that the Brazilian one has been exposed to Agent Orange, a highly toxic substance used for deforestation of the Amazonian tropical rain forest.[33, 34]

Physicians also recommend oral supplements of *Lactobacillus acidophilus*, a symbiotic acid-producing bacterium that competes with and helps control candida in the intestinal tract. One tablespoon of the liquid form three times a day should be sufficient. Use a brand made from a soy rather than a milk base.

The B vitamin biotin may also prevent candida from converting to its invasive form.[35] Biotin is essential for the metabolism of fats and proteins and is considered nontoxic. The adult required daily allowance of biotin is 150 to 300 micrograms (µg). Doses of 30 µg to 5 mg per day of biotin have been recommended for control of candida. The most concentrated source of biotin is, unfortunately, baker's yeast, which should not be taken when eliminating all yeasts to control candida. Permissible sources are dry soybeans (60 µg of biotin per 100 grams or 3 ½ ounces), walnuts (37 µg), and cauliflower, (17 µg). Other vitamins recommended for candida are vitamin A, the vitamin B complex, vitamin E, and vitamin C. Crook states that he has "found that vitamin C in large doses (2,000 to 20,000 mg or more daily) helps many of [my] patients with immune system problems."[36] Recommended minerals are calcium, magnesium, zinc, and selenium. Nonetheless, as we have said in the vitamin and mineral sections, any supplementation of these substances should be taken under the supervision of a physician knowledgeable about orthomolecular medicine.

After dietary elimination and supplementation, the second step of the candida program is to avoid antibiotics. Broad-spectrum antibiotics, in particular, kill beneficial intestinal flora while attacking pathogens. Once the flora that keeps candida in check is gone, the fungus (which is resistant to most antibiotics) proliferates and spreads rapidly. When antibiotics are unavoidable, ask your physician to use, if possible, the one most specific to the pathogen in question and least likely to disturb the normal bowel flora. You should also know that antibiotics are fed routinely to cattle and chickens. By eating beef, chicken, cheese, eggs, and milk that are not guaranteed free of these substances, you will be ingesting harmful and unnecessary antibiotics.

Step three is to avoid immunosuppressive drugs and cortical steroids (such as the hydrocortisone ointments sold over the counter for skin rashes), which weaken immune defenses, thereby decreasing the body's ability to resist chronic candida infection.

Step four, avoidance of distress, is closely related to step three. Acute distress is linked to the body's production of immunosuppressive cortical steroids. In chapter 1 we discussed the stress mechanism and touched on ways to avoid or defuse distress. Avoiding unnecessary and detrimental stress will prevent the excessive production of immunosuppressive hormones.

The fifth step of the candida program involves taking antifungal drugs prescribed by your physician. One of the most widely used and successful antifungals is nystatin (Mycostatin, Nilstat, Nystex). The drug seems to perforate the cell membrane of candida, whereby cellular components leak out and the fungus dies. Several candida strains are resistant to the drug. Nystatin is poorly absorbed through the intestinal wall and sometimes has no effect on fungus deeply rooted in intestinal tissue. Yet it is this poor absorption that makes nystatin virtually nontoxic. It does not affect beneficial flora and is well tolerated even during prolonged administration, although large oral doses occasionally can result in diarrhea, gastrointestinal discomfort, nausea, and vomiting.[37] A usual effect of the drug is a "die-off" period akin to the cleansing reactions mentioned in chapter 9, "Making the Change." As candida cells die, their toxic products are absorbed into the blood, and symptoms may temporarily worsen (called a Herxheimer reaction). Garlic and onions, which also have antifungal properties, may cause a similar discomfort.

Some physicians give ketoconazole (Nizoral) to patients who do not respond to nystatin or who exhibit systemic candidiasis. This drug also works by disrupting cellular membranes. It is a highly toxic drug, however, that can cause death from liver poisoning. Ketoconazole also has a variety of undesirable side effects, including nausea, vomiting, abdominal pain, severe itching, allergic reactions, and, rarely, anaphylactic shock.

Clotrimazole lozenges (Mycelex) are often prescribed for candidiasis of the mouth and throat. Like nystatin, clotrimazole works by altering the permeability of the fungal membrane, but it also can cause abnormal liver function, as it did in one-sixth of its clinical trial users. People who have had previous liver trouble—hepatitis, for instance—should be monitored while taking this drug. Amphotericin B (Fungizone), in cream, lotion, or ointment is used on skin and mucous-membrane candida infections and seems to possess no side effects other than possible drying reactions and localized irritation.

Intravenous amphotericin B, however, causes potentially dangerous side effects such as kidney failure, blood-clot formation, nausea, vomiting, diarrhea, weight loss, and loss of appetite. In some cases, the drug can also be immunosuppressive and toxic to the liver. Intravenous amphotericin B is therefore given primarily to people with a progressive, potentially fatal fungal infection such as systemic candidiasis in which the benefits of the treatment will outweigh the dangerous side effects.[38]

Caprylic acid, a fatty acid derived from coconut oil, seems to inhibit certain metabolic functions of fungal cell membranes; a small amount of caprylic acid chokes the fungus to death. Because the required dosages are usually low, caprylic acid has almost no side effects, except perhaps those associated with candida die-off and some mild gastrointestinal discomfort. Many physicians believe caprylic acid is more effective than nystatin and use it as the primary treatment for intestinal candida and as an adjunct in cases of disseminated infection. Although caprylic acid is available without prescription under the trade name Caprystatin, it should be used only under medical supervision.[39, 40] Gentian violet works effectively when painted on mouth lesions but looks rather messy.[41]

To stimulate immune cells to fight back, many doctors recommend immunotherapy with candida extracts—that is, vaccination—as the sixth step of the program. Candida, however, had at last count seventy-nine different antigens; each new strain of the organism adds to the number. C. Orion Truss warns in *The Missing Diagnosis* that anyone with autoimmune manifestations or who is under nystatin treatment should avoid yeast vaccines, antigen injections, and sublingual drops. In fact, an overstimulated immune system might be the precise factor that leads to AIDS immunosuppression. PWAs should therefore be wary of this sixth step.

The seventh and last step in the candida program is environmental control. Many molds in the environment cannot exist within the body but nevertheless possess cross-antigenicity with candida. If molds aggravate your symptoms, you should establish a program of mold control around your house. Keep in mind that dampness and darkness promote mold growth.

Several rooms in a typical dwelling serve as breeding grounds for molds. First and foremost is a damp basement. A dehumidifier and a few low-wattage bulbs will lessen the basement mold population. Next is the kitchen, where breeding grounds can be numerous: the area between the sink and the wall and around the bottom of the cold water pipe, wooden chopping boards, fruit and vegetable shelves in the pantry, and the water tray under the refrigerator. Maintaining good ventilation and keeping all surfaces dry, as well as immediately removing decaying matter, should make the kitchen less hospitable to mold. Mold also grows everywhere in the bathroom—on walls, drains, crevices, washcloths, towels; no place is left untouched. A preventive measure is to ventilate the bathroom completely after a bath or shower to reduce moisture. Leaving the bathroom light on also helps discourage mold. Make sure towels dry thoroughly after each use and wash them frequently. Antimold sprays can be effective, but try not to use them yourself; have someone whom the spray will not affect do it. Do not use the bathroom afterward unless it has been well ventilated.

In your bedroom, bed linen and mattress pads that are not washed frequently can breed mold. Pillows should be aired regularly in the sunshine. If you sweat at night, change bed linen regularly, since perspiration encourages mold growth. For the same reasons, do not let dirty clothes pile up. Suits and other garments that cannot be washed after each use should be aired separately before storing or else kept in a closet with a light on. An air filter that remove spores from the air can also be a good addition to your bedroom.

Other places around the house might not be as attractive to mold, yet there are always dark and damp spots where molds can take hold, such as shag carpets, old upholstered furniture, and old books and newspapers. If you have a yard or patio, keep it as clear as possible of bushes, shrubs, and trees that might promote dampness and darkness.

Part of the environmental control program is to keep chemical exposure at a minimum. Cigarette smoke, pesticides, detergents, and other chemicals can aggravate the symptoms of chronic candida infection.

⁂ ⁂ ⁂

The Missing Diagnosis by C. Orion Truss and *The Yeast Connection* by William G. Crook are two excellent books on candida. If you suspect that your current physician is not knowledgeable enough about candida, send a stamped, self-addressed envelope to the Price-Pottenger Foundation (see "Candida" in appendix H for address), which keeps a roster of physicians experienced in treating fungus-related health problems.

VIRUSES

A virus is the ultimate parasite because it depends on its host not for food, as other parasites do, but for life itself. A virus has thrown away—or never did possess—the paraphernalia of metabolism; it uses that of its host. A virus consists only of a submicroscopic protein capsule enclosing a tight core of genetic material, either DNA or RNA, that contains information on how to make more viruses.

Viruses can therefore replicate or reproduce only within living cells. This fact and the lack of metabolic activity outside cells have led many scientists to consider viruses to be nonliving biological particles; as such, they may be only stray pieces of genetic information being interchanged, for good or for worse, among cells. During the interchange, however, cell metabolism is commandeered, and the cells themselves are often destroyed. Whether or not viral infection serves to distribute genetic information among cells, it is usually detrimental to higher organisms and leads to illness.

After infection, the genetic materials of a virus and its host cell become indistinguishable. Viral illness is thus difficult to treat because parasite and host become one. Destroying the virus means destroying the cell—and usually the organism to which the cell belongs. A virus ensconced within its host cell is immune to almost all antipathogenic substances in the arsenal of modern medicine (except drugs like acyclovir, to be discussed later). The immune system is greatly challenged by viral illness and combats it much as it does cancer: the killer T cells and natural killer cells that destroy cancerous body cells also kill body cells infected by a virus. Many viruses have evolved various mechanisms to foil these immune cells. But in a disease such as AIDS the immune cells themselves cannot perform their antiviral job properly, and they allow the virus to take hold.

We have already talked about HIV, the virus that, possibly assisted by yet unidentified cofactors, opens the way to the immunosuppression of AIDS and ARC. The severe immunosuppression of AIDS in turn opens the door to other opportunistic viruses that can be fatal, the most common of which is cytomegalovirus.

CYTOMEGALOVIRUS

Cytomegalovirus (CMV) is a virus that belongs to the large family of herpes viruses. Although CMV infection is usually asymptomatic in adults, it can resemble infectious mononucleosis, eliciting fever, enlarged lymph nodes, and fatigue. In immunocompromised people, however, CMV infection can disseminate throughout the body. The virus has a special affinity for the endothelial cells lining the blood vessels. Many researchers believe that cytomegaloviral infection of endothelial cells, along with some other factor not yet identified, causes these cells and the fibroblasts surrounding them to divide out of control into the malignancy known as Kaposi's sarcoma. If this is so, cytomegalovirus would be second only to *Pneumocystis carinii* as an agent of opportunistic AIDS disease.

CMV pneumonia is common in AIDS and usually coexists with *Pneumocystis carinii* pneumonia. Disseminated CMV can also cause esophagitis, colitis, liver malfunctions, retinitis, and encephalitis. CMV involvement in these infections can often be diagnosed only after other pathogens such as amoebas and toxoplasmas have been treated or ruled out. There is currently very little treatment yet available for CMV infections, although several drugs like acyclovir show laboratory promise.

Retinitis due to CMV has been treated with vidabarine, or adenine arabinoside (Ara-A or Vira-A). This drug, however, can cause severe bone marrow suppression that will worsen any existing immune competence and may even contribute to the dissemination of cytomegalovirus through the rest of the body. There is no data showing that vidabarine is effective against CMV itself.

EPSTEIN-BARR VIRUS

The Epstein-Barr virus (EBV), another member of the herpes family, is responsible for the infectious mononucleosis that affects adolescents and young adults. Like other herpes viruses, EBV often produces no symptoms; in fact, most people in the United States will have acquired EBV by the time they reach age forty. The Epstein-Barr virus has a particular affinity for B lymphocytes and may be associated with malignant tumors of these cells such as African Burkitt's lymphoma. The carcinoma of the nose and throat widespread in China is also believed to be induced by EBV.

In people with AIDS, EBV may cause B cell lymphomas similar to Burkitt's. It is indeed the EBV origin of these non-Burkitt's lymphomas that has shed light on the possible relationship between CMV and Kaposi's sarcoma. Similar mechanisms may be at work in both malignancies. Although Burkitt's lymphoma in children is especially responsive to chemotherapy, there is no known nonimmunosuppressive treatment for severe EBV infections in AIDS.[42, 43, 44, 45]

HERPES SIMPLEX VIRUS

Herpes has become so widespread in the United States today that it would have earned the distinction of the disease of the 1980s had it not been for the appearance of AIDS. Herpes is an inflammation of the skin characterized by small blisters and is caused by two slightly different strains of the herpes simplex virus (HSV). HSV type 1 usually appears above the waistline and causes cold sores, whereas HSV type 2 is present below the waist and is the source of genital herpes infections. There has been so much crossover between the types, however, that both can be found in almost any area of the body.

In 1979 an estimated 80 to 90 percent of the population of the United States had some symptoms of oral herpes, and around six million people—12 to 13 percent of the total population—suffered from genital herpes, with half a million new cases being reported each year.[46] The spread of genital herpes has been so quick and pervasive that some researchers predict we will all have contracted the virus soon, thereby ending all worry about getting it. Genital herpes is not transmitted exclusively through sexual contact; but can be contracted nonsexually through skin cuts. HSV can survive on the plastic surfaces of exercise mats and workout benches and in hot tubs or whirlpools where the water isn't hot enough. If you are worried about catching HSV at the gym, put a towel on work benches or other workout surfaces before you lie on them, and avoid the hot tub or whirlpool.

For most people the first occurrence of genital herpes is accompanied by flulike symptoms and the appearance of blisters on the genitals, the groin, the area between the genitals and the anus, or the buttocks. The blisters turn into painful sores that disappear, along with the rest of the symptoms, in the ten to fourteen days HSV takes to become latent. During its latency, the virus hides within the ganglia, a group of nerve cells that, like other nerve cells, do not usually express enough viral antigens to elicit the attention of the immune system. The herpes simplex virus is often reactivated by even the most insignificant of factors: sunlight, fever, certain foods and drugs, and stress. Once reactivated, the virus travels down the nerves, usually to the areas of the initial lesions. Recurrent episodes vary in frequency and intensity from person to person and are often psychologically crippling to the individual. Most evidence suggests that herpes simplex is contagious only during an active episode, when sores are visible.

On-and-off genital herpes episodes nonetheless might be a sign that the immune system is in good working order. In people with AIDS, herpes appears not recurrently but chronically. In other words, the herpes infection often does not go away and ulcerates severely. Such ulcerated herpes sores can open the body to infection by other dangerous organisms. Herpes can also spread to the brain where it may cause permanent damage.[47, 48, 49, 50]

Acyclovir (Zovirax) is one of the first relatively safe antiviral

TABLE 27
Arginine-rich foods

Almonds
Barley
Beer
Brazil nuts
Chocolate
Corn, fresh cooked
Hazelnuts
Peanuts
Sesame seeds
Walnuts

Source: Nicholas Sampsidis, *Herpes:Something Can Be Done about It.* Sunflower Publishing, 1984.

drugs. The drug works by mimicking one of the genetic building blocks of the herpes virus. Fooled by the similarity, the virus incorporates the drug into its genetic structure and finally stops dead in its tracks; viral replication halts. Acyclovir, however, does not eliminate the latent virus hidden in the ganglia and therefore does not cure herpes. It only lessens the severity of symptoms and shortens the length of each episode. In fact, the sooner the drug is taken—when the telltale itching starts, for example—the less severe the symptoms and the shorter the recurrence. Ulcerative herpes in AIDS recedes under intravenous acyclovir treatment. The drug may also help prevent the virus from spreading to the brain. Because it acts preferentially on viral metabolism, acyclovir's side effects are minimal even when high doses are administered.[51]

Certain nutritional methods may help prevent a herpes occurrence. Viral particles owe their resistance to many immune agents to their tough and often highly variable protein coating, which in herpes simplex consists almost wholly of one amino acid, arginine. Cellular proteins, on the other hand, contain very little arginine. To make its coating, the virus uses excess arginine provided by foods rich in this amino acid. If foods such as peanuts, almonds, and chocolate are avoided regularly, little arginine will be available to the virus. Table 27 lists the most common arginine-rich foods.

Lysine is an amino acid whose chemical makeup closely resembles that of arginine. So close is the resemblance that the virus will try to use lysine if arginine is not available. But with lysine the virus cannot make a proper coating and is eventually destroyed. Although lysine is a common component of cellular proteins, it is its *relative* abundance, coupled with the relative lack of arginine, that serves to control herpes. Lysine supplements help maintain a beneficial lysine-to-arginine ratio, but such supplementation works better if arginine-rich foods are also minimized.

Antioxidants such as vitamins C, E, and A, biotin, selenium, and the food preservative BHT may also be helpful.[52]

HERPES ZOSTER VIRUS

The herpes zoster virus (HZV) causes chicken pox, or varicella, in children and shingles in adults. In fact, shingles are a reactivation of latent herpes zoster virus left over from childhood chicken pox. Like herpes simplex, the herpes zoster virus hides in the ganglia and resurfaces when immunity is compromised, as in the elderly, and usually during a period of severe stress.

Shingles usually start with pain along a nerve pathway (often in the face, chest, and abdomen) and then might appear to be a severe case of poison ivy or poison oak until clusters of painful blisters develop. The disease runs its course in about three weeks, but the affected nerve might cause severe pain for many months. Herpes zoster can also manifest itself in the Ramsay Hunt syndrome, in which a facial nerve is affected and partial paralysis, ear pain, and loss of taste occur.

Herpes zoster is relatively uncommon before age fifty. Before then, it usually occurs in persons with systemic lupus erythematosus or malignancies such as Hodgkin's disease and leukemia and in organ transplant patients undergoing immunosuppressive treatment. A study of thirty-three HIV antibody–positive individuals under age fifty revealed that seven (21 percent) developed AIDS within two years after the onset of shingles. This study, however, used no appropriate controls and considered a group that might have been too small to draw definite conclusions from. A retrospective study of 300 people with AIDS showed that only 8 percent had had shingles. Thus, all one can say is that shingles in someone at risk may constitute a sign of impending immune deficiency but is not predictive of either AIDS or ARC. In those with AIDS or ARC, however, herpes zoster is not uncommon.[53]

Herpes zoster is most commonly treated with acyclovir. It is extremely important to seek medical help as soon as the first signs develop. The quicker acyclovir treatment starts, the shorter the run of the disease and the less painful the nerve damage. Aspirin is frequently prescribed to prevent the latter. If you have either AIDS or ARC and you had chicken pox as a child, you might want to avoid arginine-rich foods, because the herpes zoster protein coat is similar to that of herpes simplex. An ounce of prevention is worth a pound of cure and, in this case, precludes tons of pain. By the way, since chicken pox generally confers lifelong immunity, you will not contract herpes zoster from another person if you had the childhood disease; shingles are a reactivation of your own latent virus. If you didn't have chicken pox as a child and your immunity is compromised, avoid anyone with shingles.

COLDS AND THE FLU

For people with AIDS, the common cold and even the flu usually do not represent as grave a danger as the viral infections previously discussed. A cold or the flu, however, is sometimes hard to get rid of, so contagion should be avoided. Colds and flus are transmitted primarily by hand contact with an infected person. Rubbing your nose or your eyes with your contaminated hand completes the inoculation process. Viral transmission of colds can be controlled by careful attention to personal hygiene. Wash your hands with soap and water after covering your mouth for a sneeze or a cough; after hand contact with someone with a cold, keep your hands away from your eyes and nose. Use disposable facial tissues and disinfect the house with Lysol whenever anyone in the household has a cold.[54]

CHAPTER 13

Detoxifying the body: methods

FASTING

Fasting is the act of eating little or no food. Foregoing a few meals or drinking only vegetable or fruit juices in lieu of your regular diet constitutes a fast.

Although often touted as a cure-all, fasting can be dangerous, especially when prolonged or drastic. Advocates of fasting propose that a fast diverts the energy of digestion to healing and elimination, thus helping the body get rid of toxic wastes faster. But they fail to mention that fasting itself may produce harmful toxins and cause irreversible damage through nutrient deprivation. The cells of the immune system, which have high energy and nutrient requirements, could be particularly susceptible to prolonged fasting. The extended fasting practiced by a yogi, even when accompanied by breathing exercises and meditation, is not advisable for anyone with AIDS.

This doesn't mean you should force yourself to eat if you are ill and have lost your appetite. During illness, the body often temporarily suppresses the need for eating so as to direct all its energies into healing. If illness has taken away your appetite, you could restrict your diet to liquids or to the small quantity of food your body asks for. "Many people force themselves to eat while they are sick," the McDougalls say, "even though they are not hungry. Food eaten at this time may nourish the bacteria, viruses, cancer cells, or other agents that are making them ill, but does little to help them recover."[1] Illness constitutes the one indisputable time short fasts can be appropriate. If you don't feel like eating when sick, then don't.

The duration of this kind of fast depends on the illness and individual. If you feel that your illness and lack of appetite are prolonging themselves or if you start to lose too much energy or weight, then you should consult a knowledgeable doctor for advice on nutritional supplementation. If your illness fast lasts more than one or two days, return to eating gradually, increasing your food intake by steps up to normal consumption. A diet of mostly vegetables is best when ending a fast.

MAINTAINING PROPER KIDNEY FUNCTION

The kidneys are essential for eliminating toxins from the body. But in AIDS the kidneys are often under increased stress from having to rid the body of toxins produced by pathogens or by prescribed drugs and their by-products. This extra load on the kidneys not only drains off energy that could be used for healing but also may eventually cause kidney damage. Certain drugs, such as the pentamidine used to treat *Pneumocystis carinii* pneumonia, are so toxic that they may sometimes bring about kidney failure. For people with AIDS, especially those under treatment, it is essential to maintain proper kidney function.

Although we may love soft drinks, coffee, and lots of salt, our kidneys do not. To keep your kidneys working optimally, eliminate all alcoholic beverages, soft drinks, tea, coffee, and excessive protein and fats from your diet. Also be especially cautious of over-the-counter drugs like aspirin and acetaminophen. Above certain doses these drugs may damage the kidneys. Unless your physician restricts your liquid intake because your kidneys are damaged, drink plenty of spring or filtered water every day to cleanse them.

COLONICS

Colonic irrigations are highly controversial. They are enemas of water under pressure (preferably nonchlorinated water) that last from half an hour to an hour. Colonics require a trained operator who knows how to keep the patient relaxed and the water flow under control. And this is the crucial aspect of colonics: the skill, knowledge, and training of the operator. He or she should be monitoring the process constantly and ensuring that the patient never feels discomfort.

I believe colonics should not be part of a detoxification program—especially when dealing with AIDS—because of possible injury to the intestinal mucosa and fecal contamination thereof. I include colonics here for the sake of completeness. They are sometimes recommended by bona fide practitioners and mountebanks alike, so you should be aware of their pros and cons before trying them.

Before trying colonic irrigation, read up on it. *Colon Health* by Norman W. Walker is a good introduction. You can also request information from the American Colon Hygiene Association, whose address is listed under "Colonics" in appendix H.

LIVER–GALL BLADDER FLUSH

As the name implies, this procedure involves detoxification through flushing the gall bladder. I've had firsthand experience with its good results, yet because medical complications can arise from a liver–gall bladder flush, the method should be employed only with your physician's *explicit* approval and constant supervision. There can be some pain and the definite possibility of a gall stone getting lodged in your bile duct, which could mean getting yourself rushed to the hospital for surgical intervention. Fred Rohe's *Metabolic Ecology* gives a good account of the liver–gall bladder flush.

HERBAL FORMULAS

The use of herbs for cleansing the body is as controversial as the use of colonics. There are two such herbal programs that I know of. One is outlined by Robert Gray in *The Colon Health Handbook.* Gray's herbal cleansing formula can be purchased in premeasured and premixed pills. The other program, that of John R. Christopher, is almost identical to Gray's except that you do all the mixing and measuring yourself.

The proponents of these herbal formulas claim, as do most who recommend colonics, that old feces build up in intestinal pockets and coat the entire length of the colon and the small intestine. Furthermore, Gray maintains that this intestinal buildup falls into two types: putrefactive material, which is still decaying and hardening, and postputrefactive material, which is very dry and virtually glued to the body. He claims that his herbal formula is effective against these two kinds of build-up.[2]

My research did not turn up any medical evidence to support Gray's claim. If people's intestines were indeed encrusted with these fecal accumulations, at least one autopsy would confirm this and at least one pathologist would mention such build-up. I tried to reach Gray and ask him about his sources (not included in his book), but I was unsuccessful. I then called Yerba Prima, the company that manufactures Gray's herbal formula, and asked them if they could send me a list of medical sources mentioning these questionable fecal deposits. Although they had no information at the time, they promised to send me anything they came up with. That was over a year ago; I guess they are still waiting for their material to accumulate. I suggest you devote your energy and time to more productive detoxification methods.

EXERCISE AS BODY CLEANSING

Although the importance of exercise in improving muscle tone, strength, agility, and mental health and in reducing stress is addressed at greater length in chapter 14, in this section I want to discuss its usefulness in eliminating body wastes and toxins. The skin is an important organ of excretion, and sweat from exercise is a good vehicle for waste and toxin elimination.

Vigorous walking that builds up a sweat is one of the best exercises for cleansing your body. Not only does walking help the skin release toxins, but it also manipulates the abdominal cavity that houses the intestines. Such manipulation can help regularize bowel movements.

Stretching is another exercise good for the bowels. You should sit, stand, or lie down and spend some time discovering all the muscles in your body and then use them systematically, one at a time. Lying on your back and bringing your knees toward your chest and lying on your back while make a pedaling motion with your lifted legs are two simple and effective intestinal stretches.

A word of warning on exercise: push yourself so you feel the stretch but not until you feel pain. Pain from stretching usually means that damage has occurred or is about to occur.

You can manipulate the bowel area in other ways, too. Lie on your back and roll a tennis ball over your abdomen, hard enough to make an impression but not to cause discomfort. You can also knead your abdomen using the tips of the fingers of both hands. Another method is to apply right-to-left circular pressure above the abdomen with both hands. All these methods assist the bowel in its own movements.

SKIN CARE

To help detoxify your body, you want to make sure your pores are not blocked. Daily washing is advisable for keeping your skin functioning properly as well as for maintaining a good appearance and making life nicer for friends. Hot water and a scrub with a loofah sponge work well. If you have an iron constitution—I don't—alternating hot and cold water is said to be stimulating. Briefly turning the water to cold helps contract the pores.

Avoid using soap on most of the body. Most soaps upset the skin's acid balance and strip your skin of oil, laying it open to bacteria and fungi. In places that require soap, like the underarms and the genitals, use Castile soap. Avoid deodorants and excessively perfumed soaps, which can irritate the skin and clog the pores.

You should treat your body with love; the application of chemicals, whether internal or external, is not a step in that direction. Offensive odors are defined by social convention, a fact well known by those who fill their coffers by heavily advertising all sorts of antismell preparations. Yet to live with others we often have to observe some of these conventions. If you feel you can live with just the benefits of a thorough daily bath, all the better. If you are the type who drives the zebra stampeding across the savannah when you lift your arms and you feel you have to use deodorants, do so. Try to stick to the milder ones and watch your underarms closely. If a rash develops, stop using the stuff.

Using loofah sponges while showering removes dead cells and

other wastes that solidify on the skin. Scrubbing in long, even strokes down the neck and trunk toward the lower abdomen and up the legs, arms, and buttocks gives an added benefit: it aids lymphatic circulation and waste elimination.

SAUNAS

When I go to the gym (about three times a week), I sit in the sauna for about fifteen to twenty minutes after my workout. The sauna makes me build up a sweat, cleans out my pores, and helps my body eliminate toxins. Some holistic doctors recommend a cool sauna—around 130° F—for thirty to sixty minutes at least five days a week. At around 130° F, they claim, the body releases proportionately more oils than water than it does at higher temperatures, thus helping to eliminate all the toxins, environmental poisons, and harmful chemicals that may lodge in the body's fat deposits.

Your sauna should be quickly followed by a cool shower and a glycerin soap scrub to dissolve the oils through which toxins have been excreted.[3] You should have no problem with longer saunas provided you drink plenty of water beforehand and consume a varied diet that will replace the minerals and vitamins eliminated through sweating.

HOT BATHS

To relieve stress or headaches I sit in a tub of hot water, epsom salts, and baking soda. The procedure is easy. Fill your bathtub halfway with water just a little less hot than you can bear, add a quart each of epsom salts and baking soda, and then sit down and relax. This might be a good time to practice visualization techniques. Stay in the water about thirty to sixty minutes to build up a good sweat. I usually take a cool shower and scrub myself with a loofah when I get out (for added benefit, you can brush with a dry skin brush *before* the hot bath). If you don't have access to a sauna, a hot bath is a good alternative. Epsom-salt baths can be very relaxing, but they can also be quite draining. Therefore, you should sit or lie down quietly for at least half an hour afterward or take the bath just before going to bed.

HOT TUBS AND WHIRLPOOLS

Hot tubs and whirpools should be avoided unless they are directly under your control. In health clubs they are often kept at temperatures insufficient to kill certain tough viruses, such as herpes, that resist chlorination. (HIV *cannot,* however, be gotten from a tub. HIV is extremely fragile when exposed to the environment and is transmitted only through intimate sexual contact or contaminated blood or blood products.)

CRYING

Yes, crying. Crying is typically overlooked as a method of detoxification. Just as sweating releases toxins through the pores, crying allows us to detoxify through the tear ducts. Moreover, crying helps bring repressed feelings or emotions to the surface and thus relieves tension and stress. It puts you in touch with yourself and can purge guilt, sorrow, and anger. Tears are very good overall cleansers. As anyone who has had the experience can attest, a good cry can give your respiratory, circulatory, and nervous systems a thorough workout.

Our culture, however, has taught many of us that tears—especially for men—are rarely an acceptable response to emotional or physical pain. So crying is a behavior that many people have difficulty displaying not only in public but also in private.

Many of us suppress our ability to cry, and this suppression may sometimes translate into physical illness. Richard Miles, a writer on holistic medicine, suggests that we can come down with a cold whenever we do not allow ourselves to cry. The physiological manifestations of a cold and of crying are similar: watering eyes, congested sinuses, and a flushed feeling. He proposes that the common cold might be a message that tells us we are suppressing a feeling or emotion we need to express. Since we feel society does not permit the expression of such feelings, the cold we catch becomes a convenient (and sanctioned) outlet.[4] Miles's conjecture may possess a kernel of truth worthy of psychoimmunological investigation.

Theories aside, crying is good for many other reasons. By all means, cry when you feel like it. "Life is for expression," says Shirley McLaine in *Dancing in the Light*, "so don't be judgmental of how you feel."[5] Like exercise, crying needs practice. If you are afraid someone will catch you crying, use the shower for a good, heartfelt session. Once you have experienced the calmness and sense of well-being a good cry can bring, you will become less inhibited and more able to call on this necessary function—even in public—when you need it.

CHAPTER 14

The spirit and the spark: breath and exercise

BREATH

Breath is life. We must breathe to live; if we do not breathe, we die. What is more, breathing happens automatically; we do not have to think about it because the body breathes on its own. Breath is so simple and self-sustaining that many of us often overlook how truly vital it is.

In contrast to other so-called involuntary functions such as heartbeat and blood pressure, breathing can be brought easily under conscious control by altering its rhythm, for example, or its depth. Breathing is thus a unique body function. It is the only body activity under the control of both the involuntary (or autonomic) and the voluntary (or central) nervous systems. Because of this dual control, breathing can act as a bridge between conscious and unconscious functions.

In this light, it isn't surprising that Eastern philosophers deem breathing so important that they devote decades to its study. Linking mind and body, breath becomes a valuable tool for increasing spiritual awareness and physical vitality. No other activity has a more pronounced and immediate impact on our existence. And that is why it merits some study. I recommend you read *Science of Breath,* an excellent book and a good primer on the subject.

Since the body cannot live without breathing, breath is controlled and maintained unconsciously when we choose not to control it ourselves—which for many of us is most of the time. Involuntary breathing becomes the vassal of a more primitive brain that rules through the unconscious emotions and perceptions of our distant evolutionary ancestors. These primal mechanisms can destroy the rhythm of breath and wreak havoc on the rhythm of our lives. We all have experienced the way emotions such as intense grief or fear affect our breathing, making it irregular and shallow. Yet we usually fail to recognize that the relationship between mind and breath is a two-way street: the rhythm of our breath can likewise alter our emotions. By consciously breathing smoothly and continuously, we can release tension and defuse the fight-or-flight response while achieving tranquillity and relaxation.

Rhythm and movement are primary expressions of the dynamic equilibrium of health and life, and the rhythm and motions of breath closely reflect the broader pulses of life.

When we observe and influence breath rhythm, we get a grip on our total self. Breath acts as a natural biofeedback mechanism, one that can effect deep physical and psychological changes in our bodies. Learning breath control could be a springboard to learning how to influence other usually involuntary functions of the body, possibly even those of the immune system. Control over involuntary activities can increase gradually as breath mastery is achieved.

Proper breathing begins through the nose. The nose directs, filters, warms, and moisturizes the air we inhale. Ideally, air humidity should be 30 to 40 percent. In winter, take care to adjust your indoor environment to an ideal air moisture, especially if you use forced-air heating. A humidifier helps, but if you suffer from mold problems, use it judiciously.

Low relative humidity increases susceptibility to upper respiratory infection by drying up the lining of the respiratory passages, thereby impairing their output of immunoglobulins and their immune responsiveness.[1] All body channels in contact with air, such as the the respiratory and alimentary tracts, are lined with a membrane, the mucosa, whose glands secrete mucus, a viscous mixture of water, cells, proteins, inorganic salts, and an especially sticky kind of carbohydrate—a mucopolysaccharide. Mucus in the lungs and nose traps bacteria, fungi, viruses, dust, and other debris; hairlike cilia in the cells of the mucosa propel the mucus, and whatever it traps, out of the nose and lungs and into the pharynx, where it is swallowed. In the stomach, enzymes digest the mucus and any accompanying pathogens. Immunoglobulin A (IgA) and the many phagocytic cells in the respiratory mucosa provide additional defense against pathogens.

Mucus kept continuously in motion by the epithelial cilia keeps the lungs clean of dust, bacteria, and other pathogens. When the mucosa dries out, however, or when its mucus becomes too viscous, ciliary movement stops, and microbes can then establish a foothold, multiply, and cause infection. Mucus that is too liquid and runny, on the other hand, will fail to act as an effective trap. Cigarette smoke paralyzes ciliary movement, stimulates mucus secretion, and injures the phagocytic cells of the mucosa (the smoker's cough is an attempt to get stationary mucus out of the lungs).[2] Since opportunistic organisms often establish their beachhead in the lungs of the immunocompromised, impairing the function of the mucosa by smoking makes the invasion as easy as when bunkers are destroyed and barbed wire removed before an enemy attacks.

Some people claim that diet can determine the viscosity of mucus. Dairy products, and refined starchy carbohydrates, are said to create a thicker, more viscous mucus. Although I concur with the other compelling reasons, such as the presence of antibiotics, to avoid these foods, I have yet to find support for this claim in the literature. A nasal wash is also said to help clear especially thick mucus. Such a wash, or *neti,* consists of a warm isotonic salt solution (a solution with the same salt concentration as your tears) that is poured down one nostril and allowed to flow out the other.[3] *Science of Breath* describes the procedure in detail.

We might notice the chest and abdominal movements during breathing, but few of us ever pay close attention to how these motions carry air in and out of the body. What kind of a breather are you? Sit back and relax for a moment. Place one hand on your abdomen and the other on your chest and breathe in and out normally. If your chest rises and falls while your stomach remains relatively still, then you are a chest breather.

Chest breathing is inefficient. Although it expands the thorax, increases the diameter of the chest, and causes the lungs to distend and pull air, chest breathing fills only the middle and upper parts of the lungs. It doesn't get enough oxygen to the lower lungs, however, where most of the blood is drawn by gravity.

Chest breathing is necessary at the end of a fight-or-flight situation in nature because the body quickly needs to repay the oxygen debt incurred during its surge of adrenalin. But as any runner knows, the body soon shifts from chest breathing to the more efficient abdominal respiration a few minutes after the race is over.

If chest breathing becomes the normal breathing pattern—as it has in many of us—it can bring about chronic nervous arousal. For example, feedback signals from shallow and jerky chest breathing can induce a sustained and unnecessary fight-or-flight response and disrupt mental tranquillity. On the other hand, deep, even, and steady breathing will help us achieve relaxation. This is why we sigh deeply after a moment of high stress or emotion.

Deep breathing means breathing with the diaphragm. The

diaphragm, a muscular partition that separates the abdominal and thoracic cavities, expands the lower lungs where most of the blood circulates. Diaphragmatic breathing therefore mixes more air with the blood, expending less energy in the process than chest breathing. By providing maximum oxygen to the body, deep breathing helps promote tissue healing. Continuous and rhythmical breathing from the diaphragm also gently massages the abdominal organs and improves abdominal circulation. In our society, however, a pushed-out chest and tight abdomen are considered beautiful. Diaphragmatic breathing conjures inaccurate visions of protruding abdomens, thus making it unfashionable.

Diaphragmatic breathing is easy but has to be practiced daily before it becomes automatic. Start by lying face up on your bed with one palm on your abdomen below your navel and the other on the center of your rib cage where the abdomen begins (the solar plexus). Loosen any restricting garments, relax your muscles, and empty your mind of distracting thoughts. Inhale deeply, slowly, and evenly through your nose. Make sure your mouth is closed and your tongue touches your palate. As you inhale, your abdomen should rise toward the ceiling and the lower edge of your rib cage should expand. There should be relatively little movement in your upper chest. Now exhale through your nose, drawing your abdomen toward your spine while expelling all the gases from your lower lungs. Make sure all the old air is out to make way for the new.

After learning to move the diaphragm properly, we need to develop rhythm and harmony in breath by learning to breathe deeply and constantly without forcibly holding the breath between inhalation and exhalation. Determine the maximum time you find comfortable between full inhalation and full exhalation and practice diaphragmatic breathing at this pace for at least five minutes three times a day. You can also practice during your daily routines, as I do while waiting in line at the bank or supermarket. It gives me something to do and keeps me from getting upset.

Breathing exercises can relieve as well as prevent stress. As your breathing becomes increasingly smoother, both inhalation and exhalation will become slower and deeper and last anywhere from six to ten seconds.

Breathing exercises offer a perfect opportunity to practice healing imagery. Everyone should create his or her own images. I visualize incoming breath as a broom sweeping together the waste in my lungs and outgoing breath as the broom sweeping the collected waste out of my body. You can visualize breath entering any part of the body that needs special attention. How you do this is up to you, but the more concrete the image, the better.

Through breathing you can control certain body functions, detrimental emotional responses, and the mind. As diaphragmatic breathing becomes automatic, you soon learn to recognize chest breathing resulting from fight-or-flight situations. You will also notice the times when you hold your breath to suppress feelings or emotions. This is when performing what is known as the full yogic breath will defuse tension.

The full yogic breath is a threefold process that includes diaphragmatic, thoracic, and clavicular breathing in one smooth, coordinated sequence and achieves maximum air intake. The breath begins by ballooning out the abdomen as in diaphragmatic breath. Once the lower lungs are filled, the breath is continued by moving the chest outward and expanding the middle of the lungs. Finally, the shoulders are raised and pulled back so the breath can fill the upper lungs. Exhalation is the same steps in reverse. Relax with a sigh as the air passes from your mouth. Drop your shoulders, collapse your chest, and finally, contract your abdomen, giving it a little extra squeeze at the end. Five or six of these complete breaths will be beneficial when you need to relieve stress or during heavy physical activity.

No discussion of proper breathing is complete without mention of the hazards of smoking. For proper breathing, the air you breathe must be clean and fresh. Tobacco smoke contains large amounts of carbon monoxide that combines more easily and permanently with hemoglobin than does oxygen.[4] Carbon monoxide decreases the ability of hemoglobin molecules to transport oxygen and, for all practical purposes, puts them out of circulation. Even when not smoking, a smoker may still have up to 15 percent of his or her hemoglobin tied up and useless.[5] Smoking a cigarette is akin to breathing in a closed garage with your car engine running.

We have all read the Surgeon General's warnings that tobacco smoking causes cancer, emphysema, and other respiratory and heart ailments. To enumerate all the myriad dangers tobacco poses would be beyond the scope of this book. I cannot emphasize sufficiently, however, that for those at risk of AIDS or ARC, smoking destroys the immune competence of the lungs and opens the way for opportunistic pathogens such as *Pneumocystis carinii* or tubercular bacteria.

If you smoke and want to quit, join a smoke-enders program, seek therapy, or send for a quit-smoking tape from one of the organizations listed under "Smoke-Ending" in appendix H. If you do not smoke and someone lights up in your presence, move away if possible, because secondhand smoke is also a hazard to health. If you can't leave, politely inform the smoker that smoke aggravates your physical condition. Do not even wait until after the cigarette is lit. Most smokers will refrain from smoking if you deal a gentle but effective blow to their conscience. In your home, of course, simply but courteously say no. Having no ashtrays is a subtle hint.

EXERCISE

Exercise is probably the activity in which the mind produces the most noticeable effect on the body. Although the benefits of exercise depend on the kind and quantity of activity, some common results are increased muscular strength, improved flexibility and body tone, better overall appearance, and greater stamina. While exercising, we are also improving our reflexes, balance, coordination, complexion, posture, and ability to rest during sleep. The most dramatic consequences of exercise, however, are not the most visible. Exercise strengthens support of internal organs, improves digestion and removal of wastes, increases nutrient and oxygen exchange in tissues and cells, removes cellular waste, and enhances immune functioning. Exercise can also make you feel great.

Exercise does not have to involve weightlifting marathons or injurious tests of macho endurance. Improperly performed exercise can be a source of physical stress and can cause injury, trigger heart attacks, and lower resistance to disease. Proper exercise, on the other hand, can help alleviate the stress created by improper exercise. If your goals are to have massive pectorals, big arms, and powerful legs, then weightlifting will be rewarding if you do it creatively and in harmony with your body's demands. There are quite a few people with AIDS who pursue body building.

Good exercise properly performed should suit your goals and physical condition. Goals and physical limits may change as your overall health improves. One of the ways exercise improves health is by increasing the flow of oxygen to the body's cells. Disease often develops if body cells, particularly those in the heart, lungs, and brain, do not receive adequate oxygen. Aerobic exercise, involving vigorous heart, lung, and vascular activity, is highly effective in increasing oxygen flow. Exercise also helps remove cellular waste products by promoting lymphatic circulation. Lymph is the clear liquid that bathes and removes wastes from all cells. It is also the major means of transportation for lymphocytes, your immune cells. But unlike the cardiovascular system, the lymphatic system lacks a central pump to aid circulation. Only muscle action—in your legs and arms, for example—moves the lymph along. Exercise enhances this action and gives the lymphatic system a good flushing.

Regular exercise strengthens the chest muscles and the diaphragm, allowing for deeper and richer breathing. The extra demand for oxygen during exercise induces production of more red blood cells and hemoglobin and increases the oxygen-carrying capacity of the blood.[6] Increasing the volume of blood pumped per heartbeat enhances this oxygen capacity further. Exercise produces other cardiovascular changes that decrease your chances of heart disease: it lowers blood cholesterol and increases beneficial high-density lipoproteins, increases the diameter of heart arteries and the flexibility of blood vessels, and may aid in the formation of collateral blood vessels in the heart.[7]

Moreover, exercise may help prevent cancer. Researchers have found cancer death rates to be highest among people whose daily routines entail little muscular effort and lowest among those whose activities demand greater muscular activity. Some doctors report that the most dramatic cancer recoveries occur in very physically active patients.[8] Studies on laboratory animals lend ample support to the role exercise plays in combating cancer.[9]

Many benefits of exercise derive from the elimination of stress. As discussed previously, the stress response, which among other things brings about suppression of immune activity through the release of cortical steroids, is triggered by the need for physical activity during a fight-or-flight situation. Vigorous activity brings the stress response to an end and subsequently puts the body into a state of relaxation and equilibrium.

Studies have shown that organs and tissues deteriorate steadily when animals are continuously stressed but not allowed to release their stress physically. When a physical outlet for stress is provided, however, body damage is minimal.[10] Your body is indifferent about whether such an outlet comes from fighting, fleeing, or just doing some good exercise.

When physically fit, your body releases fewer immunosuppressive corticosteroids in response to stress.[11] The fewer the corticosteroids in your blood, the greater the ability of certain phagocytes to carry out their immune function. Vigorous exercise also stimulates production of endorphins and enkephalins, two kinds of brain hormone that also enhance immune function. These hormones most likely act as chemical mediators between the nervous and immune systems, delivering go-ahead messages from the brain to helper T cells and returning acknowledgements that immune functions have been carried out. A good gym workout shortly before blood testing has been found to improve helper T cell counts and helper/suppressor T ratios in people with AIDS.[12]

Enkephalins and endorphins are also responsible for the runner's "high" and generally reduce anxiety and relieve depression. Mildly depressed patients have improved their mental states more through increased physical activity than through psychotherapy.[13]

Reduction of anxiety and depression through activity is invaluable—and essential—for those with AIDS or ARC. Writing about people diagnosed with supposedly fatal diseases in *Stress without Distress,* Hans Selye states that "those who sought relief in complete rest suffered most because they could not avoid thinking constantly about their hopeless future, whereas those who managed to go on being active as long as possible gained strength from solving the little tasks of daily life which took their minds off more sinister conditions."[14] Through the healthy effect of distraction and the action of brain hormones, exercise reduces depression and anxiety, promotes well-being, encourages a better outlook, and gives a boost to hope.

The ancients held exercise in high regard, believing that a fit mind could only exist in a fit body. Indeed, we know that physical exercise can bring about a healthier psychological profile: improved alertness and mood, enhanced self-image, higher self-worth, clearer and more flexible thinking, and a sense of being at ease with oneself and others. Above all, exercise teaches you to listen to your body and tend to its needs. The health and energy acquired from regular exercise will turn your body into a good friend and a source of pleasure. And good friends do not come prepackaged or in pill form; instead, any cherished relationship has to be cultivated and requires effort.

Exercise can be either aerobic or anaerobic. Aerobic exercise is performed at a rhythmic pace that elevates your heart rate for a period of time without creating shortness of breath. All other exercise is anaerobic. Only aerobic exercise effectively ends stress by acting out the fight-or-flight response.

What is and is not aerobic depends not only on the exercise but also on the individual and how he or she performs the exercise. Running, cycling, skating, jogging, rowing, and walking elevate the heart beat and are all aerobic. Horseshoes and croquet are not aerobic since they do not maintain an elevated heart rate for any length of time. Body building falls into either category depending on how it is done. A forty-five minute workout in which attention is given to form and breathing and in which sets and stations follow one another evenly without long pauses is aerobic, even when heavy weights are used. Lifting weights without this kind of routine is anaerobic.

What is aerobic or anaerobic depends on the individual and the shape he or she is in. A good, steady walk might keep the heart rate of someone who is physically fit where it ought to be, whereas someone who is out of shape might become breathless. The pace of the exercise is very important. An aerobic pace should make you perspire a little but still allow conversation with a workout friend. Huffing and puffing are signals that you should slow down.

Your pulse is a reliable indicator of whether or not you are maintaining an aerobic pace. For a proper cardiovascular workout, you want to keep your pulse within a range known as the aerobic target zone. You can figure out your target zone in pulse beats per minute by subtracting your age from 220 and using 70 percent and 85 percent of that figure as the bottom and top limits, respectively, or you can use a chart such as the one in table 28. Monitoring your pulse, however, can be a chore. One procedure is to stop exercising every five or ten minutes and immediately count your pulse for six seconds. (The pulse will accurately reflect your heart rate during exercise only if it is taken within 15 seconds.) Such interruptions can be annoying, however, so a better solution, budget permitting, is to get a reliable digital pulse monitor that you can read easily without interrupting your routine.

There are no ideal exercises. What matters is how regularly one exercises. Do exercises that you can comfortably and enthusiastically maintain for at least twenty minutes three or more times a week (at least every other day, with a possible two-day rest each week). Exercise is drudgery if it does not become more appealing and enjoyable as you progress. Do not embark on crash programs, which are the major reason beginners stop exercising. If you are out of shape, try working out initially for an hour at a low or moderate intensity. Then slowly shift into a higher gear. Avoid injury, which is the second reason beginners quit. Observe any warning pain or stiffness, for these can be indications that something is wrong or that you are proceeding too rapidly.

TABLE 28
Pulse target zones

AGE	TARGET ZONE (beats/minute)
Up to 29	140 to 170
30 to 39	130 to 160
40 to 49	120 to 150
50 to 59	120 to 140
60 and over	110 to 130

Note: To easily obtain a per minute figure, count the pulse beats per fifteen seconds and multiply by four.

In a body-building program, however, the line between gainful and injurious pain is difficult to define. For free weights or Nautilus equipment to be effective, repetitions should be performed until the muscle becomes exhausted. The intense soreness that signals muscle exhaustion should not be avoided if you want to gain from weightlifting. On the other hand, painful muscle tears resulting from lifting too heavy a weight improperly must be avoided at all costs. Whatever weight exercise you do—as with any exercise—observe proper form because this lessens the chances of injury.

My own two-part exercise program addresses the three components of fitness: flexibility, strength, and endurance. First, I take a forty-five minute walk three days a week. I always plan the walks ahead and wear comfortable, well-cushioned, light running shoes and thick socks to avoid foot injuries. I do not stretch before walking since I stretch every other day at the gym, but light stretching is always advisable if you feel stiff before a walk. It is pleasant to walk in picturesque, appealing surroundings. Try to walk or hike in open spaces uncluttered by the trappings of civilization. Wherever you go, observe the beauty of things; walk in the "now" and forget about past and future. Watch out for obstacles, too, since they tend to disrupt the steady pace of an enjoyable walk.

As you take a step with your right foot, bring your left arm forward, and vice versa, while maintaining a rhythmic swing of the arms. Coordination of opposite sides of the body, and thus of the opposite hemispheres of the brain, is believed to help maintain glandular balance. If nothing else, coordination makes for grace and agility.

Again, the shape you are in determines how long and how fast you should walk. Walking fifteen minutes at two miles per hour is a good start if you are out of shape. Over a month, slowly build up to an hour at four miles per hour. After a brisk walk you will notice many of the benefits of increased production of endorphins.

"Walking is the best exercise there is," says Ronald M. Lawrence, medical advisor to the U.S. Olympic Committee and the President's Council on Physical Fitness Sports. This only confirms what I have always known. I like walking because it is inexpensive and does not involve elaborate equipment. I can do it almost anywhere and anytime, and it provides numerous benefits. "It uses more of the body's muscles than any other type of exercise," adds Dr. Lawrence, "improves cardiovascular efficiency and is virtually injury free."[15] I like it, well, because I like it. You might not. It's very important to find out what works for you.

The second part of my program entails stretching and weightlifting exercises every other day. In other words, one day I walk and the the next day I go to the gym. At the gym I first do slow stretches with a high bar. I find that stretching helps my coordination, increases my range of motion, and just feels good. Then for five to ten minutes I perform a series of stretches and body movements to quicken my heart rate (Bob Anderson's *Stretching* offers good direction and advice). For the next two hours I alternate between these body stretches and weightlifting, thereby keeping my heart rate moderately high for an extended period of time without physically exhausting myself.

Some people believe that those who have AIDS or ARC should not lift weights, because weightlifting does not promote health. I must vehemently disagree. These people are often so immersed in Eastern philosophy that they reject any kind of Western exercise. They associate a body builder's physique with the fabled Castro clone (a mythical San Francisco inhabitant who in the age of AIDS has turned into a convenient scapegoat for gays and straights alike). One should not be blinded by ideology or personal likes or dislikes. Dogma traps the mind. AIDS research, in fact, documents improved lymphocyte counts after weight or Nautilus exercise.

Throughout most of my life, I have often been labeled skinny. Recently, however, I have been able to build, with free weights and Nautilus equipment, muscle that I never even knew existed. I always used to think "Who am I to have money? Who am I to have love? Who am I to deserve this or that? Who am I to have a beautiful body?" Well, now that I am getting that beautiful body, my sense of self-worth in other areas is growing, too. Or maybe my body is becoming more beautiful from body building because my general self-worth is improving; these processes work reciprocally. If having a muscular, well-defined body helps me build self-esteem and self-love, then body building cannot be anything but health-promoting. If weightlifting does not feel right for you, however, find an exercise that does.

Yoga is one of my favorite disciplines. Although yoga's main objective is to achieve a balance between body and mind and thus open a path toward self-realization and inner peace, the discipline can also produce a high level of physical fitness. The kind of yoga that deals with the physical is hatha yoga, a system of directed postures and organized stretches called *asanas.* Hatha yoga exercises increase oxygen flow and reduce carbon dioxide levels in the body, aid in the cleansing of the digestive tract, and give greater control over both voluntary and involuntary muscles. For those desiring an even greater degree of muscular competence, Iyengar yoga offers a stricter and more demanding approach that employs prolonged and almost gymnastic *asanas.*

Iyengar yoga is best done under the instruction of a qualified teacher; regular hatha can be practiced at home (Richard Hittleman's *Introduction to Yoga* is a good primer). You should practice yoga on a large towel, pad, or mat either before or at least two hours after meals. The practice room should be quiet and well ventilated. Wear light clothing to allow complete freedom of movement without restricting breath or blood flow.

Tai ji quan (t'ai chi ch'üan) is another system of exercises that promotes self-discipline and a sense of well-being. A traditional Chinese discipline, *tai ji* encourages meditation and works toward uniting body and mind. Its movements, derived from the Chinese concept of nature, seek to restore contact with the natural world. To achieve its goal of strength without strain, *tai ji* often visualizes the body as a firmly rooted tree that derives its energy from the ground. Breath, which is deep and natural, is seen as the tree's gentle swaying in the breeze. *Tai ji* encourages very slow, natural movements that calm both body and mind and increase body energy. It therefore is well suited not only for those whose health is good but also for the weak, the ill, the old, and the very young.[16]

Exercises like jogging, handball, squash, and tennis may be too strenuous and might cause knee, ankle, or foot damage. You may want to avoid them. Jogging, for instance, exerts tremendous force on the feet, a pounding that eventually injures 55 percent of all running enthusiasts in the United States.[17] The morning or afternoon jog is a self-punishment routine well suited to compulsive personalities. Transformed into a machine, a person joylessly chugs along faster every day, looking neither left nor right, all for the experience of relief at the end of the run. Such strenuous exercises could become truly life-threatening if your immunity is already compromised.

Look for an exercise program that feels right for you, whether it is walking or belly dancing. But *exercise,* even if it means just walking around your bed. If your body cannot muster enough energy for physical activity, use your mind—all exercise is first in the mind, and then in the body. Visualize yourself doing the physical activities you enjoy. Put a strong desire into it. You just might convince your body to perform.

CHAPTER 15

Body manipulation

POSTURE

Many of the changes produced by proper breathing, good exercise, and adequate sleep are basically changes in how we carry ourselves; in other words, they are changes in posture. Chronic poor posture can have many causes, but a very common one is lack of self-worth. Many of us belittle ourselves. If we feel uneasy about asserting our presence in the world, we bend and curl up our bodies so they take as little space as possible.

Incorrect posture is sometimes a legacy of childhood. A series of scary but otherwise harmless falls, for example, can make a child hold on to a particular posture—hunched shoulders and a caved-in chest—in anticipation of other falls. Though the falls stop, the incorrect posture might persist for life. Even as adults, we hold our bodies incorrectly in anticipation of dangers that may never come. The startle reflex, an initial manifestation of the fight-or-flight response, causes muscles to tense and breathing to become quicker. Muscles can often become locked in tension during the startle reflex. It is not uncommon, for example, to develop a stiff neck after quick head movements during a sudden fright.

There is an intimate relationship between what we think and

how we position our bodies. Many thoughts are automatically translated into muscular movements and body stance. These gestures, or body language, serve in turn to reinforce the particular feeling, emotion, or attitude that produced them. As anyone who has caught a person lying can attest, body language is an accurate gauge of mental state; it takes great skill to make the body lie. To repress an emotion, we force the muscles away from the position the emotion wants them to take. When this becomes habitual, the muscles become frozen in place and trap the emotion. Tension, stress, and other dysfunctions occur because we are, in effect, wrestling with ourselves.

Besides being unattractive, poor posture makes the body expend energy fighting gravity rather than in other more beneficial ways. Fatigue, tension, and even chronic pain may result from having to hold the body in an unnatural, energy-consuming position. Poor posture also prevents proper breathing, creating shortness of breath and chronic anxiety that might set off the immune-suppressing stress response. Poor posture means being disconnected from your body and, as such, might reinforce an attitude of hopelessness.

Good posture, on the other hand, aids circulation and respiration and thus increases vitality and alertness while decreasing distress. As Chinese medicine proposes, good posture eases the flow of life energy throughout the body. Our body is our home. How we fit into that home and occupy space in the world often indicate whether or not we feel good about being alive. Among the greatest benefits of good posture are a better attitude toward ourselves, increased self-confidence, and a greater ability to deal with the world.

Besides the breathing, exercise, stretching, and stress-management routines discussed in the last chapter, there are several things you can do to improve your posture: Stand up straight. Try to sit upright as much as possible without slouching, sprawling, or slumping. Work on your body language. Avoid fumbling, for example, or covering your face with your hands. Try to make your body communicate the self-confidence and strength you want to achieve.

Sometimes it takes more than the above steps to correct posture, especially when chronic poor posture has frozen into a permanent pattern. Detecting and correcting such dysfunctions may call for the expertise of bodywork professionals. Bodywork, or body manipulation techniques, usually involves but is not restricted to massage-like therapies.

Depending on its approach and method, bodywork can be classified under one of three schools: the mechanical, the psychological, and the energetic. Although their emphasis and techniques vary, all three traditions hold that health, which depends on proper body function, can be achieved through retraining the body's posture and movements to a natural balance or equilibrium. Which bodywork technique is best for you is a highly individual matter. It may be that none is satisfactory by itself, so you may find that using several simultaneously is best.

MECHANICAL

The mechanical school of bodywork is mainly concerned with body mechanics. Practitioners of this tradition regard the body as an interconnected system of levers, hinges, pulleys, and plates that requires adjustment whenever stress and tension cause misalignment or wear. Although mechanical bodywork deals mainly with the skeletal and muscular systems, it can often produce results beyond those of purely physical adjustments. The different techniques deal with different aspects of the body's mechanical components.

MASSAGE

Most bodywork utilizes some kind of massage as a tool, making massage a natural starting point for our discussion of body manipulation. Massage is the rubbing, pressing, stroking, tapping, and kneading of flesh with the bare hands. You can massage yourself or have someone else massage you. It is ideal to combine the two.

During your daily shower, firmly draw your hands along your body towards the lower abdomen, that is, upward from the legs and thighs and downward from the shoulders and chest. This will help lymph to circulate. Self-massage can be beneficial when sitting in a bus, train, or plane for a long time. Using little grasping motions, knead up and down the length of each arm two or three times. Move with the grain of the muscle, not against it. Vary hand placement on each cycle to cover the whole arm area. Similar methods can be used on your legs. Put your imagination to work.

There's nothing quite like having someone massage you. Another person will be able to reach parts of your body not accessible to you. His or her touch can be a luxurious experience—it will make you feel pampered and offer a powerful boost to your self-confidence. As you would with anyone whose services you pay for, check out the qualifications of your masseur or masseuse.

TRAGER PSYCHOPHYSICAL INTEGRATION

This style of bodywork, developed over thirty years by physician Milton Trager, works on releasing tension from body joints using various gentle, rhythmic massages and stretching movements. The shaking, swinging, pressing, bouncing, and rocking of limbs and body go way beyond regular massage in producing lasting relaxation and restfulness.

ALEXANDER TECHNIQUE

The Alexander technique, developed by Australian actor F. M.

Alexander at the turn of the century, bases its methods on the realization that certain dysfunctional movements come not from reflexes but from learned habits and can therefore be unlearned. By means of spoken instructions, demonstrations, and light touch, an Alexander practitioner can show people how to replace these detrimental motions with beneficial ones.

Plagued by a vanishing voice that threatened his stage career, Alexander discovered that an unconscious backward head motion depressed his larynx and made him suck his breath in, resulting in his voice-loss problem. He began to see that his problem was not local but, rather, concerned his whole posture. For ten years he experimented with various methods until he developed the techniques used today by many actors, opera singers, performers, and even body builders.

An Alexander session is difficult to describe because the movements involved are often so subtle that they escape notice. For example, a small, almost imperceptible adjustment of the head slightly forward and up can make one's body immediately feel wonderfully relaxed. Alexander called the area where head and neck meet the "primary control." Alexander practitioners use no special exercises, preferring to work with the everyday movements of a person while guiding through gentle words and touch.[1,2]

FELDENKRAIS METHOD

The Feldenkrais method is based on the concept of a two-way connection between body and brain: not only can the brain tell the body what to do, but the body can reprogram the brain by acting out the easiest and most effective ways to move. The method was developed by engineer Moshe Feldenkrais as an outgrowth of techniques he had used to cure a chronic knee problem caused by soccer. The Feldenkrais method fosters learning from the biofeedback of everyday movement. Although the method teaches awareness through movement and does not deal directly with pain relief, flexibility, relaxation, or fitness, the discovery of habitual movement restrictions can nevertheless produce these results as well as engender a new sense of pleasure through movement.

There are two forms of Feldenkrais bodywork: one-on-one tablework sessions, called Functional Integration (FI), and movement re-education group classes, called Awareness Through Movement (ATM). During Functional Integration, the practitioner observes body movements of which the subject is habitually unaware and helps the person become more conscious of and comfortable with these. There is no one standard of movement everyone must conform to; functional integration depends on what the individual wants. The more formal "Awareness Through Movement" classes strive for awareness using a series of gentle anaerobic motions. A participant learns to search for tension areas in the body and compare limbs as clues to imbalances. The lessons have built-in variations to avoid dullness and are reminiscent of the processes babies use when learning how to move their bodies. The sessions can be quite demanding nonetheless and often produce results similar to those of sitting meditation—increased energy and an altered state of consciousness, for example. ATM sessions are also much cheaper than FI, although the individually tailored approach of the latter is sometimes invaluable. In my one encounter with ATM I found no instant miracles, yet I developed an awareness of numerous body imbalances that could be corrected with time and guidance.[3,4]

CHIROPRACTIC AND APPLIED KINESIOLOGY

Chiropractic is concerned with neuromechanical structure, the interrelationship between the skeletal, muscular, and nervous systems. The nervous system is the master system of the body, processing information from all other body systems to achieve homeostasis. How well the nervous system performs depends on how well it receives or delivers this information. Chiropractic holds that the disruption of this data flow can lead to dysfunction and eventually to disease. Therefore, chiropractic seeks to maintain the functional and structural integrity of the nervous system.

Vertebral subluxation is an example of such a disruption in a nervous pathway. A subluxation results when one or more bony segments, or vertebrae, in the spine become dislodged from normal position and impinge on the nerves running from the spinal cord to various body organs. Since most body functions and tissues are controlled by nerves, a subluxation alters the normal configuration of the nervous system and interferes with the natural forces that maintain order in the body. This interference can lower tissue resistance and make it more susceptible to damage and disease.

Chiropractic does not employ surgery or drugs to restructure nerve pathways; rather, it uses manipulation and adjustment of the soft tissues and joints of the body, especially the spine, as its primary therapy. Most chiropractors prefer holistic approaches that deal with the nutritional, physiological, emotional, and spiritual needs of the whole person.

Many chiropractors use applied kinesiology as a primary diagnostic tool. The theory of applied kinesiology maintains that certain dysfunctions are associated with specific points of weakness in muscles and that finding and correcting those weak points will therefore alleviate dysfunction. The practice of applied kinesiology is less convincing than its theory. To test for organ weakness or intolerance to food or drugs, the practitioner asks the patient to extend one arm while resisting downward pressure. This resistance test is repeated with the patient's other hand on and off various body parts or substances. Organ weakness or food and drugs intolerance supposedly produce a decrease in muscle resistance. The practice of applied kinesiology is so subjective that it is hard to tell whether the technique actually reveals information about the body or just works by subtle suggestion between practitioner and patient.[5]

Sacro-occipital technique (SOT) is a method of both diagnosis and treatment that focuses on the relationship between structural distortion and abnormal physiological function. SOT gently adjusts the bones and cranium, manipulates soft tissues (muscles and organs), and employs reflex treatments. This chiropractic technique is an effective preventative that can diagnose and treat many illnesses before any clinical symptoms—often too tardy—surface.

Although I have never been in a car accident or taken any bad falls, I agree with the chiropractic dictum that undisturbed flow of information between the body and the brain is essential for health, so I decided to visit a chiropractor. He found two vertebrae out of alignment, which were subluxing the nerves leading to my thymus gland and kidneys. I decided to follow through with treatment, and I derive great benefit from these visits. Chiropractic has enhanced my sense of responsibility for my body's health. For example, I learned that something as simple as putting my wallet in my back pocket and sitting on it could have led to my misaligned vertebrae and subluxed nerves.

A visit to a competent chiropractor should benefit anyone, especially those whose immune system cannot afford to be further impaired by a structural nervous dysfunction. Make sure your chiropractor is well versed in sacro-occipital technique and uses a holistic approach to healing. *Touch for Health* by John F. Thie is an excellent practical guide to chiropractic.[6,7,8]

OSTEOPATHY

Whereas chiropractic is neuromechanical, osteopathy is osteomechanical, that is, it deals with the manipulation of bone. Osteopathy extends this manipulation to include not only the vertebrae, as chiropractic does, but all bones and joints in the body. Osteopaths perform surgery and occasionally use drugs. In fact, osteopathy seems to be adopting so many of the techniques of traditional medicine that the distinctions between the two are becoming increasingly blurred.[9]

ROLFING

Rolfing has developed an opposite body manipulation approach from osteopathy. Whereas the latter manipulates the rigid bone and joint structures, the former reshapes the more plastic deep fascia, or connective tissue, that surrounds muscle. While other bodywork methods describe ideal posture through standardized relationships (the knees vertically above the ankles, the hip joints vertically above the knees, and so forth), Rolfing states that verticality, or straight posture, is more individual. According to founder Ida Rolf, Rolfing strives to achieve a balanced, symmetrical posture that is the outward expression of deep structural relationships inherent in a person's body design. In other words, your posture is not necessarily determined by your bone structure as much as by how your muscles relate to—how they shape and maintain—that structure. Rolfing does achieve a very recognizable type of posture, however.

Repression of grief, fear or anger seeks a bodily outlet in muscle. These physical manifestations of repressed emotion reshape the plastic fascia and alter the body's basic structure. When a repressed emotion becomes a habitual pattern, the unnatural muscular arrangements it causes become set; the body deviates from true verticality. Being out of alignment with the vertical, it also becomes out of alignment with gravity, a vertical force. When this happens, the body fights rather than uses gravity, and as a result its energy is diminished.

Rolfing brings deviant muscles closer to their optimal location and then requires them to move in that less energy-consuming position. Rolfing manipulations can be intense and sometimes painful, often eliciting strong emotions or triggering floods of suppressed memories. But the results of Rolfing can be striking: improved posture, increased energy, better health, greater awareness of your body, and a better rapport with others.[10]

ASTON PATTERNING

Aston patterning brings the theme of postural individuality to its logical conclusion. After being treated by Ida Rolf for auto accident injuries and learning Rolfing herself, Judith Aston became uneasy about the fact that Rolfed bodies seemed to look alike. She also believed that Rolfing was needlessly painful. Parting from the idea that three-dimensional movement is asymmetric, Aston patterning fosters cooperation among moving body parts, no matter how they move.

Aston patterning includes massage to relieve chronic stress (the touch can be light to intense, depending on individual need), re-education of an individual's movements, and redesign of his or her environment by changing daily objects to suit their user better. The massage and the movement re-education work together to show a person immediately how tension release in one part of the body can elicit a new way of moving.[11] For those unwilling or unable to get Rolfed, Aston patterning offers an attractive alternative.

PSYCHOLOGICAL

Unlike the mechanical tradition, the psychological school of body manipulation is concerned not with proper body function per se but with the healthy functioning of the mind. By removing psychological blocks manifested in tissue, this tradition views the body as the entry point to the mind. Although it is reminiscent of

Rolfian principles, the psychological tradition traces its roots to the work of psychoanalysts Wilhelm Reich during the 1940s and Alexander Lowen in later years.

REICHIAN THERAPY

Wilhelm Reich, a clinical assistant to Sigmund Freud in the 1920s, eventually took issue with the Viennese father of psychoanalysis by stating that all neuroses—and neurosis is the rule, not the exception, in American society—are based on an inability to achieve "full orgiastic potency." The strongest prohibitions in our society are those against sex and eroticism, and these taboos emerge early in our lives. Infants are promptly weaned from the warmth and sensuality of suckling and cuddling, toddlers are quickly taught anxiety and disgust for excretion (formerly experienced as blissful release), little boys' and girls' crotches become private parts too nasty to be seen in public, and sex, when puberty arrives, comes veiled in secrecy, shame, and guilt. For gay men and lesbians, this sexual repression is greatly compounded by societal scorn.

According to Reich, proper orgasm entails a great energy buildup followed by a sudden release. The body's muscles contract and relax like surging waves; ego awareness is lost and replaced by deep fulfillment, peace, relaxation, and tenderness towards one's partner. You do not have to reach sexual orgasm in your analyst's office, however, to achieve the full orgiastic response sought by Reichian therapy. Rather, full Reichian orgiastic response entails achieving the uninhibited wavelike convulsions, breathing patterns, and melting and flowing sensations necessary to total orgasm.

Reich believed that because of society's prohibitions on sex, we resist the massive, primal energy flow of orgasm, massively contracting our bodies in compensation. The ensuing pain and frustration bring on strong feelings of sadness and anger, which, in turn, we seek to suppress by yet more bodily contraction. The heavy contractions make us stiffer and duller and squelch the spontaneity we possessed as children, all of which leads to suppression of emotions in general.

Reich believed that emotions are not solely phenomena in the brain but are also impulses toward action. Sadness, for example, entails an impulse to cry, an urge to enact a very specific set of breathing patterns, vocalizations, and body movements. Suppression of this urge means voluntarily locking the muscles in place. When suppression of emotion becomes habitual, muscle contractions become chronic and persist even in sleep. All these chronic, spastic contractions constitute a body armor that protects and isolates us from inner feelings and external perceptions.

The Reichian therapist—preferably a psychotherapist or psychoanalyst—seeks by means of direct, nonsexual body contact to help remove the armor in a person's customary posture, carriage, gait, gestures, mannerisms, facial expressions, and tone of voice, thereby allowing the underlying true character to surface. Proper breathing is important for reasons different from those of yoga. In yoga, deep breathing is directed toward inward spiritual growth; in Reichian therapy it is directed toward the outward unlocking of the muscular armature that traps feelings and emotions. Reichian therapy ends when the individual can express full, uninhibited orgiastic response.[12] Reichian therapy and bioenergetics (described next) could prove powerful in healing those emotional and psychic components of AIDS arising from guilt-laden and repressed—or misdirected—sexuality and misplaced self-love.

BIOENERGETICS

It is more likely you will find an analyst trained in bioenergetics than in Reichian therapy, which lost its popularity during the

McCarthy years after Reich lost a long battle with the FDA and died in jail. Reich's disciple, Alexander Lowen, known better for his formulation of the body language concept, expanded and transformed Reich's work into a new therapy called bioenergetics.

Like Reich, Lowen thought that the primary energy of the individual is sexual and that its repression results in neuroses and body armature. Nonetheless, Lowen's approach to therapy differed considerably from Reich's. He believed Reich's method of attacking sexual hang-ups head on generally failed to yield results because of strong societal taboos on sex . Lowen got better results working on personality problems that went beyond sexual anxieties and hang-ups as well. He continued character-analysis work abandoned by Reich and established correlations between psychological states and the physical behavior patterns popularly known as body language.

Whereas Reichian therapy takes place on the analyst's couch, bioenergetics makes a person stand up and move about. Bioenergetics, like Feldenkrais or Alexander technique, teaches a person to move in the ways for which the body was designed.

In spite of its beneficial effect on the body, bioenergetics remains basically a therapy for the psyche. Sooner or later, body rigidities yield their long-repressed feelings or emotions. When this occurs, the psychoanalytic side of bioenergetics comes into play. Therefore, one should seek a psychotherapist trained in bioenergetics rather than a bioenergetics practitioner who knows nothing about analysis. "Bioenergetics," Lowen states, "aims to help a person open his heart to life and love. This is no easy task."[13] Bioenergetics seeks to bring down the formidable defenses that encase a person's heart and to re-establish a free flow of feeling and an inner harmony. These goals translate to freedom, grace, beauty, and the ability to love.

HELLERWORK

Whereas Reichian therapy and bioenergetics use body manipulation to cause psychological change, Hellerwork uses psychological techniques to achieve changes in body posture. Hellerwork was developed by former aerospace engineer Joseph Heller after he studied under Ida Rolf and spent seven subsequent years in Rolfing practice. Hellerwork uses the same deep tissue manipulations as Rolfing but also encourages a person to delve into the past for the time and place a particular improper posture first began. Besides massage work that can be as intense and painful as Rolfing, Hellerwork includes movement re-education. A typical course lasts for eleven sessions. For people who feel unsure about grappling with their psyche, Hellerwork offers a good sneak preview of psychotherapeutic techniques along with postural benefits similar to those of Rolfing.[14]

ENERGETIC

Whereas the psychological tradition deals with proper flow of feeling or emotion, the energetic tradition generally deals with a more indefinite vital force that is called, for lack of a better term, body energy. Most schools in this tradition recognize the inadequacy of the term *energy* in describing an elusive but real component of life and do not equate it with physical phenomena such as electromagnetic waves or electric currents. Each school defines this energy differently, but all are concerned with its proper flow through the body. The energetic tradition encompasses long-standing Oriental therapies such as acupuncture and shiatsu, some Western practices such as reflexology and polarity therapy, and also the therapeutic touch, an old healing technique now being rediscovered by modern medicine.

ACUPUNCTURE

Acupuncture presupposes a life energy, *qi* (or *ch'i,* meaning breath or steam), that flows along pathways, or meridians, in the body. Chinese medicine in general sees the body as a dynamic system in which the active principle, or *yang,* must be kept in equilibrium with the passive one, or *yin.* Illness results if these energies are blocked or out of balance. The acupuncturist unblocks *qi* by inserting very fine needles at specific points on appropriate meridians, of which there are fourteen major ones. Acupressure uses finger pressure instead of needles.

Chinese healing practices go much further than just acupuncture or acupressure. In fact, Chinese medicine is a highly complex synthesis of philosophy, ethics, science, clinical data, and herbology used for diagnosis, prevention, and therapy. Westerners might recognize many of its techniques, but may often be baffled by much of the reasoning behind its methods. For most chronic disorders, for example, Chinese doctors will understandably prescribe herbs, breathing exercises, and changes in diet. Sometimes they will also recommend a series of highly integrated and refined exercises such as Taoist yoga. The latter prescription would have provoked giggles among Western doctors a few years ago, although it seems perfectly reasonable nowadays, since the work of Herbert Benson on the therapeutic uses of meditation.

A retrospective study of thirty-four men with ARC and thirty-seven with AIDS who underwent acupuncture at Lincoln Hospital in New York reported that those with ARC experienced increased energy and calmness, a sense of well-being, decreased size of lymph nodes, and less night sweats and diarrhea. Increases in absolute helper T cell counts and helper/suppressor T ratios were noted in some of the men. The positive results were similar in the men with AIDS but also included increased appetite, weight gain, and less toxicity from chemotherapy. There is one report of a man who, after a cryptosporidial diarrhea of two and a half years, experienced relief of symptoms and showed negative stool exams after fifteen acupuncture treatments. The appearance of KS lesions, however, did not seem to be affected by acupuncture.

The authors of this preliminary study warn that these are tentative results, subject to change during controlled research, but believe that "acupuncture has had a long-term preventive and protective value for [their] patients based on the seemingly low incidence of relapse and on longer survival."[15] Acupuncture has no side effects; the worst part is getting to and from the acupuncturist.

I go to a Chinese acupuncturist and doctor regularly. I first went to her with congested lungs. She did her work and predicted my lungs would begin to clear the day after—and they did. Today, after a number of visits, my energy level has improved, I am able to carry out more demanding tasks, and I feel calmer. I believe everyone should visit a competent acupuncturist, preferably a Chinese doctor and herbologist. Make sure he or she has several years of clinical experience, is proficient at pulse diagnosis, and possesses a license or certificate and, for those trained in Asia, a diploma from a traditional Chinese medical college. Some of the best acupuncturists are not fluent in English, but they usually have assistants who are.[16]

For a scientific explanation of how acupuncture works and an overview of the traditional principles of Chinese medicine, I recommend *Acupuncture* by Felix Mann.

SHIATSU

Shiatsu or acupressure, used in Japan for over one thousand years, consists in finger pressure applied to acupuncture points with varying degrees of pressure and for different lengths of time. There are several varieties of shiatsu. Zen shiatsu uses the weight of the body, stretches, and leverage. In barefoot shiatsu the practitioner uses the sole of the foot to lean his or her weight into the recipient.

Acu-yoga combines finger pressure, posture, and breathing. Yoga postures are used before treatment to break down body armor and after treatment to further its effectiveness. Certain yoga postures are also used to press naturally against pressure points. Do-In, a self-acu-massage, combines several massage techniques to stimulate points and also includes stretching, breathing, and body awareness exercises.

Acupressure might appeal to those who feel uneasy about the thought of a needle. However, although an acupuncture needle is not nearly as painful as a hypodermic one, a little prick actually might have therapeutic value for those who feel that medicine should either hurt or taste bad to be effective.[17]

Two introductory books on acupressure and acu-yoga are *Acupressure Way of Health: Jin Shin Do* by Iona Marsaa Teeguarden and *Acu-Yoga* by Michael Reed Gach and Carolyn Marco.

REFLEXOLOGY

Reflexology is a latter-day Western variation on pressure-point therapy that focuses exclusively on the feet. The underlying theory states that points on the bottom of the feet are linked to specific body organs. Massage of a specific point should promote health in the corresponding organ. If nothing else, this therapy is effective in relieving tension.

POLARITY THERAPY

Polarity therapy, developed by Dr. Randolph Stone, seems to be a Westernized version of certain Eastern medical ideas. Practitioners of polarity therapy believe that diet, exercise, body manipulation, and "right thinking" increase and balance the flow of energy for physical, emotional, and mental well-being. In a theory that echoes the Chinese concept of meridians, Dr. Stone proposes that the body's vital energy follows certain interlinked channels that reflect the condition of particular body parts. But he postulates a dualism different from the Chinese *yin* and *yang*. According to Dr. Stone, life energy moves between positive and negative poles—the head and feet, respectively—through energy channels that sweep through all the vital organs and glands. Naturally, health results from the balanced alignment of positive, neutral, and negative energies, which can be re-established and strengthened by the body manipulation, the yogalike exercises, the cleansing diet of fresh fruits, vegetables, and other natural foods, and, above all, the program of self-improvement that constitute polarity therapy.[18] If you want to learn more about polarity therapy, *Your Healing Hands: The Polarity Experience* by Richard Gordon is a good introduction.

THERAPEUTIC TOUCH

Therapeutic touch—plain and simple human touch—is one of the oldest and most widely used healing techniques. Successful physicians know the therapeutic value of touching their patients. Humans are social animals that have evolved around body contact. Touch was probably the principal means of communication among our ancestors for millions of years. In many societies—and ours is no exception—being declared an untouchable is considered worse than death.

Touch is life-giving. Premature babies who are not handled enough by nursing attendants are less likely to survive than those who are. Therapeutic touch enhances life forces in adults, too. Studies show that touch stimulates the production of endorphins and other substances that play an important role in health.[19] The need for touch is built into our genes.

Dolores Krieger is well respected by physicians and laypeople alike for having reintroduced the idea of the therapeutic touch to the medical community. Although she believes that all healthy people have an abundance of life energy, Krieger maintains that only the true healer can direct this vital energy to the ill. She sees this energy as a force that binds all visible, invisible, tangible, intangible, mental, and physical manifestations. In 1971 she performed a controlled pilot study that confirmed an increase in subjects' hemoglobin after a laying on of hands.[20]

AIDS can be a very alienating and dehumanizing experience. But there is no reason why it must be, except for prejudice and ignorance. Increasing the amount of touching and hugging among friends still remains the ultimate bodywork technique. Touching can also be fun. I highly recommend Krieger's *The Therapeutic Touch: How to Use Your Hands to Help or Heal*.

CHAPTER 16

Looking at the whole of health

A self-help health book cannot be complete without a summary of what you can do to achieve health. If this means a set of step-by-step instructions on what to do about AIDS, however, I'm afraid this book must be incomplete. At this point in time, AIDS remains a confounding disease for which oversimplified solutions can be as deadly as no solution at all.

Even though AIDS remains devastating, however, we need not remain helpless. Diet, exercise, alternative therapies, nonimmunosuppresive drug treatments, visualizations, and a positive approach to life, for example, may help us prevent the downward spiral of immune suppression and, in some instances, bolster immunity. Many of the approaches discussed in this book may help us improve the quality of our lives, and thus bring us a measure of health. Progress is being made against the disease: combinations of immune-enhancing and anti-HIV substances, that are opening promising avenues of treatment may become available not too distantly.

How should this book be used? No matter how comprehensive it appears, it presents only what I have discovered about my disease. The book is a resource guide, not a bible, and thus points, not dictates, *one* possible way to your own discoveries. Trying to keep constantly in mind all the myriad details presented here is unnecessary. Reject anything you feel doesn't enhance your immunity, maintain your health, or improve the quality of your life. Simplify your life, and avoid organizing it around minutiae. Look at the whole of your health. Feeling that your health depends only on one particular fact, another's intervention, or one hard-to-get substance may help you feel powerless against your disease. There is always something you can do, even if it seems small and inconsequential at the moment. Hope should never be abandoned.

But feeling that your health depends solely on you is also unrealistic and possibly detrimental. Assuming responsibility over what you can do should not imply feeling guilt for your disease. Nor should you feel defeated if you have tried everything and nothing seems to work—the realities of the virus are, after all, undeniable and there are many things in life over which we seem to have no control. At times the best course of action is to let things be. Death is a part of being alive; one cannot help but to always choose life.

I wish I could offer you something more substantial than these three-hundred-odd pages. As it is, I can only offer you my hand, my embrace, and, above all, my love.

May you grow.

Appendixes

APPENDIX A

A comprehensive psychosocial and nutritional approach to the treatment of AIDS*

by Keith D. Barton, M.D.

The following is an outline of an integrated program designed by Russell Jaffe, M.D., for the treatment of AIDS. The underlying objective of the program is to strengthen the healing capacities of the person with AIDS in as many different ways as possible. Presumably, these various capacities will work together and reinforce one another in restoring health and well-being.

An initial group of nineteen persons with AIDS started this program about two years ago. The results are promising. Eighteen of these original participants are living, and most show significant improvement.

This outline is intended to provide the reader with a detailed picture of Dr. Jaffe's program. If a person with AIDS chooses to use this approach to dealing with his or her illness, he or she will need some skilled assistance in implementing various portions of the program.

If the scope of the program seems exhaustive or impossible, rest assured that it is not intended to be done all at once. The usual portions to start with in the first month have been set in SMALL CAPITALS inthe

*Adapted by permission of the author from *A Comprehensive Psychosocial and Nutritional Approach to the Treatment of AIDS*, an unpublished manuscript released for patient use in April 1985.

outline: I. A, B, C, D, E, F, and G; II. A, B, C, D, E, and F; III. A, B.1, B.2 and B.3, and III. C. Other parts that can be added later as time, energy, and interest permit are enclosed in parentheses.

Section I concerns the initial evaluation of the person with AIDS by a physician. Because this information is fairly technical and tedious for the general reader, it has been abridged in this version.

If this program looks like an exciting adventure in self-discovery, then further exploration is in order. If it appears burdensome or bizarre, however, then it may not be the program to undertake at the present time. This program engages the head, the heart, the stomach, and the feet. If any of these balks at what is required, then the whole process is likely to go awry. If they are willing to work together, then the progress can be impressive and lasting.

Please note that this article is an abbreviated outline of a complex approach to treating a complex disease. Such an outline is therefore incomplete and may contain inaccuracies. This treatment program should be undertaken only under competent medical supervision by a sympathetic physician.

* * *

I. BASELINE EVALUATIONS performed by a physician to monitor progress and guide therapy:
   - A. MEDICAL HISTORY AND PHYSICAL EXAM with psychosocial history, occupational and drug exposures, and dietary assessment.
   - B. PHOTOGRAPHIC RECORD including KS lesions.
   - C. IMMUNE SYSTEM PARAMETERS including helper/suppressor T lymphocyte ratio.
   - D. BLOOD SYSTEM TESTS: complete blood count, platelet count, sedimentation rate, and blood clotting tests.
   - E. LIVER TESTS: liver enzyme levels; test of conjugating ability (the liver's ability to remove certain toxins).
   - F. DIGESTIVE SYSTEM TESTS including a careful search for amoebas and other parasites, and tests for digestive capacity and efficiency.

G. HORMONE LEVELS including blood levels of adrenal hormones.
H. Measurement of toxic substances stored in the body:
1. Urinary test for toxic metals such as lead, cadmium, mercury, aluminum, and arsenic.
2. Sweat test for organic toxins such as insecticides, PCBs, and other fat-soluble hydrocarbons. Sweat is collected on clean paper and sent to a laboratory that can test for tiny amounts of these substances.
I. Chinese medical evaluation including a pulse reading.
J. (Psychological assessment to determine the degree of motivation, initiative, mood, and relative balance of depression and optimism.)

II. Psychosocial part of treatment program (designed to create and maintain positive self-image, attitudes, and expectations):
   A. GATHERING AND CREATING AN ORGANIZED SUPPORT SYSTEM.
      1. The support system should provide ongoing support to the patient for both material and emotional needs, as well as feedback and guidance in navigating the treatment program.
      2. The support system should consist of four to eight friends or relatives who are dedicated to seeing the patient through the duration of the illness and can meet regularly with the patient, individually or as a group.
      3. The members of the support system should become familiar with the treatment approach and actively participate with the patient. The members should delegate and divide tasks.
   B. REGULAR COUNSELING several times a week to work on expressing feelings that arise during the course of the program. A form of peer counseling—either permissive co-counseling or re-evaluation co-counseling—is most advantageous. Professional counseling may be utilized, however.
   C. Training in methods of DAILY RELAXATION. The simplest is to soak in a hot bath daily.
   D. Training in the SIMONTON DAILY VISUALIZATION METHOD.
   E. Training in methods to promote self-esteem. Options include

re-evaluation co-counseling; a study group of *A Course in Miracles;* the Center for Attitudinal Healing in Tiburon, California; and a study of the Vedanta or of Ericsonian hypnosis.

F. Keeping a personal journal of emotional insights and psychic or spiritual changes.

G. (Visual body-language feedback using videotape and camera so the patient can see his or her own appearance and demeanor. To be done during the third, fourth, and fifth months of treatment program.)

III. Nutrition and supplements:

A. DIET:

Ideally, one should first determine whether one has a sensitivity to certain foods and then exclude those foods from the diet. Food sensitivities are common and can be detected by special time-consuming food-challenge diets or by blood tests that take less time and cause less trouble but are somewhat less reliable than the diet tests. After food sensitivities are determined, the person can proceed with the following sequential diet, designed to restore the bowel to proper functioning. Whenever possible, all food should be organically grown and all water be bottled spring water.

1. (In extremely weakened individuals, intravenous hyperalimentation may be necessary for one to three weeks.)
2. First week: OBSERVE A SIMPLE LIQUID DIET: hatcho miso broth; fresh vegetable broths; vegetable juices such as carrot, celery, cucumber, watercress, beet, and melon; lentil broth; herbal teas; and spring water.
3. Second week: ADD COOKED FRESH, ORGANIC VEGETABLES to the liquid diet.
4. Third week: ADD COOKED GRAINS (brown rice, millet, barley, and buckwheat, for example), selecting those not in the patient's usual diet to avoid allergic reactions. Also ADD MEAT BROTHS.
5. Fourth week and beyond: Gradually ADD OTHER ORGANICALLY

GROWN OR RAISED FOODS INCLUDING MEAT AND FISH, watching for any unfavorable reactions to the new items.

6. During first four weeks, INCLUDE A SOURCE OF PREDIGESTED PROTEIN such as free amino acids or hydrolyzed lactalbumin (NOT protein powder). Start with 10 to 20 grams daily and increase to at most 40 to 50 grams daily, as tolerated. Gradually taper off the amount of predigested protein as more foods are added to the diet during the third and fourth weeks.

B. Vitamins and minerals:

1. Perque™ formulation of VITAMINS, MINERALS, ANTIOXIDANTS, AMINO ACIDS, AND LIPOTROPICS. This is a formulation with low allergenicity and high bioavailability. One dose consists of two tablets of Perque 1, two tablets of Perque 2, and one tablet of Perque 3 (formulas follow). The patient is to take one dose daily for the first week, two doses daily for the second week, and three doses daily for the subsequent four to twelve weeks, and then start to taper off to one dose daily. (Note: If the D-glucaric acid level remains elevated at twelve weeks, continue with three doses of Perque daily until this value normalizes. See V. E. 2.)
2. HIGH-DOSE ASCORBIC ACID (VITAMIN C): 80 to 180 grams daily by I.V. infusion. This can usually be administered at home by a visiting nurse or by the patient himself or herself (a subclavian vein catheter greatly facilitates administration of the ascorbate). The vitamin C can be administered as sodium ascorbate (from Bronson's Pharmaceuticals) or as a mixture of sodium, potassium, magnesium, and calcium ascorbates (from Sigma Lab) in a concentration of 60 grams per liter prepared in sterile water and passed through a 0.2-micron millipore filter. The vitamin C is given intravenously for three weeks and then by mouth every one or two hours, except during sleep, in the maximum amount the person can tolerate without developing diarrhea or other gastrointestinal distress

(that is, to bowel tolerance). The oral vitamin C should be taken in a buffered form. This reduces the acidity of the vitamin and also provides other minerals the body needs. The recommended product is called "C-Salts" (available from Wholesale Nutrition Club, P. O. Box 3345, Saratoga, CA 95070). Unbuffered vitamin C taken for several months can dissolve tooth enamel. Rinse the mouth with plain water after each dose of vitamin C.

3. OMEGA-3 AND OMEGA-6 FATTY ACIDS: These are essential nutrients required for the synthesis of certain hormones called prostaglandins and can be obtained from several natural oils. These oils are easily inactivated by exposure to heat and oxygen; therefore, they should be refrigerated at all times. Ideally, the bottle should be made of brown glass, and there should be some sediment at the bottom, indicating that natural tocopherols (vitamin E) are present. Unless a person is sensitive to a particular oil, two tablespoons daily of each of the following oils should be taken:
   a. edible linseed oil (Aubrey Organics recommended)
   b. cod liver oil (Dale Alexander or Schiff's recommended)
   c. sesame oil
   d. grape seed oil (check a French foods supplier for this oil).
4. (L-carnitine is given if the creatine/creatinine ratio is elevated [see sections I.E and VI.D.1]. Dose is 400 mg twice a day for three days, off for seven days, then 800 mg twice a day for three days, and finally tapering off as symptoms indicate. Twin Labs brand is recommended.)
5. (Biotin is given to promote beneficial bacterial growth and discourage yeast in the bowel. Take 1 mg a day, increasing gradually to 5 mg unless abdominal cramps develop. (The recommended brand is Bronson's Pharmaceuticals.)

C. Acidophilus is given to promote beneficial bacterial growth and discourage yeast in the bowel. One teaspoon three times a day of Maxidophilus brand is recommended. (If the patient is allergic or sensitive to milk, a soy-based brand such as Vitaldophilus can be used). The powder is mixed in a liquid and taken with meals to prevent destruction by stomach acids. Sugar-free yogurt, if tolerated, is a satisfactory source of acidophilus and can be used after the fourth week of the diet.

D. Herbal preparations: Certain herbs, called "adaptogens," enhance the body's ability to adapt to stress.
   1. A tea made of chopped ginger root is highly recommended. Brew a concentrated tea with two cups of water and three linear inches of ginger root chopped into small pieces. One cup of this tea, diluted to taste, should be taken daily over the course of the day. Fresh ginger can also be juiced with the vegetables in III.A.2 or cooked with the vegetable broth.
   2. Chinese ginseng extract, prepared by the Fmali Company in Santa Cruz, California (408/ 423–7913), may be taken in a dose of one ampoule per day.
   3. Shiitake mushroom powder, prepared by Scientific Consulting in Oakland, California (415/ 632–2370), may be taken by persons not sensitive to this mushroom. The recommended dose is take two capsules once or twice a day boiled for five minutes as a tea or cooked with food (heat helps release the active ingredients).
   4. *Echinacea augustifolia* or *E. purpura* taken in capsules or prepared in an infusion or tincture may be a general immune stimulant. The amount to take varies with the different preparations. Three capsules a day of freeze-dried *Echinacea* prepared are recommended.
   5. (Schizandra and ma huong are two other Asiatic herbs with adaptogenic properties. Ideally, these and other Asiatic herbs should be prescribed by someone skilled in Chinese herbology.)
   6. (A tea prepared from the bark of the pau d'arco tree, also known as taheebo, may be of benefit in suppressing candida overgrowth in the bowel or mouth. Amounts vary according to brand. The tea should be taken three times a day. Brew

enough tea for two days and refrigerate. Fuji Tea Company ([415] 457–5406) is a recommended brand.)

IV. Detoxification program:

A. TREATMENT OF PARASITIC INFESTATIONS if detected during the baseline evaluation. A particular herbal preparation containing *Artemesia annua* and *Valerian officinalis* is the preferred course of treatment. Cost is around $50 plus the cost of repeat parasite tests.

B. If the initial baseline tests showed elevated levels of organic toxins such as PCBs or insecticides, then a cool sauna (130° F) is recommended for thirty to sixty minutes at least five days a week.Immediately After the sauna, a cool shower should be taken, with vigorous cleansing of the skin to remove oils that may contain these fat-soluble toxins.

C. Chelation of heavy metals detected by baseline tests. Use either D-penicillamine or N-acetyl-penicillamine, 500 mg peroral four times a day, on alternate days, for two months; then repeat urine tests for heavy metals to evaluate treatment. [Editor's note: Long-term use of penicillamine can cause severe bone-marrow suppression and immune disorders. Although the D-form of the drug (DPA) is reported as less toxic, the value of DPA for heavy-metal chelation in people with AIDS may be marginal compared to its risks.—A. G. N.]

V. Ongoing monitoring:

A. The person undergoing treatment needs to MAINTAIN A DAILY LOG OF ACTIVITIES, DIET, VITAMIN AND HERBAL INTAKE, BODY WEIGHT, AND TEMPERATURE.

B. One week after starting high-level ascorbate intake, CHECK URINE FOR OXALATE AND CREATININE LEVELS during a twenty-four hour period. If elevated, monitor urinary oxalate daily or discontinue ascorbic acid. (In practice, the recommended level of ascorbic intake produces such an intense osmotic diuresis that the likelihood of renal lithiasis is remote at best. [Editor's note: The volume of urine is such that the formation of kidney stones from oxalates is unlikely.—A. G. N.]).

C. Every two weeks or so:
   1. PHYSICIAN SHOULD EXAMINE PATIENT and record weight, note size of KS lesions, palpate lymph nodes, record the occurrence of any infections, and note patient's sense of well-being and degree of compliance with treatment plan.
   2. OBTAIN COMPLETE BLOOD COUNT AND SEDIMENTATION RATE.

D. Every month or so:
   1. TEST FOR LIVER FUNCTION, SMAC, CREATINE/CREATININE RATIO (and optionally for beta-2 microglobulin and D-glucaric acid).
   2. Obtain Chinese pulse reading.

E. At three months and as indicated thereafter:
   1. REPEAT T-LYMPHOCYTE SUBSET TESTS.
   2. Repeat tests for neutrophil phagocytic index, platelet aggregation, D-glucaric acid urine catecholamines, stool fat, serum cortisols, and growth hormone levels *if* initial values were abnormal.
   3. Repeat toxin assays of sweat and urine.
   4. (Repeat MMPI, Eysenek index, Maslow actualization scale, and POMS.)

F. Other tests as indicated by the clinical condition of the patient.

VI. (All the following modalities are entirely optional and may be done if they sound worthwhile or interesting.

A. Breathing exercises are the easiest and the most important adjunct to the core program above. These exercises confer various benefits such as physical and mental relaxation, internal massage of the abdominal organs, and regulation of the autonomic nervous system. They should be performed for ten minutes two or three times a day and may be combined with other exercises.

B. Regular hatha yoga practice. Hatha yoga strengthens the body without producing exhaustion and stimulates the circulation of blood and, according to yoga pundits, of the *prana* or the body's vital energy, calming the mind and rejuvenating the body. The Iyengar variety of hatha yoga is especially recommended.

C. *Tai ji* (or *t'ai chi*), a Chinese discipline that combines movement and meditation.

D. Traditional Chinese acupuncture, provided it is performed by an experienced practitioner. Inexperienced practitioners and experimental forms of acupuncture may be deleterious.

E. Massage improves blood flow, relaxes muscles, produces a feeling of connectedness, and promotes self-worth and self-esteem.

F. Philosophical or religious inquiry to reduce fear of death and restore confidence and hope.

G. Art or music therapy. Participating in beauty can promote the will to live.

H. Humor can improve mental outlook and attitudes. Avoid the negativity of the daily newspapers.)

* * *

PERQUE FORMULATIONS

PERQUE 1

AMINO ACIDS

L-glycine	250 mg
L-phenylalanine	100 mg
L-methionine	100 mg
L-cystine + L-cysteine	250 mg
L-glutathione	1 mg

LIPOTROPICS

Choline	250 mg
Inositol	250 mg

PERQUE 2

VITAMINS

A	(Beta-carotene)	5,000 IU
B_1	(Thiamine)	100 mg
B_2	(Riboflavin)	50 mg

B_3	(Niacin + niacinamide)	100 mg
B_5	(Calcium pantothenate)	100 mg
B_6	(Pyridoxine)	200 mg
B_{12}	(Cyanocobalamine)	200 μg
Folic acid		800 μg
C	(Ascorbate, buffered)	100 mg
D_4	(OH-cholicalciferol)	400 IU
E	(Mixed tocopherols)	200 IU
F	(Octacosanol)	500 μg
K	(Phylioquinone)	0.5 mg
P	(Bioflavonoids)	10 mg
MINERALS		
Potassium		100 mg
Calcium		100 mg
Magnesium		200 mg
Zinc		25 mg
Chromium		200 μg
Manganese		100 μg
Selenium		50 μg
Vanadium		100 μg
COFACTORS		
Aspartate		100 mg
Betaine HCL		50 mg

PERQUE 3

LECITHIN	700 mg
Phosphatidylcholine	
Phosphatidylserine	
Phosphatidylethanolamine	

The Perque formulations can be ordered from EHI, 249 E. 48th St., Suite 7H, New York, NY 10017 ([212] 355–2347) and cost $75 for 100 doses as described in III.B.1 above. [Editor's note: One can substitute any other low-allergenicity, high-bioavailability formula or combination of vitamins that meets or exceeds the Perque dosages.—A. G. N.]

APPENDIX B

Drugs used in AIDS or ARC

DRUGS USED IN TREATING OPPORTUNISTIC INFECTIONS

Many of these drugs are the sole treatment for the disease in question even though they are not invariably effective and may exhibit serious side effects.

SEVERELY IMMUNOSUPPRESSIVE

DRUG	TRADE NAME	MAIN USE	OTHER SIDE EFFECTS
Adriamycin/ bleomycin/vinblastine	ABV	KS	Cf. bleomycin, vinblastine and vincristine
Cyclosporin A	Sandimmune	ARC	Kidney failure, anaphylaxis
Chloramphenicol	Chloromycetin	Salmonellosis	
D-penicillamine (DPA)	Cuprimine, Depen	ARC, HIV infection	High liver/kidney toxicity
Etoposide (VP-16-213)	VePesid	KS	
Pyrimethamine	Daraprim	Toxoplasmosis	Vomiting, CNS reactions
Vinblastine	Velban	KS	Death, hair loss
Vincristine	Oncovin	KS	Death, hair loss

MILDLY, OCCASIONALLY, OR REVERSIBLY IMMUNOSUPPRESIVE

DRUG	TRADE NAME	MAIN USE	OTHER SIDE EFFECTS
Azidothymidine	AZT	Antiviral for HIV	Anemia
DFMO		Cryptosporidiosis,PCP	Gastrointestinal
DHPG	Gancyclovir	Cytomegalovirus (CMV) infections	Thrombocytopenia, skin rashes
Flucytosine	Ancobon	Candidiasis, cryptococcosis	Liver impairment, nausea, diarrhea

DRUG	TRADE NAME	MAIN USE	OTHER SIDE EFFECTS
Isoniazid	INH tablets, Laniazid, Rifamate	Mycobacterium avium–intracellulare (MAI)	Nervous system reactions and liver toxicity
Rifampin	Rifadin, Rifamate, Rimactane	MAI	Kidney toxicity
Sulfadoxine-pyrimethamine	Fansidar	PCP	Fatal allergic reactions
Trimethoprim–sulfamethoxazole	Bactrim, Septra	PCP	Nervous system reaction, hypersensitivity to sulfonamides in AIDS

WITH OTHER SIDE EFFECTS

DRUG	TRADE NAME	MAIN USE	OTHER SIDE EFFECTS
Acyclovir	Zovirax	Herpes simplex and zoster infections	Some nausea, vomiting, and headache
Amphotericin B	Fungizone	Aspergillosis, candidiasis, MAI crytoccocal meningitis	Kidney toxicity
Azimexon	Investigational new drug (IND)	ARC (increases T cell count & ratio)	Hemolytic anemia
Bleomycin sulfate	Blenoxane	KS (27 percent stable remission rate)	Possible pulmonary failure, death
BW301	Under study	Toxoplasmosis	Folic acid antagonist reactions
Ciprofloxacin		Salmonellosis	No side effect data
Clindamycin	Cleocin Phosphate	Central nervous system (CNS) toxoplasmosis	Sometimes fatal colitis
Cycloserine	Seromycin	MAI	CNS reactions
Dapsone	Dapsone USP	PCP (in conjuction with other drugs)	Red blood cell loss, CNS reactions
Ethambutol	Myambutol	MAI	Loss of visual acuity
Ethionamide	Trecator–SC	MAI (in conjuction with other drugs)	Gastrointestinal, increases side effectsof other drugs
HPA 23 (Antimony tungstate complex)	IND.	HIV infection	Thrombocytopenia and kidney toxicity
Ketoconazole	Nizoral	Candidiasis	Liver toxicity
Metronidazole	Flagyl	Amebiasis, giardiasis	Neurotoxicity, gastrointestinal troubles
Miconazole	Monistat	Mycetoma caused by *Petriellidium boydii*	Phlebitis, pruritus, nausea sea, fever, chills, and rash
9-deazainosine	Under study	PCP	
Pentamidine isethionate	Pentam 300	PCP	Kidney toxicity

DRUG	TRADE NAME	MAIN USE	OTHER SIDE EFFECTS
Pentamidine, aerosol		PCP	Less toxic than IV pentamidine
Phosphonofarmate	Foscarnet	CMV infection, ARC, and KS	Kidney toxicity
Ribavarin	NDA as Virazole, IND for AIDS/ARC	HIV infection	Anemia, CNS toxicity, and inactivation of AZT
Rifabutin (available from CDC)	Ansamycin	MAI, ARC	Mild toxicity
Spiramycin	IND	Cryptosporidial diarrhea	No side effect data
Streptomycin		MAI	Hearing loss
Trimetrexate	Under study	PCP	Safe when used with a folinic acid supplement

EXPERIMENTAL DRUGS FOR UNDERLYING IMMUNODEFICIENCY

Drugs licensed by the Food and Drug Administration as investigational new drugs (INDs) have not been approved for sale and can be legally obtained only by participating in controlled clinical trials. An IND has to be proven safe and effective against a particular disease before the FDA grants it the new drug approval (NDA) status that permits marketing. Moreover, the FDA will allow testing an IND in humans only if satisfied by the results of animal toxicity tests, the nature of the proposed clinical trials, and the qualifications of the investigators.

Not every IND licensee can afford the costly three-phase process that brings a new drug to market. Phase I, usually a small-scale trial in a carefully selected group of patients, determines whether a drug is effective, and in what dosages, and uncovers unacceptable toxicities. Phase II, often double-blind tests on a larger number of patients, confirms phase I successes on a bigger and more reliable scale, deepens knowledge about the drug's therapeutic action, and documents most of its side effects. Phase III, distribution of the drug to all patients that meet trial criteria, gathers clinical and side-effect data from as many people as possible before the drug is released. Some small manufacturers who may be financially unable to bring a drug to market will submit detailed plans for the three trial phases anyhow and obtain an IND license, hoping that the initial small-scale trial of a promising drug will attract investment by the stock market or the partnership of larger drug companies.

A physician should prescribe a drug only for its FDA-approved use. A doctor who uses a drug against conditions other than those for which it was tested might not be breaking the law, but could be violating ethical standards and opening the door to a malpractice suit for nonstandard practice. In AIDS and ARC, however, fully effective treatment does not yet exist—there is no standardized practice—and the ethics of not letting a patient die often override those of using a drug in an unapproved or nonstandard way. Such de facto use of drugs is rather common in AIDS and ARC, often gathering impressive clinical data to justify more extensive and rigorous testing. In what could be either a move to sanction such practice or a response to appeals for compassion, the FDA is considering changing its regulations so as to make investigational new drugs available to patients of immediately life-threatening diseases.

As for drugs the FDA has not approved, no physician can prescribe these without getting into serious legal trouble, but he or she can monitor the progress of those patients who obtain the unapproved drug from outside sources, usually from countries that permit its use.

USED AS ANTIVIRALS OR IMMUNE ENHANCERS

DRUG	DESCRIPTION	ACTION AND SIDE EFFECTS	DRUG STATUS
AL 721	Lipid mixture from egg-yolk lecithin	Antiviral and immune enhancer.No observed side effects	IND. Phase II
Anti-inteferon immunoglobulin	Antibodies against acid labile alpha interferon	Immune enhancement by neutralizing this hyperproduced interferon. No observed toxicity.	IND. Phase I
Bestatin	An antiprotease compound	Unexplained immunoresto rative action with no observed side effects	Under study in France
Carrysin	Polymannoacetate, purified from an extract of the *Aloe barbadensis* plant.	Antiviral and immunomodulator producing reduced HIV antigen expression and improved clinical condition.	IND. Protocol development

DRUG	DESCRIPTION	ACTION AND SIDE EFFECTS	DRUG STATUS
CL 246,738	A heterocyclic compound related to coal-tar dyes.	Induces interferon and augments NK cell activity and B an d T cell function. Toxicity unknown	IND. Phase I
CS-85	Dideoxiethyluridine, an analogue of AZT	May be less toxic than AZT	Pre-clinical
Deoxythymidine	A nucleoside derivative	Synergistic antiviral effect even with marginal doses of dideoxycytidine. Toxicity unknown	Unknown
Dideoxicytidine	A nucleoside analogue	Antiviral activity similar to yet greater than that of AZT. No discernible bone-marrow suppression observed	IND. Phase I
Exovir-HZ gel	A combination of alpha interferon and the spermicide nonoxynol-9	May prevent HIV transmission	In vitro effectiveness and human toxicity trials
Gamma globulin		Immune modulator used in pediatric AIDS	Open study
Gamma interferon	White blood cell immunoregulator	No clinical improvement in AIDS, ARC, or KS	IND
Glucan	A biological response modifier isolated from brewer's yeast	Proliferates and activates macrophages and their lymphokines. Transient chills, fevers, and headaches	IND. Open study
GM-CSF	Human recombinant granulocyte and macrophage colony stimulating factor	Increases granulocytes and macrophages but also confers anti-HIV properties on bone marrow stem cells.	IND. Phase I
Guanosine derivatives	C-8 substituted guanine ribonucleotides: 8-bromoguanosine, 8-mercaptoguanosine	In vitro HIV inhibition and enhancement of induced lymphocyte proliferation	Pre-clinical
HIVA	Human immune virus antiviral reportedly produced by microrganisms	Press and stock market reports describe HIVA as a potent transcriptase inhibitor	Pre-IND. Pre-clinical
Imreg-1	A leukocyte-derived polypeptide immunoregulator	Helps remaining T cells produce more lymphokines and mount delayed reactions to recall antigens. No toxicity	IND. Phase II random blind
Imreg-2	Immunoregulator		IND.

DRUG	DESCRIPTION	ACTION AND SIDE EFFECTS	DRUG STATUS
	similar to Imreg-1	Noa data at this time	Open study
Interleukin-2	A lymphokine that proliferates activated T cells	In HIV-infected T cells, IL-2 produces no clinical improvement and may worsen condition.	IND. Phase I ended
Lamprene	A leprosy drug	Antiviral being tested in 225 AIDS patients. No other data	
Methionine-enkephalin	An opioid compound produced by the body	Increases NK number and activity, IL-2 production, and helper T cell count. Side effect data not available	IND. Pilot study
Neurotropin	Nonprotein extract from rabbit skin tissue infected by vaccinia virus	T-cell potentiator that may have produced a rise in helper T cell in AIDS and ARC. Flulike side effects	No IND. Japanese pilot study
Peptide T	The part of the HIV glycoprotein envelope that may attach to helper T cells	Blocks HIV infection of T cells by competition or by antibody stimulation. May require continuous IV treatment	IND submitted
Rifabutin (Ansamycin)	A rifamycin-derived antibiotic alsoused for MAI infections	Inhibits HIV replication by binding to reverse transcriptase. Good cell penetration. Reversible liver toxicity.	IND for AIDS/ARC Phase I/II
Silicotungstate (ST)	Antiviral similar to HPA-23	In vitro HIV inhibition	
Suramin	A drug used against African sleeping sickness	In vitro HIV inhibitor, failed to produce clinical or immunologic improment and had unacceptable toxicity	Studies closed
Thymic humoral factor	A hormone that establishes and maintains cellular immune function	Increase in count and mitogenic response in helper T cells	Clinical testing in Israel
Thymosin alpha-1 antisera	An antiserum that neutralizes HIV and blocks its replication		Pre-clinical
Transfer factor	A polypeptide from peripheral blood lymphocytes of cell-mediated immunity	Transfers immunological specificity to nonsensitized T cells thus producing modest immune enhancement	IND. Pilot study
Xanthate compound D609	A xanthic acid derivative combined with an ionic detergent for penetration	In vitro antiviral activity that does not affect mitotis in uninfected control cells	Pre-clinical in Germany

USED IN AIDS-RELATED KAPOSI'S SARCOMA

DRUG	DESCRIPTION	ACTION AND SIDE EFFECTS	DRUG STATUS
ABPP	A pyrimidine derivative	Stimulates NK cell activity and macrophage mediated cytotoxicity. Some nausea, vomiting, and tachycardia	IND. Phase I
Alpha interferon		Tumor regression in 30 percent of KS patients. Fatigue, fever, chills, myalgias, and headaches	IND. Phase I
DNCB	Dinitrochlorobenzene-	Increase in helper T cell counts in some patients	Not approved
MT-PE	Muramyl tripeptide, also known as CGP 19835A, when lipid encapsulated	Stimulates tumoricidal action of monocytes and macrophages, known to be deficient in KS. Nontoxic when encapsulated in dipalmitoylphosphatidyletha nolamine (PE)	IND. Phase I
Protein A column	(Prosorba) Extacorporeal plasma filtration through through an immunosorbent protein column	Removal of IgG, immune complexes and autoantibodies has produced tumor shrinkage and increased platelets.	Approved medical device. Open pilot study

USED IN ARC OR PROGRESSIVE GENERALIZED LYMPHADENOPATHY (PGL)

DRUG	DESCRIPTION	ACTION AND SIDE EFFECTS	DRUG STATUS
Ampligen	A mismatched, double-stranded RNA molecule	Antiviral eliciting production of RNase L, which degrades double-stranded RNA in a cell including HIV genome	IND. Phase I
Immuthiol (DDTC)	Sodium diethyldithiocarbamate, a low molecular weight sulfur compound	Induces T cell diferentiation and increases helper T cells and delayed type hypersensitivity. Antabuse-like side effects	IND approved
Isoprinosine	A synthetic immunopotentiating agent	Has produced increased NK cell activity, helper T cell count, and helper/suppressor ratio. No notable toxicity	IND Double blind placebo
Lithium carbonate	An antipsychotic drug with possible immune enhacing properties	No clinical data yet available	IND for psych use
Naltrexone	A narcotic antagonist with possible immune enhacing properties	Increases lymphocyte opium receptors andtheir sensitivity	

DRUG	DESCRIPTION	ACTION AND SIDE EFFECTS	DRUG STATUS
		thus enhancing endorphin enkephalin inmmune regulation No side effects at dosage for AIDS/ARC	NDA as narcotic antagonist Random double-blind
Thymopentin (TP-5)	A synthetic peptide with immunoregulating activity similar to that of thymopoietin	Induces maturation of T cell precursors and immature T cells both in vitro and in vivo	IND. Double blind
Thymostimulin (TP-1)	A partially purified extract of calf thymus gland	No data at this time	
Zinc gluconate	A chelated esssential mineral	In France, doses of 125 mg twice daily for three weeks produced increased helper T cell count and helper/supresser ratio. No observed side effects	

Sources:

Michael S. Gottlieb, Michael H. Grieco, Lucy N. Painter, and Seymour Bernstein, editors.
AmFAR Periodical Directory of Experimental Treatments for AIDS and ARC.
American Foundation for AIDS Research (AmFAR), 15 March 1987.

CDC AIDS Weekly :3, 9 February 1987.
Experimental AIDS therapies: Drug and treatment wrap-up.

Martin S. Hirsch and Joan C. Kaplan.
Antiviral therapy.
Scientific American 256(4):76, April 1987.

1987 Physician's Desk Reference.

APPENDIX C

Vitamin C in the treatment of acquired immune deficiency syndrome (AIDS)*

by Robert F. Cathcart , III, M. D.

ABSTRACT

My previous experience with the utilization of ascorbic acid in the treatment of viral diseases led me to hypothesize that ascorbate would be of value in the treatment of AIDS (acquired immune deficiency syndrome). Preliminary clinical evidence is that massive doses of ascorbate (50–200 grams per 24 hours) can suppress the symptoms of the disease and can markedly reduce the tendency for secondary infections. In combination with usual treatments for the secondary infections, large doses of ascorbate will often produce a clinical remission which shows every evidence of being prolonged if treatment is continued. This clinical remission is achieved despite continuing laboratory evidence of helper T-cell suppression. There may be a complete or partial destruction of the helper T-cells during an initial infection that does not necessitate a continuing toxicity from some source to maintain a permanent or prolonged helper T-cell suppression. However, it is possible ascorbate may prevent that destruction

*Reprinted, with changes, from Robert F. Cathcart, III, "Vitamin C in the treatment of acquired immune deficiency syndrome (AIDS)," *Medical Hypotheses* 14:423-433, 1984, by permission of Longman Group UK, Ltd. Copyright 1984 by Churchill Livingsone.

if used adequately during the prodrome period. Emphasis is put upon the recognition and treatment of the frequent intestinal parasites. Food and chemical sensitivities occur frequently in the AID syndrome and may aggravate symptoms considered to be part of the AID syndrome. A topical C-paste has been found very effective in the treatment of herpes simplex and, to a lesser extent, in the treatment of some Kaposi's lesions. Increasingly, clinical research on other methods of treating AIDS is being "contaminated" by patients taking ascorbate.

INTRODUCTION

I had previously described that the amount of ascorbic acid which can be tolerated by a patient without producing diarrhea, increases somewhat proportionately to the toxicity of his disease (1,2,3,4). Among the roughly 80% of persons who tolerate ascorbic acid very well, *bowel tolerance* will be reached when in excess of 10 to 15 grams of ascorbic acid dissolved in water is taken in 4 to 6 divided doses per 24 hours. The astonishing finding was that when that same person is acutely ill with a mild cold, that tolerance may increase to approximately 50 grams per 24 hours. A severe cold can increase tolerance to 100 grams; an influenza, even up to 150 grams; and mononucleosis or viral pneumonias, to as much as 200 grams per 24 hours. These higher doses may have to be divided as frequently as hourly.

These large amounts of ascorbate are being drawn off the GI tract at a rate sufficient to prevent significant amounts from reaching the rectum and producing diarrhea. Measurements of ascorbate in urine, saliva, or serum indicate that if sufficient doses of ascorbate are not given when the patient is ill, the body level of vitamin C drops rapidly. In such a case, there is not enough vitamin C left in the body, particularly in the cells directly involved by the disease, to guarantee all the known housekeeping functions of the vitamin. Those functions known to be dependent on vitamin C, including several metabolic reactions necessary for proper functioning of the immune system, are put at risk of malfunctioning. I call this *acute induced scurvy*.

PREMIERE FREE RADICAL SCAVENGER

The reason ascorbate ameliorates so many conditions in that it functions as the *premiere free radical scavenger* (5). This function is not because it is the most powerful free radical scavenger, but because it is possible to saturate every cell of the body with more molecules of ascorbate than any other free radical scavenger. The reason that it takes such massive doses for optimal effect is because high concentrations of ascorbate must be driven into the cells directly affected by the disease process sufficient to neutralize all of the free radical produced by that process, and have some left over for vitamin C housekeeping functions. When a disease process involves free radicals, that disease process is capable of being ameliorated by massive doses of ascorbate. In the case of many infectious diseases, the relief from free radical suppression of the immune system, allows for more effective attack on the pathogen by that immune system.

Note: this premiere free radical scavenger function has little to do with nutrition but is a pharmacologic effect of ascorbate when utilized in unnatural amounts for humans.

Actually, the complete neutralization of free radicals requires several steps involving other substances, e.g. glutathione. However clinically, the most frequent limiting factor in the reduction of free radicals is ascorbate. In certain conditions such as chemical allergies, certain other limiting factors may become critically important, e.g. selenium and glutathione. Some have worried that a buildup of dehydroascorbate would be toxic in certain of these conditions. Clinically, this consideration has not created a problem when very large doses of ascorbate are used. Perhaps it is the large ratio of ascorbate to dehydroascorbate, I am careful to maintain in these patients, that protects against any temporarily accumulating dehydroascorbate. Further, I should like to point out that the dehydroascorbate formed should not be as toxic as that free radical the ascorbate reduces as it itself is oxidized into dehydroascorbate.

In a way, it is unfortunate that this free radical scavenger and vitamin C are the same substance. When ascorbate is destroyed in the process of destroying free radicals, the vitamin C stores, particularly in the cells directly involved in the disease process, are so depleted as to cause disorders of known housekeeping functions of vitamin C.

It is certain that AIDS causes this depletion. The sicker the patient is, the more ascorbate will be destroyed by the disease process. This depletion certainly contributes to the terminal events and probably plays a key role in the increased susceptibility of AIDS patients to various pathogens.

ASCORBATE VS. AN AIDS SUPPRESSOR FACTOR

A recent article describes the discovery of a *suppressor factor* in AIDS patients. This suppressor factor was found to be neutralized in the test tube by concentrations of ascorbate equivalent to that which would be achieved in a man who ingested 10 to 20 grams of ascorbate a day. It was thought that this amount was *"far too toxic"* to use in humans and that a less toxic antioxidant should be found (6).

Actually, 10 to 20 grams/24 hours of ascorbate is easily tolerated and is not toxic (1,2,3,4,7,8,9,10,11,12,13,14). Unfortunately, clinically I have shown that the AIDS disease process destroys even larger amounts of ascorbate than the 10 to 20 grams because bowel tolerance is regularly increased to the range of 40 to 185 grams of C per 24 hours in the patient who has moderate Kaposi's lesions and/or moderate lymphadenopathy. *Therefore, the 10 to 20 gram equivalent of ascorbate in the test tube will not be adequate in vivo.*

PRELIMINARY STUDY

Because of the hypothesis that AIDS patients would benefit from large doses of ascorbate, I began the actual treatment of AIDS patients and have found that ascorbate is indeed very valuable when used in conjunction with certain conventional treatments.

The following preliminary recommendations are based partly upon an anecdotal group of approximately 90 AIDS patients who sought medical care from physicians but who also took high doses of ascorbate on their own. Additionally, it is based upon 12 of my AIDS patients, 6 of whom were given intravenous ascorbate for a short period of time. Most of these patients have had considerable improvement in their condition. This improvement seems somewhat proportional to the amount of ascorbate taken by the patient relative to the severity of his disease. If the patient tolerates enough ascorbate to "neutralize the toxicity" of his disease and if the secondary infections are treated; his condition will go into remission. Subjectively, symptoms decrease and increase inversely with how closely the patient titrates to bowel tolerance.

The only death has been in a patient who had previous chemotherapy, interferon, and total body X-ray therapy. Additionally, his veins were so destroyed be previous treatment that intravenous vitamin C therapy could not be continued under the existing circumstances.

Such a preliminary report of recommendations is justified only because of the urgency of the problem and because in San Francisco and now New York, news of the ascorbate treatments is spreading rapidly. Ascorbate is being used by an increasing percentage of the AIDS patient population but without much guidance. There have been many requests by physicians for the treatment protocol.

ASCORBATE TREATMENT PROTOCOL FOR AIDS PATIENTS

The following protocol is recommended for AIDS and AIDS related conditions including lymphadenopathy, idiopathic thrombocytopenia purpura, and Pneumocystis carinii pneumonia.

As predicted, AIDS patients are usually capable of ingesting large doses of ascorbate. It is desirable that the amount of ascorbate taken orally be maximized. Patients are *titrated to bowel tolerance* (the amount that almost, but not quite, causes diarrhea). A *balanced ascorbate* mixture is utilized which is made up of approximately 25% buffered ascorbate salts (calcium, magnesium, and potassium ascorbate) and 75% ascorbic acid. This mixture is dissolved in a small amount of water and taken at least every hour. The purpose of the frequent doses and this balanced mixture is to maximize the amount of ascorbate tolerated without producing diarrhea. Patients are permitted to vary the percentage of ascorbate salts to straight ascorbic acid according to taste. The usual amount tolerated initially is between 40 and 100 grams per 24 hours. *Doses in excess of 100 grams per hour may be necessary with secondary bacterial and viral infections.* As the patient's condition improves, bowel tolerance will decrease.

When intravenous ascorbate is found necessary because the toxicity of the condition exceeds the ability of the patient to take adequate amounts of ascorbate to scavenge all of the free radicals created by the primary AIDS infections and the various secondary infections, the following intravenous solutions should be utilized. Sodium ascorbate buffered to a pH 7.4 and without preservatives is added to sterile water in a concentration of 60 grams per 500 cc. This concentration is twice the concentration I have recommended before because it is well tolerated in young males with large veins. Patients with small veins may be best treated with solutions of 60 grams per liter. The time of the infusions should be over at least a 3 hour period, preferably longer. As much as daily administration of 3 bottles, 180 grams per 24 hours, may be necessary in acutely ill patients, e.g. Pneumocystis carinii pneumonia, disseminated herpes, disseminated cytomegalovirus, and atypical pneumonia. Enough ascorbate should be administered to detoxify the patient regardless of the amount needed. Additionally, oral doses of ascorbate should be taken simultaneously with the intravenous ascorbate. *Do not let the patients become lazy and discontinue bowel tolerance doses of ascorbate while the intravenous ascorbate is being administered.*

INTESTINAL PARASITES

If the AIDS patient has intestinal parasites, he must be treated for them. There is a very high percentage of male homosexuals infected with intestinal parasites. These intestinal parasites are themselves very immunosuppressive. The prognosis for an AIDS patient is greatly enhanced by proper treatment of these parasites. *Entamoeba histolytica,* especially, and *Giardia lamblia* must be treated. Intestinal parasites, ordinarily considered *nonpathogens,* should be treated. If negative, repeated stool examinations for ova and parasites should be taken if there is the slightest clinical sign of intestinal parasite infection. Samples should be fresh, not over one-half hour old. Laxatives may increase chances of discovering the parasites. Additional samples may have to be taken through a sigmoidoscope if other specimens are negative for ova and parasites. With treatment, Herxheimer's reactions should be expected frequently. Symptoms, including Kaposi's lesions, may be exacerbated, despite the ascorbate, during treatment for intestinal parasites.

CANDIDA ALBICANS

Candida should be sought and treated. It should be emphasized to patients that they owe it to themselves and society to treat the candida consistently because of the possibility of breeding resistant strains. The possibility of candida in the gut, mouth, esophagus, skin, etc. should be considered. In patients who clinically appear to have candida but in whom candida cannot be cultured, sensitivities to candida should be suspected and treatment of especially the bowel should be considered. Herxheimer's reactions, when antibiotics against candida are employed, should be considered one indication that candida is a problem. In these sensitive patients, foods and vitamins containing yeasts should be avoided. Lactobacillus in large amounts should be fed to these patients in an attempt to normalize bowel flora. Sugar and refined carbohydrates should be avoided because candida thrives on them.

There is a high incidence of food and chemical sensitivities associated with candida sensitivities (15,16,17) and candida must be suspected whenever such sensitivities are discovered.

FOOD AND CHEMICAL SENSITIVITIES

Food and chemical sensitivities, both IgE mediated allergies and enzymatic deficiency allergies (EDAs), are common because of the disorders of the immune system and the severe stress imposed by the AID syndrome. This increased incidence of sensitivities may be associated with candida, as discussed above, but may also be a result of the AIDS infection. Rashes, edema, phlebitis, etc. caused by corn, yeast (including yeast containing vitamins), molds, house gas, automobile exhaust, certain herbal formulas, cosmetics, formaldehyde, insecticides, paint, glues and cigarette smoke have all been observed in my small group of patients. Conditions such as Kaposi's lesions, lymphadenopathy, and probably idiopathic thrombocytopenia purpura, conditions which would otherwise just be considered part of the AID syndrome or AIDS related, have been seen to be aggravated by food and chemical sensitivities. These sensitivities should be anticipated and offending substances should be removed from the patient's diet and environment. Ascorbate may not block these sensitivities significantly; however, ascorbate may decrease the intensity and duration of the reaction in such a way as to make clinical discovery of the offending substance easier.

This increased incidence of food and chemical sensitivities is very important to understand because apparent adverse reactions to vitamin C may occur. These reactions are almost never due to the ascorbate itself. Most ascorbate is made from corn. Minute amounts of chemicals used in the manufacture of ascorbate may remain. Residuals of these substances are almost invariably the cause of the sensitivity reactions. Ascorbates made from sego palm or from tapioca and which presumably are manufactured with some different chemicals, are often tolerated. Different brands should be tried. It is almost always possible to find some ascorbate that is tolerated. This sensitivity problem is very important to deal with because patients frequently feel their life depends on taking adequate amounts of ascorbate and they may be correct in this feeling.

Many time gastrointestinal discomfort and excessive gas can be alleviated by changing to the sego palm ascorbate or changing brands of ascorbate.

OTHER CONSIDERATIONS

Bacterial infections should be treated with appropriate antibiotics but large amounts of lactobacillus should be administered with foods if there is the slightest tendency to candida infections or sensitivities. Ascorbate administration should be intensified during treatment for bacterial infections. Intravenous ascorbate may be necessary.

Viral infections should be treated with intensification of the ascorbate treatment. Intravenous ascorbate may become necessary.

Immunosuppressive therapy should not be utilized.

Sugar and processed foods, foods with chemicals, recreational drugs, cigarettes, alcohol, etc. should be avoided. Obvious nutritional deficits should be sought and corrected. Additional supplementation with especially zinc and selenium may be helpful.

All sharing of body fluids and fecal material should stop (18). Repeated exposures, not only to possible AIDS infection, but to the secondary infections, especially intestinal parasites and candida should be avoided.

HELPER SUPPRESSOR CELL RATIO

With this protocol, it may be anticipated that a large percentage of patients will slowly go into an extended clinical remission. Patients must be on guard to sense any impending infection, colds, etc. The patient should begin the additional large doses of ascorbate within minutes. At the dose levels that have been possible under circumstances imposed, a slow improvement of the total number of T-lymphocytes may occur but helper/suppressor cell ratios may remain suppressed. It appears that ascorbate may assist the immune system, but that in addition, there are mechanisms whereby ascorbate acts against pathogens, especially viruses and bacteria by mechanisms which do not depend on the T-cells. For this reason, I would suggest using the ascorbate portion of this protocol on children who have to be permanently isolated from the slightest exposure to infections (bubble babies).

MONITORING VALUE OF ASCORBATE "BURN"

Roughly to the degree that a patient clinically perceives himself to feel toxic (the amount of malaise, fever, pain, how swollen the lymph nodes, how much anxiety, etc.), the more ascorbic acid can be tolerated orally without it producing diarrhea. The amount tolerated becomes a rough measurement of something that represents the immediate toxicity of the condition. I use the expression "100 gram cold" to mean that at the peak of the cold a patient tolerated 100 grams per 24 hours of ascorbic acid without diarrhea. In cases where I am not sure what is causing an increased tolerance or if a person is multiply ill with several secondary infections, I refer to the processes going on which are using up the ascorbate as the *"burn."* Note that the amount of ascorbic acid tolerated is only a good measure of this burn if it is the amount determined by titrating to "true" bowel tolerance, i.e., diarrhea caused by ascorbic acid in a patient who otherwise tolerates ascorbate well; not limits set by "too much gas", "don't like the taste", "stomach too acid", etc.

The amount of this burn has some practical and prognostic values; e.g., a patient with a burn much over 25–30 grams almost inevitably has something the matter with him and a thorough diagnostic workup is indicated. A lover of one of the AIDS patients had a burn of 100 grams. It was found that his helper/suppressor T-cell ratio was 0.7 but he had no other signs of disease. Over a six month period, the burn dropped to 25 grams. AIDS has not been diagnosed in this patient but there is good reason to suspect that he has a pre-AIDS condition. The AIDS patient himself has had his burn drop from 125 grams to 35 grams. His lymphadenopathy has improved considerably.

AIDS POSSIBLY INVOLVING A PERMANENT OR PROLONGED LOSS OF T HELPER CELLS

One patient who managed to eliminate all signs of Kaposi's lesions while taking ascorbic acid had had his burn down to 15 grams a day for 6 months despite the helper/suppressor T-cell ratio remaining at 0.2. There had been some slight increase in the absolute number of helper and suppressor cells. Previously detected shedding of CMV (cytomegalovirus) had apparently stopped. This patient had 3 Kaposi's lesions (diagnosed as Kaposi's sarcoma on biopsy) recur on the right foot following a cold, herpes simplex, and influenza, all within a 2 month period. The burn markedly increased, peaking at 185 grams per 24 hours. In 2 weeks time, the patient had managed to eliminate all signs of the lesions on the foot. The ascorbate burn slowly has lessened; now 2 months later, the burn is at 25 grams and decreasing.

This case, plus the previous two cases, strongly suggest that the basic AIDS infection, probably caused by a virus, is no longer active in these cases and that subsequent ascorbate burns and various later manifestations of the AID syndrome are caused by secondary and opportunistic infections. One is reminded of the permanent damage of certain viral infections in association with certain predisposing factors initiating an immune response to the beta cells of the islets of Langerhans and causing juvenile-onset diabetes (19).

ASCORBATE AND THE POSSIBLE PREVENTION OF AIDS

Morishige has demonstrated the effectiveness of ascorbate in preventing hepatitis B from blood transfusions (20). A similarity exists between AIDS and hepatitis B. It has been my experience that patients treated with large doses of ascorbate during the acute phase of hepatitis will not develop chronic hepatitis. My experience with herpes simplex has been the same. Although ascorbate is helpful to a degree with chronic viral infections, it is in the treatment of acute viral diseases that it is most effective.

It is on this basis that I recommend that all persons who fear exposure to AIDS and certainly anyone receiving blood transfusions or other products which could in the most remote way have been obtained from an AIDS carrier, be put on bowel tolerance doses of ascorbate.

CONTROLLED STUDIES OF OTHER SUBSTANCES CONTAMINATED WITH ASCORBATE

As a result of publications in periodicals concerned about the AID syndrome, (21,22) a rapidly increasing number of AIDS patients in the San Francisco Bay Area are taking large doses of ascorbate. The same practice is starting it New York and elsewhere. I would suggest that physicians conducting controlled experiments on interferon, and shortly with interleukin 2, be sensitive to the fact that their patients are, and will be contaminating the experiment with massive doses of ascorbate. Statistical analysis of the results of such trials will probably be valueless. Ascorbate has been contaminating cancer treatment studies for some time as a result of orthomolecular literature (23,24,25). I estimate that a significant increasing percentage of cancer patients in California and other parts of the world are taking massive doses of ascorbate. Most of these patients are hiding this fact from their oncologist.

POSSIBLE ELIMINATION OF THE AIDS SYNDROME

Practical considerations (lack of money and lack of hospital facilities) have prevented me from administering the doses of ascorbate which I think might *possibly* eliminate the probable viral infection initiating the AID syndrome. I suggest that the helper/suppressor T-cell ratios should be carefully monitored while at least 180 grams/24 hours of ascorbate is administered intravenously. At the same time bowel tolerance doses of ascorbate should be taken orally. This program should be followed over an extended period of time (minimum 2 weeks) to find out if there is any direct effect on the process causing the AIDS.

I have preliminary evidence in one patient in which the above program was tried that while the secondary problems were markedly suppressed by the ascorbate (7 lbs 11 oz in 14 days) that the basic AIDS condition was not reversed. This case plus the cases implying the permanent or prolonged suppression of the immune system make it essential to treat the prodrome stages of AIDS with ascorbate.

If there is not a complete elimination of the basic AIDS process, bowel tolerance doses of ascorbate and the rest of the described protocol will probably have to be maintained for life.

My experience (1,2,3,4) and the experience of other researchers (10,11,12,13,14,20,26,27) is that acute self limiting viral diseases can be reliably cured with massive doses of ascorbate. Viral diseases that have become chronic seem to involve pathologic processes which are not quite as susceptible to ascorbate but which nevertheless are ameliorated, sometimes seemingly cured. It is hoped that funds will be made available for such a project.

C-PASTE

Herpes simplex lesions can usually be made to more rapidly heal or be prevented at the outset by increasing the doses of oral ascorbic acid and the application of C-paste. C-paste is made with either ascorbic acid or sodium ascorbate with water applied directly to the skin and covered with a bandage. Frequently, one application will suffice for herpes. Care should be taken not to irritate intact skin too much in sensitive skin areas, especially under adhesive bandages. Frequently applications to intact skin where the patient perceives an outbreak is about to occur will completely abort the attack. Several applications may be necessary to penetrate through the intact skin.

C-paste has also been useful on early Kaposi's lesions. It should be applied up to 4 times a day. Alternatively, soaks of 20% sodium ascorbate or ascorbic acid (1 gram per 5 cc of water) for 15–30 minutes, 4 times a day may be helpful. Be careful not to irritate the skin too much even with these solutions. Keep ascorbic acid out of the eyes; a 20% *sodium ascorbate* solution can be used in the eyes with care.

KAPOSI'S LESIONS

Kaposi's lesions have been described as behaving like an infectious disease closely associated with CMV (28). With ascorbate treatment, Kaposi's lesions may be made to go away if the patient takes enough ascorbate and the patient is not burdened by multiple opportunistic infections. In patients with multiple problems, there tend to be outbreaks of the Kaposi's lesions associated with colds, parasites, herpes, or emotional stress and particularly associated with a letdown in the amount of C taken. Even in patients with multiple lesions, individual lesions can frequently be seen to lose color and flatten with the local application of ascorbate soaks.

CONCLUSIONS

Ascorbate does ameliorate the AID syndrome to a significant degree. I want to emphasize, however, the absolute necessity of massive doses. Additionally, one must avoid or treat opportunistic infections. Multiple infections, lack of understanding in the use of C, or inability to tolerate the doses prescribed, all result in a poor prognosis. The success of treatments with ascorbate entirely depends on consistent administration of C sufficient to neutralize the free radicals produced by the various diseases.

The use of ascorbate is increasing in the male homosexual population of the San Francisco Bay Area and spreading across the United States. It will be very interesting to see if there are any otherwise unexplained decreases in the rate of increase of new cases of AIDS and associated deaths starting in San Francisco. The use of C is contaminating otherwise thought to be controlled studies of other therapeutic measures. Other considerations plus the potential application of ascorbate as part of the treatment of all infectious diseases, makes the clarification of the usefulness of ascorbate to the medical profession essential.

CAUTION

If these oral solutions are used over a long period of time, care should be taken to keep them off the teeth by using a straw in order to avoid enamel damage. Sickle cell anemia and G-6-PD deficiencies should be ruled out where indicated. In any condition requiring prolonged administration of large amounts of any nutrient, I would advice seeking the advice of a specialist to avoid induced deficiencies in other nutrients.

REFERENCES

1. Cathcart, R. F. Clinical trial of vitamin C. Letter to the Editor, *Medical Tribune*, June 25, 1975.
2. Cathcart, R. F. The method of determining proper doses of vitamin C for the treatment of disease by titrating to

bowel tolerance. *J. Orthomolecular Psychiatry*, 10:125–132, 1981.

3. Cathcart, R. F. Vitamin C: titrating to bowel tolerance, anascorbemia, and acute induced scurvy. *Medical Hypotheses*, 7:1359–1376, 1981.
4. Cathcart, R. F. C-vitaminbehandling till tarmintolerans vid infektioner och allergi. *Biologisk Medicin*, 3:6–8, 1983.
5. Cathcart, R. F. Vitamin C function in AIDS. Current Opinion, *Medical Tribune*, July 13, 1983.
6. Laurence, J. The mystery factor that's destroying immunity. *American Health*, May/June 1983.
7. Stone, I. *The Healing Factor: Vitamin C against Disease*. Grosset and Dunlap, New York, 1972.
8. Pauling, L. *Vitamin C and the Common Cold*. Freeman and Company, San Francisco, 1970.
9. Pauling, L. *Vitamin C, the Common Cold and the Flu*. Freeman and Company, San Francisco, 1976.
10. Klenner, F. R. Virus pneumonia and its treatment with vitamin C. *J. South. Med. and Surg.*, 110:60–63, 1948.
11. Klenner, F. R. The treatment of poliomyelitis and other virus diseases with vitamin C. *J. South. Med. and Surg.*, 111:210–214, 1949.
12. Klenner, F. R. Massive doses of vitamin C and the virus diseases. *J. South. Med. and Surg.*, 113:101–107, 1951.
13. Klenner, F. R. Observations on the dose and administration of ascorbic acid when employed beyond the range of a vitamin in human pathology. *J. App. Nutr.*, 23:61–88, 1971.
14. Kalokerinos, A. *Every Second Child*. Keats Publishing, Inc., New Canaan, 1981.
15. Truss, C. O. Tissue injury produced by *Candida albicans:* Mental and neurologic manifestations. *J. Orthomolecular Psychiatry*, 7,1:17–37, 1978.
16. Truss, C. O. Restoration of immunologic competence to *Candida albicans*. *J. Orthomolecular Psychiatry*, 9,4:287–301, 1980.
17. Truss, C. O. The role of *Candida albicans* in human illness. *J. Orthomolecular Psychiatry*, 10,4:228–238, 1981.
18. Mavligit, G. M., Talpaz, M., Hsia, F. T., Wong, W., Lichtiger, B., Mansell, W. A., Mumford, D. M. Chronic immune stimulation by sperm alloantigens. *JAMA*, 251:237–241, 1984.
19. Notkins, A. L. The causes of diabetes. *Scientific American*, 241,5:62–73, Nov. 1979.
20. Murata, A. Virucidal activity of vitamin C: Vitamin C for the prevention and treatment of viral diseases. *Proceeding of the First Intersectional Congress of Microbiological Societies*, Science Council of Japan, 3:432–42, 1975.
21. Cathcart, R. F. Vitamin C function in AIDS. *Bay Area Reporter*, p. 18, Nov. 17, 1983.
22. Cathcart, R. F. Vitamin C treatment protocol for AIDS. *Bay Area Reporter*, pp. 14–15, Jan. 5, 1984.
23. Cameron, E. and Pauling, L. Supplemental ascorbate in the supportive treatment of cancer: Prolongation of survival times in terminal human cancer. *Proc. Natl. Acad. Sci. USA*, 73:3685–3689, 1976.
24. Cameron, E. and Pauling, L. The orthomolecular treatment of cancer: Reevaluation of prolongation of survival times in terminal human cancer. *Proc. Natl. Acad. Sci. USA*, 75:4538–4542, 1978.
25. Cameron, E. and Pauling, L. *Cancer and Vitamin C*. The Linus Pauling Institute for Science and Medicine, Menlo Park, 1979.
26. Belfield, W. O. Vitamin C in the treatment of canine and feline distemper complex. *Veterinary Medicine/Small Animal Clinician*, pp 345–348, Apr. 1967.
27. Belfield, W. O. and Zucker, M. *How to Have a Healthier Dog*. Doubleday & Company, Inc., New York, 1981.
28. Siegal, F. P. and Siegal, M. *AIDS: The Medical Mystery*. Grove Press, Inc., New York, 1983.

APPENDIX D

Food additives

It is quite common for toxic chemicals, such as the nitrogen trichloride used to bleach flour before 1948, to be used in food for twenty or more years before they are discovered to be harmful. We now know that nitrogen trichloride reacts with methionine, an amino acid present in flour, to produce methionine sulfoxamine, a substance that produces convulsions in laboratory animals.

In 1960 Congress banned the use of Red Dye No. 3, a coal-tar dye used to color maraschino cherries, because tests showed it caused cancer in both animals and humans. But the *Washington Post* mentions in an editorial titled "A Lipstick You Can Live With" (National Weekly Edition: July 15, 1985) that about ten coal-tar dyes remain on the market to this day because the U.S. Department of Health and Human Services believes they "pose only a very small risk to humans" despite their carcinogenic effects on laboratory animals.

Polyoxyethylene compounds, which are the emulsifiers in ice cream and first cousins to the polyethylene from which plastic trash bags are made, have produced several types of cancer in mice. The FDA originally banned but later reapproved them after a long court battle and under increased pressure from their manufacturers. The National Academy of Science committee that reviewed the data for the FDA declared that since these compounds were not a *direct* cause of cancer, they were not carcinogenic. Such an argument is akin to asking leniency in court for the murderer of a couple, their seven children, and their cat and dog since it was the bullets, and not the murderer, that did the actual killing.

Monosodium glutamate, the sodium salt of the plant amino acid known as glutamic acid, may produce severe head discomfort, numbness, and cold sweats in many people and has been shown to cause brain lesions in the young of several primate species. It has been taken out of baby food but remains in numerous foods as a flavor enhancer, whether listed, unlisted, or under the guise of "hydrolyzed vegetable protein" on the label. Researchers at the Albert Einstein School of Medicine in New York have discovered that BOAA, a substance chemically related to MSG, causes nerve damage similar to that in Lou Gehrig's disease.[1]

APPENDIX E

Allergy tests and elimination and rotation diets

If you believe you are allergic to certain foods, chemicals, or other environmental substances, there are several tests that can identify the offending substance. But some of these, such as the skin-reaction tests, might not be particularly effective in discovering food sensitivities.

Skin tests such as the scratch, or patch, test and the intradermal test are among the most common allergy tests. The scratch test involves making a small scratch on the skin of the inner arm or back and placing a drop of the allergen on it. A patch of swelling and redness—hence the name *patch test*—usually occurs in five to fifteen minutes when a common allergy is present. The test, however, seems to detect only those allergies that are very strong, and not the more subtle ones.[1]

In the intradermal test a tiny amount of the allergen is injected under the skin, usually into the upper arm. If there's an allergy, the injection raises a small round bump, or wheal, within fifteen minutes. Size comparisons can indicate the severity of the reaction. This technique accurately indicates allergies to airborne substances like pollen or dust but might be ineffective in indicating sensitivity to foods and chemicals.

The Miller test improves upon the intradermal technique and seems to be a more reliable indicator of food and chemical allergens. Whereas the intradermal test uses an allergen concentrate, the Miller test employs a series of stepwise salt-water dilutions. The first dilution is five times weaker than the concentrate, the second one five times weaker than the first dilution, and so on. And if the allergen concentrate does not provoke a reaction, one of the Miller dilutions often will. This is an observed phenomenon for which there's yet no explanation.

The Miller test not only is diagnostic but also can be therapeutic. After the first reactive dilution, further dilutions are injected at half-hour intervals. Eventually, one of them produces no whealing and almost instantaneously switches off allergic symptoms in the patient. A drop of this "switch-off" dilution, placed under the tongue, enables a person to eat small amounts of the offending food. This switch-off therapy is very specific—the dilution works only for one particular food, not even for related foods.

The patient might also develop other sensitivities that have to be tested and switched off. One of the primary tools of clinical ecology clinics, the Miller test can be a useful, although somewhat cumbersome, diagnostic. Your insurance may cover this test.

The commonly used radio allergo-sorbent test (RAST) checks the blood for IgE antibodies against allergens. Because it identifies what an immunologist would call a true allergy, it is the only test many doctors use for diagnosis. Nonetheless, doubt has been cast on the value of the RAST. Not only has the test uncovered antibodies against common foods in people with no sensitivities, but it has also identified allegedly offending foods, removal of which from the diet of sensitive people results in no improvement. RAST, although covered by most insurers, is very expensive, up to $30 per antigen.[2]

Cytotoxic tests, also called leukocytotoxic or Bryan's tests, employ the hypothesis that sensitivity-inducing foods and chemicals also damage or destroy white blood cells in blood samples collected after fasting. The FDA disapproved cytotoxic testing in 1984, agreeing with the American Academy of Allergy and Immunology that "there is no proof that it is effective for diagnosis of food or inhalant allergy."[3] But there might be variants of cytotoxic testing in use that have escaped FDA notice. Most insurance thus does not cover this kind of test.[a] Other ineffective or controversial tests are the sublingual provocative test and the subcutaneous/intracutaneous provocation/neutralization test. The auricular cardiac reflex and electrodiagnosis, or Vega, tests show some promise but require so much testing skill that an indication of their effectiveness is still a few years away.[4]

ELIMINATION DIET TESTS

Elimination diets, the oldest and perhaps most definitive of food sensitivity tests, are commonly employed by clinical ecologists. In its most extreme form, an elimination diet subjects patients to individual food after a thorough fast has emptied the gastrointestinal tract.

The simplest elimination diet consists in eliminating one particular food one week and reintroducing it the next, while keeping accurate records of how one felt when the food was removed and added back. This is an easy and cost-free way of discovering food sensitivities and is appropriate for individuals whose health problems are not severe but whose financial limitations are.

A more drastic elimination method is for the healthy and well-off financially. It requires medical supervision and a two- to three- week stay in an ecology clinic or the clinical ecology unit of a hospital. Most insurance covers neither elimination-diet testing nor hospitalization.

Ecology units are free of offending chemicals such as certain paints, plastics, detergents, and synthetic fibers. While drinking six to eight glasses of spring water a day, the patient fasts for about four and a half days—or longer if he or she has used drugs or medication—until the gastrointestinal tract is empty. Symptoms of withdrawal from addictive foods might show up as early as the the first day of the fast. Common withdrawal symptoms are an overbearing craving for a particular food, diarrhea, excessive sweating, headaches, light-headedness, depression and weakness. Symptoms usually peak on the third or fourth day and subside when the intestines are completely empty.

Liquid chemical-free foods are then reintroduced one at a time at each meal. Less common foods are eaten first since common foods are more likely to cause a reaction—eating them first could mean going without food for too long a period. Reactions are observed during the few hours between meals. When they occur, the GI tract is usually emptied with a laxative and another food is tested; otherwise, hypersensitivity to foods might cease for about twenty-four hours.[5] This procedure is repeated until all foods are tested and sensitivities have been determined. Consumption of solid foods is resumed slowly over at least a week's time.

Several drugless methods can be used singly or in combination to control discovered allergies. The first and seemingly easiest is complete avoidance of the offending food or chemical. Avoidance of a food for three to six months can re-establish the body's ability to tolerate it intermittently. Complete avoidance (cutting down doesn't work) is often difficult since the offending food might be surreptitiously present in many edibles. Eating safely therefore might be impossible when eating out at a restaurant or at a friend's house. Furthermore, just the thought of the sacrifice can be overwhelming. Nevertheless, complete avoidance is by far the most effective control of food sensitivities.

I suggest that you wait three months before reintroducing forbidden foods, one by one, to which you had a minor reaction. Eat one of these foods for breakfast and do not eat any other foods at that meal.

A second treatment for allergies is desensitization by introducing the diluted offending substance in subcutaneous injections or drops under the tongue. As mentioned in the discussion of the Miller test, these methods are not always effective. They are useful, however, in expanding diets severely restricted by multiple food sensitivities. Desensitization can also substantially shorten rotation or avoidance periods.[6]

ROTATION DIETS

By preventing the frequent exposure that causes sensitivity to foods, rotation diets help maintain tolerance to commonly eaten, nonoffending foods, as well as the small amounts of offending foods that a person is able to consume after an avoidance period. Rotation diets thus prevent new sensitivities that will gradually restrict the number of allowed items in a diet. After avoidance periods or desensitization, rotation diets might even allow for increased variety in one's diet.

The rotation diet is an all-or-nothing enterprise that requires discipline and dedication. There's no use in trying a rotation diet for a short while. Menus have to be planned and written down; records of changes have to be kept. It is almost impossible to remember what one ate four days ago or should eat four days hence if it isn't on paper. Before beginning the rotation diet, some knowledge of the taxonomic families to which the various foods belong is essential.

The minimum length of a rotation is typically four days. If you eat a particular food on day one, you cannot have it again until day five. The strict approach extends prohibition to all members of the same food family. If you have rice, for instance, then you cannot eat wheat, rye, corn, or bamboo shoots—all members of the grass family—until the fifth day. Fish, on the other hand, belong to various families, so it is possible to have fish every day. This strict approach is used when existing sensitivities are particularly severe and debilitating. But limiting one particular food, rather than the whole family, is more common.[7] A compromise between the two methods is to leave at least one day between consumption of related foods.

Formerly forbidden foods for which a degree of tolerance has been acquired should be reintroduced on a seven-day rotation for two or three weeks. If there is no reaction during this time, the food may be eaten every four days. One must keep in mind, however, that frequent exposure can mask sensitivities. If any reaction occurs, reintroduction of the offending food should be postponed at least another six months.

In the case of substantial sensitivities, single-food meals might be necessary initially. In any case, limiting the number of foods per meal and the number of meals per day while increasing the size of the serving might help make the diet easier to follow. What is important is not how much but how often foods are eaten.

Planning and executing a rotation diet can be tough but can offer worthwhile rewards. A properly followed rotation diet might eventually allow a cautious return to the favorite foods you had to give up. In addition, the improvement of allergic responses may afford a period of rest to a battered immune system, allowing its remaining forces to gather strength for their proper job: healing your body.

APPENDIX F

The use of herbs in AIDS and ARC

by Misha Cohen, O.M.D., C.A.

Correct usage of herbs is a useful complement to all therapy for AIDS and AIDS Related Complex (ARC). Yet herbs, as well as other plant substances mentioned in this article, do not cure disease. They help the body recuperate its self-healing abilities. Herbs must be therefore used only as part of a comprehensive treatment and healing program.

Herbal medicine has been used for thousands of years as primary or adjunct therapy within many cultures in Europe, Asia, Africa, and the Americas. The indigenous peoples of North America have long employed herbal remedies for healing and preventing all types of illness. Yet while many have used natural remedies through the centuries, there has been a great resurgence of natural medicine throughout the world during the last fifteen years. At many clinics and healing centers, we are finding more and more individuals turning to natural medicine first rather than going through conventional or allopathic treatment. This is increasingly so in AIDS, ARC, and immunodefiency in general where certain combinations of indigenous North American and Chinese herbs can be highly valuable.

Traditional North American herbal medicine discovered through trial and error specific herbs to treat specific symptoms. The Chinese, on the other hand, developed their sophisticated system of herbal medicine in a more systematic way, taking into account the physiological action of the herbs, the meridians[a] they affect, and especially what happens when herbs are combined. Some herbalists in the United States are beginning to apply these Chinese principles of herb combination to native herbs. We can use, for the first time, certain combinations of indigenous herbs geared specifically toward the illness of a particular individual. Using herbs grown in the United States gives us better quality control over herbal preparations. Unfortunately, imported herbs are not as pure as we would like. The United States Department of Agriculture requires that all herbs be sprayed with insecticides and fungicides before entering the country, so we cannot use imported, traditional Chinese herbs in people who are allergic to these pesticides.

I have found two herbal formulas developed in the United States to be particularly effective in AIDS and ARC. These balanced preparations have the widest therapeutic effect with the least amount of toxicity. This is often not so with herbs such as goldenseal that are strongly effective but are toxic in the long run.

Although these two formulas are very similar as to the action of their herbs, one uses mainly North American herbs while the other employs only Chinese ones. A combination of these two formulas can work rather well, as I have seen over and over in clinical practice. Several of the herbs in the formulas are under clinical trial in the United States, China, and Japan.

The first formula, developed by Brian Weissbuch of KW Botanicals in Fairfax, California, is a tincture or alcohol extract[b] of yerba mansa, echinacea, dandelion, burdock, figwort, *wuchaseng* or Siberian ginseng, cleavers, red clover, chaparral, yarrow, kelp, *pau d'arco*, althea, and astragalus. The preparation stimulates immunity, tones up the glands, cleanses the lymph system, strengthens the kidney and liver, and clears infection and inflammation. It is primarily used when there are systemic or local symptoms of immune deficiency.

The first ingredient of the Weissbuch formula, yerba mansa, is a little-known herb that is nevertheless important in building cellular immunity. Because yerba mansa's effects are cumulative, people who use it preventively need not take it over long periods of time. It works well with other immune-building herbs, and is often used by herbalists on people with lymph-gland problems or cancer.

Echinacea has long been shown to slow down the rate of viral and bacterial growth and allows the body to regain homeostasis. It is recommended in the Jaffe protocol as an adaptogen, a substance that helps the body adapt to environmental stresses.[1,2]

Wuchaseng or Siberian ginseng (*Eleutherococcus senticosus*) is used extensively in China where research has shown it to be as effective as ginseng but with lesser side effects. It is particularly useful in building white blood-cell counts after chemotherapy, radiation therapy, or debilitating illness. Because of its beneficial effect on the heart, *wuchaseng* is used in people with chronic heart disease. Traditional Chinese medicine utilizes *E. senticosus* as a tonic for the kidney, lung, and heart.

Red clover and chaparral have been used traditionally by native Americans to treat various cancers. Weissbuch states that research in Great Britain showed that this combination brought about an 80 percent remission rate in melanoma or fatal skin cancer.[3]

Pau d'arco, a Central American herb, is known mainly for its antifungal properties and has been quite useful in the treatment of candida infections throughout the body. It is extensively employed in remedies for ecological illness (a condition in which a person develops allergies to a great many substances in the environment).

The final herb in Weissbuch's formula, astragalus, is also the main ingredient of the second preparation I have found useful in AIDS and ARC, the astragalus eight- herb formula or *ba wei huang qi pian.* Although this second formula is traditionally Chinese in ingredients, it was only recently created by Subhuti Dharmananda, Director of the Institute for Traditional Medicine and Preventive Health in Portland, Oregon, who combined traditional Chinese medical concepts with the results of his modern herb research.[4] The preparation includes astralagus, ligustrum, schizandra, Siberian ginseng, ganoderma and white atractylodes mushrooms, codonopsis, and licorice.

Astragalus is a dried root known in Chinese as *huang qi* and belongs to the *qi*-tonic[c] herbs such as ginseng and codonopsis used in Chinese medicine to strengthen the body's overall energy. According to Dharmananda, in clinical trials astragalus doubled the survival rates of cancer patients. It also increased the number of IgA and IgG antibodies and induced the formation of interferon in people susceptible to cold viruses.

Astragalus is specifically used in Chinese medicine to strengthen the spleen and lungs. It increases overall energy, eliminates toxic substances, stops both nightsweats and excessive day sweating, helps injured tissue to heal, and increases red blood-cell count. Astralagus also helps the digestion and absorption of food and increases appetite. In combination with other herbs, it helps fight infection and build up resistance to viruses and bacteria. Astragalus also aids in the discharge of pus from hard-to-heal wounds.

Ligustrum is a fruit used in particular to strengthen the kidney, especially its *jing* and *yin*,[d] and as a tonic for people who are debilitated and wasting away. Known to the Chinese as *nu zhen zi*, ligustrum is used traditionally for symptoms such as dizziness, floating spots in the visual field, low-back pain, premature greying of hair, ringing in the ears, and fever from tuberculosis. Ligustrum works primarily as an immune enhancer, as do many other herbs classified as kidney tonics by traditional Chinese medicine.

Schizandra has been found very effective for strengthening the liver and works well against hepatitis. The herb lowered SGPT[e] levels in 72 percent of 102 patients with hepatitis during an average period of twenty-five days. Schizandra acts strongly on the central nervous system, strengthening and quickening reflexes and helping to overcome stress and fatigue.

Traditional Chinese medicine classifies schizandra as both a *qi* and kidney tonic, and uses it to stop coughing and asthma. Because of its astringent properties, it helps stop the diarrhea commonly found in people with AIDS or ARC. Schizandra is also used to treat frequent urination, or excessive urination or seminal emission at night, and is very good for stopping excessive day or night sweating. Chinese medicine prescribes the herb to calm the mind and help memory, functions traditionally thought to be governed by the heart.

Ganoderma, known in China as *ling zhi* and in Japan as *reishi,* is a mushroom whose active ingredients lie pricipally in the spores. Ganoderma mushrooms have been used successfully in treating viral hepatitis where they have both lessened symptoms and decreased SGPT levels. The immune-enhancing effects of this mushroom as well as those of the Japanese shiitake mushroom are under current research in the United States, Japan, and China. In traditional Chinese medicine, ganoderma is a *qi* tonic that increases energy and reduces the effects of chronic infection. It is all right to take this mushroom for candidiasis as it has no known adverse effects.

The white atractylodes mushroom increases white blood-cell count and so is used traditionally in immune-enhancing formulas. Atractylodes can also be beneficial in cardiovascular problems by retarding clotting through a reduction in platelet aggregation. Because of these blood-thinning properties, I would warn people with idiopathic thrombocytopenia, a diminution in blood platelets that is sometimes AIDS-related, to be careful with this mushroom and watch platelet levels while using it. Chinese medicine holds that white atractylodes, or *dang shen,* strengthens the spleen and stomach, eliminates dampness, alleviates diarrhea, improves appetite, helps digestion, calms the nerves, and increases weight and energy.

Codonopsis is an herb often used instead of ginseng to increase body energy, for although it tones up *qi,* it is not considered as "hot" as ginseng by traditional Chinese doctors. It strengthens the lungs and spleen and is especially good for problems such as lack of appetite, fatigue, tired limbs, vomiting, shortness of breath, and chronic, sputum-producing cough. This herb brings about an increase in red blood-cell numbers, so it could be especially beneficial to those people with AIDS or ARC who have red blood-cell anemia. Codonopsis is said also to enhance T-cell transformation, although it does not increase the total number of white blood cells.

The last herb in the astragalus eight-herb formula is the well-known and widely used licorice root, recently found to exhibit anti-HIV properties in the test tube.[5] Licorice, or *gan cao,* is used to harmonize the herbs in Chinese formulas because it enters all the body's meridians. Aside from being a *qi* tonic itself, licorice thus enhances the total *qi*-toning properties of any formula. Licorice is also used traditionally for weak spleen conditions. It serves to stop pain and spasms, and decreases the effect of toxic substances in the body. Licorice root is a powerful anti-inflammatory frequently used for arthritis and gastric ulcers.

In prolonged doses, however, licorice can be toxic, causing high blood pressure and water retention, reduction in thyroid function and decrease in the basal metabolic rate. Licorice root should be used with care.

There are other herbs and plant substances that can be used effectively in AIDS and ARC, but these vary according to the needs of the individual. A proper discussion of these is outside the scope of this article. Herbs in general can be powerful because they contain powerful drugs. Thus, although the correct use of herbs can enhance the quality of life, their misuse can lead to serious problems. You should always consult your practitioner before embarking on any herbal protocol.[6]

APPENDIX G

A macrobiotic dietary plan

by Ellen Lipsius

This is a preliminary cleansing diet. As your body achieves a greater health balance, you can develop a more elaborate general diet.

BREAKFAST

MISO SOUP

Miso soup is traditionally made from a wakame seaweed base. To prepare the wakame for cooking, soak a five-inch piece for ten minutes in a small bowl of water. Then spread it out on a cutting board and cut away the tough spine down the center.

Cut the wakame leaf into one-inch squares and cook for five to six minutes in a quart of water. Add other vegetables according to their cooking times. These may include but not be limited to shiitake mushrooms, carrots, or small blocks of bean curd. Vegetables should be well but not overly cooked.

Four minutes before the soup is ready, add half a teaspoon of miso for every cup of liquid. Dissolve the miso in a cup with a small amount of broth and add to the soup.

You can prepare a larger quantity and store in the refrigerator, where it will keep for several days. Variety is essential to macrobiotic balance, so make sure you vary the vegetables each time you prepare the soup.

BROWN RICE

Cooked brown rice is a good complement to morning miso soup. You should only serve yourself enough to satisfy your appetite and not force yourself to eat.

Wash thoroughly one cup of organically grown, medium-grain brown rice. Place in a saucepan with a three-inch piece of kombu seaweed, add two cups of water, and allow to soak for one hour. Add a pinch of sea salt, bring the water to a boil, lower the heat, cover, and simmer at low heat about fifty to fifty-five minutes until the water has evaporated and the kernels are tender. Pressure cooking is even a better method for cooking rice [see the "Cooking" section in chapter 10, "Living with Food"].

You can season the rice at the table with gomasio, kombu-sesame powder, powdered beefsteak or shiso leaves, a vegetable sauce, or cooked vegetables. You could also make a larger quantity and refrigerate it.

MIDDAY MEAL

The midday meal should include the following:

1. a serving of grain
2. two or three vegetables
3. a small serving of seaweed
4. one tablespoon of pickles
5. a pressed salad
6. a small serving of beans, or tempeh or seitan
7. a serving of fish or chicken

Brown rice should be eaten once a day. If you had rice during breakfast, your lunch could include millet, buckwheat (during cold-weather months), barley, whole oats, whole wheat berries, or cornmeal.

You should vary not only your vegetables but also the way you prepare or cook them.

Sea vegetables that you can use regularly are kombu, wakame, arame, hijiki, and nori. Agar-agar can be used for making jellied molds or thickening sauces (for a thickener, you can also use kudzu root). Try eating a sheet of toasted nori daily.

Homemade pickles and pressed salads are easy to prepare and improve digestion.

The beans, in combination with the grains, are the "meat" of the diet, consisting of high-quality protein. You should regularly use aduki and black soy beans and chick peas. Always soak beans overnight to improve their digestibility and prevent flatulence problems. Examine the beans for stones and broken pieces, wash thoroughly, and soak in three cups of water for every cup of beans. A three-inch piece of kombu will assist the soaking process.

Tempeh and seitan are protein fermented foods used as an alternative to beans. They are more easy to digest than beans and are also very nourishing.

Free-range chicken, white-fleshed sea fish such as halibut, sea bass, turbot and cod, and shrimp are acceptable animal protein sources. Because excessive animal protein is not necessary, you should consume only small quantities. In cooking, you can use tamari soy sauce, ginger, and natural herb seasonings to enhance flavor.

EVENING MEAL

Because you should not tax your body energy unduly during sleep, the evening meal should be lighter in terms of quantity, because it is before bedtime, but should also be the richest in terms of calories, so it will provide your body energy to last the night. This is why it should include some of the sweeter vegetables as well as whole-grain macrobiotic noodles made of buckwheat (soba) or whole wheat (udon) that are rich in complex carbohydrates. Choose the rest of your evening foods from the categories listed under the midday meal.

DESSERTS

You should eat sweets for dessert only once or twice a week and then only as those fruits grown in your climate. Local fruit can be eaten raw or cooked. If you live where cold weather precludes the availability of local fresh fruit during winter, you can make unsweetened fruit compotes or agar jelly molds from the unsulphured dried fruits available in your area.

BREAD

The best bread should be homemade without leavening or yeast. Whole-grain sourdough is perfect, and even commercial sourdough is all right if no yeast has been added. An occasional whole-wheat pita or chapati is okay.

SNACKS

If you are hungry between meals while on this cleansing diet, try to rely on the leftover grains and vegetables you have prepared. An occasional rice cake or a handful of toasted pumpkin seeds, however, is fine.

APPENDIX H

Resources

ACUPUNCTURE

THE GREEN CROSS
1512 U St. N.W.
Washington, DC
(202) 938-7360

QUAN YIN ACUPUNCTURE AND HERB CENTER OF SAN FRANCISCO
Misha Cohen, Director
513 Valencia St.
San Francisco, CA 94110
(415) 861-1101

NAOMI RABINOWITZ, M.D.
32 W. 32nd St., Suite 503
New York, NY 10001
(212) 967-9736

MICHAEL SMITH, M.D.
Lincoln Hospital Acupuncture Clinic
349 E. 140th St.
Bronx, NY 10454
(212) 993-3100

AIDS COMPLIMENTARY THERAPY, INFORMATION

Berkeley, CA

IMMUNE ENHANCEMENT PROJECT
2016 10th St.
Berkeley, CA 94710
(415) 841-7019

Boston, MA

AIDS ACTION COMMITTEE
661 Boylston St., Suite 4
Boston, MA 02116
(617) 437-6200; In-state Hotline: (800) 235-2331

Los Angeles, CA

HAY HOUSE
3029 Wilshire Blvd., #206
Santa Monica, CA 90404
Send $10 for a copy of Louise Hay's visualization tape, "AIDS: A Positive Approach."

Minneapolis, MN

THE ALIVENESS PROJECT
5307 Russell St.
Minneapolis, MN 55410
(612) 929-8256

New York, NY

HEAL (HEALTH EDUCATION AIDS LIAISON)
P. O. Box 60
New York, NY 10014
(212) 243-1858

NEW YORK AIDS ACTION
263A W. 19th St.
New York, NY 10011
(212) 807-0699

San Francisco, CA

AIDS ALTERNATIVE HEALING PROJECT
(415) 668-1611

AIDS INTERFAITH NETWORK
1995 Turk St., #2
San Francisco, CA 94115
(415) 928-HOPE

PROJECT INFORM
25 Taylor St., Suite 618
San Francisco, CA
(415) 928-0293; State: (800) 822-7422; National: (800) 334-7422

National

AIDS TREATMENT NEWS
c/o John S. James
P. O. Box 411256
San Francisco, CA 94141
(415) 282-0110
Biweekly. Subscription costs $25 per quarter.

AMFAR PERIODICAL DIRECTORY OF EXPERIMENTAL TREATMENTS FOR AIDS & ARC
American Foundation for AIDS Research (AmFAR)
40 W. 57th St., Suite 406
New York, NY 10019
(212) 333-3118

AIDS COMPLIMENTARY THERAPIES, SUPERVISION

KEITH BARTON, M.D.
Berkeley Holistic Health Offices
3099 Telegraph Ave.
Berkeley, CA 94705
(415) 845-4430

ROBERT F. CARTHCART III, M.D.
127 2nd St.
Los Altos, CA 94022
(415) 949-2822

ROBERT GORTER, M.D.
San Francisco General Hospital
Ward 86
995 Potrero Ave.
San Francisco, CA 94110
(415) 821–8830

RUSSEL M. JAFFE, M.D.
c/o Sera Corp./Advanced Cell Technologies
2177 Chain Bridge RoadVienna, VA 22180
(703) 938-7360

MICHAEL JANSON, M.D.
Cambridge Center for Holistic Health
2557 Massachusetts Ave.
Cambridge, MA 02140
(617) 661-1225

JIM JOHNSON, M.D.
The Green Cross
1512 U St. N.W.
Washington, DC 20002
(202) 265-0100

EMMANUEL REVICI, M.D.
164 E. 91st St.
New York, NY 10128
(212) 876-9669

RICHARD SHAMES, M.D.
232 E. Blithedale
Mill Valley, CA 94941
(415) 383-1262

CHARLES WILLIAMSON, M.D.
45 Castro St., Suite B-200
San Francisco, CA 94114
(415) 863–3366

AIDS NATIONAL RESOURCES

AIDS LEGAL RIGHTS HANDBOOK
National Gay Rigts Advocates
540 Castro St.
San Francisco, CA 94114
Free with SASE.

MOTHERS OF AIDS PATIENTS
c/o Barbara Peabody and Miriam Thompson
P. O. Box 89040
San Diego, CA 92138

PWA COALITION *NEWSLINE*
263A W. 19th St., #125
New York, NY 10011
Free to PWAs and PWARCs, $20 to all others.

WOMEN'S AIDS NETWORK

c/o San Francisco AIDS Foundation
333 Valencia St., 4th floor
San Francisco, CA 94103
(415) 864–4376

WORLDWIDE MOMENT OF PRAYER/MEDITATION

AIDS Interfaith Network
(415) 928–HOPE

ALTERNATIVE CANCER THERAPY

COMMONWEAL

P. O. Box 316
Bolinas, CA 94924
(415) 868-0970

CANDIDA

PRICE-POTTENGER FOUNDATION

P. O. Box 2614
La Mesa, CA 92041
Write for a referral list of physicians

COLONICS

AMERICAN COLON HYGIENE ASSOCIATION

7770 East Camelback Road, Suite 23
Scottsdale, AZ 85251

ENVIRONMENTAL MEDICINE

AMERICAN ACADEMY FOR ENVIRONMENTAL MEDICINE
P. O. Box 16106
Denver, CO 80216

HOLISTIC MEDICINE

AMERICAN HOLISTIC MEDICAL ASSOCIATION
2727 Fairview Ave. E., #D
Seattle, WA 98102
(206) 322-6842
Send a self-addressed, stamped envelope and $2 for a list of holistic physicians in your area.

HOMEOPATHY

NATIONAL CENTER FOR HOMEOPATHY
1500 Massachusetts Ave. N.W.
Washington, DC 20005
(202) 223-6182

HOMEOPATHIC EDUCATIONAL SERVICES
2124 Kittredge St.
Berkeley, CA 94704

MACROBIOTICS

WORLWIDE MACROBIOTIC DIRECTORY
The East-West Journal
P. O. Box 1200
Brookline, MA 02147
Send $2 for a list of macrobitic centers and intructors.

MAIL-ORDER VITAMINS

THE APOTHECARY
5415 Cedar Lane
Bethesda, MD 20814
(301) 530-0800

BRONSON PHARMACEUTICALS
4526 Rinetti Lane
La Canada, CA 91011
(213) 790-2646
Best deal on vitamin C salts.

WHOLESALE NUTRITION CLUB
P. O. Box 1113
Sunnyvale, CA 94088
(408) 867-6368

MAIL-ORDER WHOLE-FOOD COMPANIES

EREWHON
236 Washington St.
Brookline, MA 02146
(617) 738-4516
Extensive variety.

GARDEN SPOT DISTRIBUTORS
Route 1, Box 729A
New Holland, PA 17557
(800) 292-9631 in Pa., (800) 445-5100 in the Northeast,
(717) 354-4936 elsewhere.
Extensive variety.

JAFFE BROTHERS

P. O. Box 636
Valley Center, CA 92082-0636
(619) 749-1133
Grains, nuts and seeds, oils and dried fruits

KENNEDYS' NATURAL FOODS

1051 West Broad St.
Falls Church, VA 22046
(703) 533-8484
Extensive variety.

LUNDBERG FARMS

P. O. Box 369
Richdale, CA 95974
(916) 882-4551
Grains and grain products.

MOUNTAIN ARK

120 S. East Street
Fayetteville, AR 72701
(800) 643-8909, toll free
They carry reliable brands like Chico-San, Lima-Belgium, Eden, and Lundberg.

PAUL'S GRAINS

Route 1, Box 76
Laurel, IA 50141
(515) 476-3373)
Grains and grain products

NUTRITION INFORMATION

NUTRITION ACTION HEALTHLETTER
Center for Science in the Public Interest (CSPI)
1501 16th St. NW
Washington, DC 20036
(202) 332-9110
The newsletter is available to members of CSPI for an annual membership fee.

ORTHOMOLECULAR MEDICINE

THE HUXLEY INSTITUTE FOR BIOSOCIAL RESEARCH
900 N.. Federal Highway, Suite 330
Boca Raton, FL 33432
(305) 393–6167; (800) 847–3802
Ask for a referral list of orthomolecular physicians.

PEOPLE-WITH-AIDS ORGANIZATIONS

Boston, MA

BOSTON PWA/PWARC
c/o Seth Newman and Allan Kuconis
Boston AIDS Action Committee
661 Boylston St.
Boston, MA 02116
(617) 437–6200

Dallas, TX

PWA COALITION – DALLAS
c/o Mike Meridan
3905 Cedar Springs, #C8
Dallas, TX 75219
(214) 520–7254

Houston, TX

PWA COALITION – HOUSTON

c/o Billy Burton
4300 Montrose Ave., #700
Houston, TX 77006
(713) 522–7569

Indianapolis, IN

PHOENIX

c/o Robbie Richards
P. O. Box 44347
Indianapolis, IN 46224
(317) 925–8703

Minneapolis, MN

THE ALIVENESS PROJECT

c/o Steven Katz
5307 Russel South
Minneapolis, MN 55410
(612) 929–8256

New York, NY

PEOPLE WITH AIDS COALITION – NEW YORK

263A W. 19th St., #125
New York, NY 10011
(212) 627-1810

Portland, OR

LIFELINK

c/o James Chase
P. O. Box 02681
Portland, OR 97202
(503) 234–0193

San Francisco, CA

PEOPLE WITH AIDS – SAN FRANCISCO
519 Castro St.
San Francisco, CA 94114
(415) 553–2509

Washington, DC

NATIONAL ASSOCIATION OF PEOPLE WITH AIDS
c/o Michael Hirsch and Griff Gold
1012 14th St. N.W., Suite 601
Washington, DC 20005
(202) 347–1317

West Hollywood, CA

BEING ALIVE
c/o Ron Rose
8235 Santa Monica Blvd., #311
West Hollywood, CA 90046
(213) 656–1107

SMOKE ENDING

For address of the Smoke Enders' group nearest you, call (800) 828–4357

WATER QUALITY

ENVIRONMENTAL PROTECTION AGENCY
Water Supply Division
Washington DC 20460
Ask for *Water Quality Improvement in the Home*
by Frank Bell, Ervin Bellack and Joseph Cotruvo
and for *Is Your Drinking Safe?* March 1985, 170 35–61–OPA.

Glossary

adrenal cortex – the part of the *adrenal glands* that produces steroid hormones necessary for carbohydrate metabolism (cortisol), the body's salt and mineral balance (aldosterone), and the regulation of the sex glands (estrogens and androgens).

adrenal glands – two endocrine glands each located over a kidney and divided into two functional parts: an outer portion called the *adrenal cortex* and an inner one called the *adrenal medulla*.

adrenal medulla – the part of the *adrenal glands* that produces two related hormones, epinephrine and norepinephrine.

adzuki bean – a small, angular red bean related to the kidney bean and widely cultivated in Japan.

aflatoxins – carcinogenic toxins produced by the mold *Aspergillus flavus*, which is invariably found in peanuts and sometimes in almonds, Brazil nuts, pecans, pistachios, and walnuts.

autoimmune disease – a group of diseases in which antibodies react against the body's own cells, causing localized or bodywide damage. See *idiopathic thrombocytopenia purpura, rheumatoid arthritis*, and *systemic lupus erythematosus*.

antimitotic – a substance that prevents cells from undergoing mitosis, or dividing, and is therefore used against rapidly proliferating cancer cells. These substances often do not distinguish between cancerous and normal cells and so can produce toxic side effects.

antioxidant – a subtance, such as vitamin C or E, that regulates the harmful combination of organic substances with oxygen, thus prolonging their usefulness to the cells.

autonomic nervous system – the part of the nervous system that controls involuntary functions such as heartbeat, glandular secretion, and the movement of food through the gastrointestinal tract.

basophil – a *granulocyte* whose cytoplasmic granules stain blue when exposed to a basic, or alkaline, dye. Although their precise function is unknown, basophils ingest some foreign particles and may act as blood *mast cells*, releasing histamine and heparin into the blood during allergic reactions.

B cell – A *lymphocyte* that originates in the bone marrow and that upon stimulation by helper T cells matures into a plasma cell whose main function is to produce antibodies.

blood-brain barrier – an anatomical barrier that surrounds the *central nervous system* and isolates it from the blood, slowing or preventing the passage of certain chemical compounds and disease-causing organisms such as viruses. For a drug to work in the brain, it needs to penetrate the blood-brain barrier.

burdock – a hardy plant, with a long, dark root, that grows through most of the United States. Known as *gobo* in Japan.

central nervous system – the division of the nervous system that consists of the brain and spinal chord. It processes all information and coordinates and controls the entire body.

cerebral cortex – a thin layer of gray matter on the surface of the cerebral hemispheres that integrates higher mental functions, general movement, visceral activity, perception, and behavior.

cofactor – any agent, substance, or environmental factor that activates or furthers the action of an agent of disease.

daikon – a long, white, and mild radish popular in Japan.

endocrine gland – a ductless gland; that is, a gland whose cells secrete hormones directly into the bloodstream and not through a duct. The endocrine glands include the pituitary, the thyroid, the *adrenal glands*, and the ovaries and testes. Glands that secrete through a duct are called exocrine glands (e.g., the pancreas).

eosinophil – a *granulocyte* whose cytoplasmic granules stain heavily with the acid dye eosin. Although their precise function is poorly understood, eosinophils can ingest foreign particles and are involved in allergic responses. They are present in large numbers in all lining or protective surfaces within the body.

epinephrine – also known as adrenaline; mainly controls circulation, muscle tone, and sugar metabolism during the stress response.

granulocyte – any of several white blood cells that show a granular cytoplasm when stained with special dyes. A granulocyte, also called a *polymorphonuclear leukocyte*, can be further classified as a *neutrophil*, *eosinophil*, or *basophil* depending on the pH of the dye that stains it best.

hypothalamus – an area of the brain that controls the peripheral autonomic nervous system, endocrine secretion, and other body functions such as body temperature, sleep, and appetite.

idiopathic thrombocytopenic purpura – an *autoimmune disease*, often seen in people with AIDS or ARC, in which antibodies attack the blood platelets that mediate clotting, reducing their numbers and resulting in multiple bruises, tiny purple or red skin spots, and hemorrhage into the tissues.

Kupffer's cell – a fixed *phagocyte* lining the numerous small blood vessels of the liver. Kupffer's cells filter bacteria and small foreign proteins from the blood and are involved in the formation of bile.

large granular lymphocyte – the *natural killer cell*, so called because it possesses some of the characteristics of a *lymphocyte* and the granular cytoplasm of a *granulocyte*. Large granular lymphocytes form a distinct category of white blood cells.

limbic system – a set of connected areas in the brain that are associated with emotions and feelings such as anger, fear, sadness, pleasure and sexual arousal. The limbic system is under *cerebral cortex* control and is connected to the *hypothalamus*.

leukocyte – any white blood cell.

lymph – a clear, watery, often faintly yellowish liquid, containing white blood cells and some red blood cells, that travels through the *lymphatic system*, removes bacteria and certain proteins from the tissues, tranports fats from the intestines, and supplies lymphocytes to the blood.

lymphatic system – the system of interconnected spaces and vessels between tissues and organs through which lymph circulates in the body. The lymphatic system includes the *lymph* vessels and lymphoid tissue: the lymph nodes, *thymus, spleen,* and tonsils.

lymphocyte – a white blood cell, or *leukocyte,* originating in the *lymph* or lymphoid tissue. *T cells* and *B cells* are regular lymphocytes. *Natural killer cells* fall into a separate category: the large granular lymphocytes.

macrophage – any of several large, scavenging phagocytes present, either fixed or free, in connective tissue and many major organs and tissues such as the bone marrow, lymph nodes, spleen, liver (see *Kupffer's cell),* and central nervous system (see *microglia).* In the blood, free macrophages are also called monocytes.

mast cell – a large connective-tissue cell that contains the chemicals heparin, histamine, and serotonin and releases them during inflammation and allergic rection.

microglia – a nonnervous cell of the central nervous system that acts as a *macrophage.*

miso – a fermented soybean purée that should be used only unpasteurized in soups and as a flavor enhancer.

natural killer cell – a nonspecific, *large granular lymphocyte* that destroys cancer cells and certain virus-infected cells.

neutrophil – a kind of *granulocyte* that ingests bacteria and removes and destroys cellular debris and solid particles, thus performing a major immune function that is independent from helper T cell regulation. A neutrophil is also a *phagocyte.*

norepinephrine – or noradrenaline; mainly serves as the chemical through which the nerve cells of the sympathethic nervous system communicate with each other.

"nude" mice – a strain of hairless mice with atrophied thymus glands and depressed immune function.

parasympathetic nervous system – a division of the *autonomic nervous system* that acts to protect, conserve, and restore body resources, often as an antagonist to the sympathetic nervous system.

peripheral nervous system – all of the nerves and ganglia, or nerve bundles, outside the brain and the spinal cord.

phagocyte – any cell that can engulf and digest microorganisms and cellular debris. A phagocyte can either be free, circulating in the blood, or fixed, not circulating. See also *Kupffer's cell, macrophage, microglia,* and *neutrophil.*

polymorphonuclear leukocyte – a *granulocyte.* This alternate name derives from the various forms granulocytic nuclei can assume.

rheumatoid arthritis – an *autoimmune disease* that attacks the collagen in the articular capsule that surrounds a freely movable joint, causing painful joint swelling that may lead to deformation and loss of joint use.

shiitake mushrooms – medicinal, dried mushrooms, usually imported from Japan and whose active ingredient, lentinen, possesses in vitro anti-HIV and possibly anticancer properties.

spleen – a lymphatic organ located between stomach and diaphragm in the left side of the body and acting as a major center of phagocytosis and white blood cell production and as a blood volume regulator during severe hemorrhage.

sympathetic nervous system – a division of the *autonomic nervous system* that acts to accelerate heart rate, constrict blood vessels, and raise blood pressure, usually during fight-or-flight reactions.

systemic lupus erythematosus – an *autoimmune disease* that attacks the connective tissue in blood vessels, skin, and nervous system, causing severe inflammation of the blood vessels, lesions of the skin, renal failure, and severe neurologic abnormalities.

tamari – natural soy sauce, as distinguished from the commercial, processed variety.

tannier – the starchy, edible tuber of a tropical American plant that is related to the calla lilly. Also called *yautía*.

taro – the starchy, edible rootstock of a widely cultivated tropical plant with large leaves like elephant ears.

T cell – a *lymphocyte* that, after maturation in the thymus or thymus-equivalent tissue (hence the name T[hymus] cell), is responsible for cell-mediated, specific immunity. There are three kinds of T cells: helper, killer (or cytotoxic), and suppressor T cells.

tempeh – a pressed soybean cake, made from split soybeans, water, grains, and special bacteria and allowed to ferment several hours.

thymus – the primary central gland of the *lymphatic system*, where *T cells* mature before migrating to the lymph nodes and the spleen. T-cell maturation is mediated by the hormone thymosin produced by the thymus.

tofu – fresh soybean curd made from soybeans, water and nigari, a natural sea-salt coagulant.

Notes

All explanatory notes, which contain complimentary material not necessary to understanding the text, are referenced by lowercase letters in alphabetical order and have been placed at the beginning of each chapter section. Reference notes, which give sources for data, citations, and quotations, are numbered and follow the explanatory notes. This system permits readers to distinguish between the two kinds of notes before having to turn to the back of the book.

Reference notes follow the more succinct style of scholarly citation advocated by Mary-Claire van Leunen in *A Handbook for Scholars* (Alfred A Knopf, 1979). Because *Living with AIDS: Reaching Out* is intended for the general public and not as a scholarly work, however, data is not pinpointed to specific pages in the sources. Of course, page number are provided for direct quotations so that the reader may check for accuracy or context.

INTRODUCTION

a. The Embarcadero Center is an office and shopping complex in downtown San Francisco.

b. It is for these survival stories and not necessarily its dietary recommendations that I strongly recommend you read the book.
c. In no way should this book take the place of any course of treatment prescribed by a physician. Its recommendations should be followed only under the advice of a sympathetic doctor.

CHAPTER 1. LEARNING ABOUT HEALTH

a. HIV was formerly called HTLV–III/LAV, for human T cell lymphotropic virus, type III, and lymphadenopathy-associated virus. I use the name HIV only for convenience, since it is less of a mouthful than the older one. The name HIV seems to imply that the virus is the sole agent of immune deficiency in AIDS, an implication not supported by epidemiologic data.
b. These T cell chemicals, as well as the one produced by the macrophages, are called lymphokines, substances produced by white blood cells to prod other white blood cells into action. The lymphokine produced by macrophages at the site of infection is interleukin-1, which causes helper T cells to multiply, raises body temperature to enhance immune-cell activity, and breaks down muscle protein to provide energy for immune functions. Helper T cells in turn produce gamma interferon, which keeps macrophages at the site of infection, allows them to digest engulfed pathogens, and enhances the activities of other immune cells. Without gamma interferon, a macrophage would just lie around bloated and unable to digest an ingested invader, which would eventually gain the upper hand. The macrophage would die from food poisoning.
c. A helper T cell primed by a macrophage produces gamma interferon and interleukin-2. Gamma interferon attracts macrophages and allows them to digest pathogens. Interleukin-2 attracts more helpers and other kinds of T cells to the site of infection and causes them to multiply.
d. These substances comprise the B cell growth factor (BCGF) that

causes B cells to multiply and the B cell differentiation factor (BCDF) that induces some B cells to start antibody production.

e. The world of immune intrigue also places little trust on spies and their ilk. The immune system spies on its spies and sabotages its saboteurs through a group of antibodies that work specifically against antibodies, the anti-idiotypic antibodies. These get rid of any supernumerary antibodies left in the field and, in the process, conveniently neutralize themselves. But no system is perfect. Because production of anti-idiotypic antibodies often lags behind that of antibodies, the latter might not always be completely neutralized.

f. These are the Langerhans' cells. They present antigens to the appropriate T cell. Other skin cells called keratinocytes produce the necessary interleukin-1.

g. Epinephrine and norepinephrine are also known as adrenaline and noradrenaline.

h. Cortisol is a steroid better known as hydrocortisone and found in man-made form in some first-aid ointments.

i. In the tooth-and-claw stituations out of which the fight-or-flight response evolved, suppression of inflammation and immunity enhanced survival because an animal had to channel all its energies into not getting eaten. Risking wounds and infections was preferable to ending up as someone else's dinner.

j. Many new–age gays insist that considering ourselves gay limits us, that we should see ourselves just as people. Let's all grow into our full potential as humans, they say, and I agree. But to graduate into high school we have to pass elementary school first. Our gayness is as much a part of our personhood as a heterosexual's straightness is a part of his or hers. We cannot put our gayness aside without denying a large portion of our humanity. We can grow *from* the gay experience, but we can never grow *out* of it. What these new age gays propose smacks of denial.

k. Why not say "conscious" instead of "analytical" and "unconscious" instead of "deep"? The terms *conscious* and *unconcious*, as understood in popularized Freudian psychology, often add little to our understanding of the mind. Although all analytical or verbal thought is necessarily conscious, not all conscious thought is necessarily analytical or verbal—that is, capable of being put into words. Similarly, although all unconscious processes are deep within the mind, not all deep mental processes are unconscious. The transcendental awareness often achieved through contemplation or meditation and sometimes associated with alpha brain waves is both conscious without being analytical or verbal, and deep without being unconscious.

l. Seeing health processes in terms of information exchange is more productive than seeing them in terms of energy, for then one doesn't need to focus on how one kind of energy is transformed into another (the neurochemical into the cellular or the mental into the spiritual, for example). Informational exchange is likely to be more important than energy exchange. The energy involved in viral infection, for instance, is almost insignificant, whereas the information introduced by the viral genes can severely interfere with normal function in the host.

m. I use "spirit" here not in the formal religious sense but to mean the feeling of belonging to an order that transcends all other orders.

* * *

1. Christopher M. Walker, Dewey J. Moody, Daniel P. Stites, and Jay A. Levy. CD8[+] lymphocytes can control HIV infection in vitro by suppressing virus replication. *Science* 234 (4783):1563, 19 December 1986.
2. Buck Nunes and Chuck Frutchey. *Coping with ARC.* San Francisco AIDS Foundation, 1986.
3. Richard L. Ederson and Joseph M. Fink. The immunologic function of skin. *Scientific American* 252(6):46, June 1985.
4. Donald V. Belsito, Miguel R. Sanchez, Rudolf L. Baer, Fred Valentine, and G. Jeanette Thorbecke. Reduced Langerhans' cell Ia antigen and ATPase activity in patients with the acquired immunodeficiency syndrome. *The New England Journal of Medicine* 310(20):1279, 17 May 1984.

5. Steven B. Mizel and Peter Jaret.
In Self-Defense.
Harcourt Brace Jovanovich, 1985.
6. Linus Pauling.
How to Live Longer and Feel Better.
W. H. Freeman and Company, New York, 1986.
7. Frederick P. Siegal and Marta Siegal.
AIDS: The Medical Mystery.
Grove Press, 1983.
8. Nicholas R. Hall and Allan L. Goldstein.
Neurotransmitters and the immune system.
In Robert Ader, editor, *Psychoneuroimmunology*, pages 521–543. Academic Press, 1981.
9. H. O. Besedovsky and E. Sorkin.
Immunologic-neuroendocrine circuits: physiological approaches.
In Robert Ader, editor, *Psychoneuroimmunology*, pages 545–573. Academic Press, 1981.
10. Hans Selye.
Stress without Distress, page 14.
New American Library, 1975.
11. Steven Locke and Douglas Colligan.
The Healer Within: The New Medicine of Mind and Body, page 62.
E.P. Dutton, 1986.
12. Andrew A. Monjan.
Stress and immunologic competence in animals.
In Robert Ader, editor, *Psychoneuroimmunology*, pages 185–228. Academic Press, 1981.
13. Locke and Colligan, *Healer Within*.
14. Joan Borysenko.
Psychoneuroimmunology: Behavioral factors and the immune response.
In J. D. Matarazzo, editor, *Behavioral Health: A Handbook of Health Enhancement and Disease.* John Wiley and Sons, 1984.
15. George F. Solomon.
The emerging field of psychoneuroimmunology with a special note on AIDS.
Advances 2(1):6, Winter 1985.
16. Solomon, Emerging field of psychoneuroimmunology.
17. Locke and Colligan, *Healer Within*.
18. Borysenko. Psychoneuroimmunology.
19. Andrew Weil.
Health and Healing: Understanding Conventional and Alternative Medicine.
Houghton Mifflin, 1983.
20. Alastair Cunningham.
Information and health in the many levels of man: Toward a more comprehensive theory of health and disease.
Advances 3(1):32, Winter 1986.

21. Garrett Porter and Patricia A. Norris.
Why Me? Harnessing the Healing Power of the Human Spirit.
Stillpoint Publishing, Walpole, New Hampshire, 1985.
22. Kenneth Pelletier.
Mind as Healer, Mind as Slayer: A Holistic Approach to Preventing Stress Disorders.
Dell, 1977.
23. Michio Kushi and Alex Jack.
The Cancer Prevention Diet: Michio Kushi's Nutritional Blueprint for the Prevention and Relief of Disease.
St. Martin's Press, 1983.

CHAPTER 2. NURTURING HEALTH

a. This is not a euphemism but the politically acceptable term. Many people with AIDS feel that the word *victim* is condescending (a victim is someone for whom we should feel pity) and the word *patient* is inaccurate (one is only a patient while in the hospital or at the doctor's). The use of AIDS victim or AIDS patient depersonalizes a person with AIDS.

b. This exercise is better described by the Simontons in their book *Getting Well Again.*

c. We often stand to lose by achieving a goal. In graduating from college and obtaining a degree, for example, we lose the freedom afforded by the student life.

d. Laughter can be very effective against the anxiety attacks that often haunt us in these days of AIDS. Norman Cousins used laughter and comic movies as part of his cancer self-healing program. Smiling can be of greater value. It gets all the right chemicals going in our bodies, yet we do it too infrequently. Try a five-minute smiling session in front of the bathroom mirror every morning. It does wonders!

* * *

1. Ken Coupland.
The vitamin C resistance.
San Francisco Sentinel 12(14):7, 17 January 1985.

2. Locke and Colligan, *Healer Within*.
3. Van R. Ault.
Louie Nassaney's survival strategies.
San Francisco Sentinel 14(13):11, 4 July 1986.
All quotations of Louie Nassaney are from this source.
4. Carol Reuben.
Striking the word "incurable" from the media's vocabulary.
Heartland Journal, Spring 1986.
5. Kathy Butler.
Three who beat the odds.
The San Francisco Chronicle 122(123):44, 9 June 1986.
6. Keith Barton.
A Comprehensive Psycho-social and Nutritional Approach to the Treatment of AIDS: An Introduction.
Unpublished manuscript intended for patient use, April, 1985.
Keith Barton is one of several physicians implementing the Jaffe protocol in the San Francisco Bay area. For address, see AIDS Complimentary Therapies, Supervision, in appendix H. Appendix A contains an adaptation of this article for this book.
7. Michael A. Weiner.
Maximum Immunity, page 207.
Houghton Mifflin, 1986.
8. Norman Cousins.
Human Options, page 210.
Berkley Books, 1981.
9. Viktor E. Frankl.
Man's Search for Meaning.
Pocket Books, 1984.

CHAPTER 3. OTHERS AND YOUR HEALTH

a. Prompting a fictional twenty-third-century physician, *Star Trek*'s Dr. McCoy, to shout "Spanish Inquisition!" when he inspected the latest twentieth-century medical facilites at a San Francisco hospital.

b. Homeopathic remedies are stepwise dilutions. The first dilution used in homeopathy, the 1X, consists of one part of the full-strength substance in nine parts of diluent. A 2X dilution, one part of the 1X dilution in nine parts of diluent, would be 100 times weaker than full strength; a 3X, one part of the 2X in nine parts of diluent, 1000 times weaker; and so on. Remedies of 200X dilution, which the homeopathic "less is more" dictum would hold as quite powerful but which the laws of chemistry say do not contain even a single atom of the original substance, are not uncommon in homeopathy.

c. Vaccines are a case in point. Although there might be reasons to avoid some of the vaccines produced from the serum of horses, cows, and other animals, many holistic practitioners seem to reject all vaccines, which are by definition homeopathic, just because they are one of the bastions of conventional medicine's "war against disease." Now that recombinant DNA technology has come up with vaccines that utilize not foreign agents but substances that are indistinguishable from those your body uses to immunize you, the argument is that it might not be good to mobilize the body's defenses too much. Yet isn't mobillizing the body's own defenses one of the basic premises of holism?

* * *

1. Mike May to Tom O'Connor and Ahmed González–Núñez, 17 November 1986. Unpublished letter in the authors' possession.
2. Stephanie Matthews Simonton and Robert L. Shook. *The Healing Family: The Simonton Approach for Families Facing Illness.* Bantam, 1984.
3. Weil, *Health and Healing.*
4. Pauling, *How to Live Longer.*
5. Sandra Dowie. My search for the golden cure. *Medical Self-Care* (32):38, January-February 1986.
6. Norman Cousins. *The Healing Heart,* page 117. Avon, 1984
7. Cousins, *The Healing Heart.*
8. Tom Shealy. How to find a great doctor. *Prevention* 38(4):130, April 1986.
9. Irving Oyle. *The Healing Mind,* page 19. Celestial Arts, Millbrae, California, 1979.

CHAPTER 4. THE HARD CHOICES OF DRUGS

a. If you are taking sulfa drugs, you should avoid excessive sunlight.

b. Bactrim and Septra are trade names for co–trimoxazole, a combination of the sulfonamide sulfamethoxazole and the antiseptic trimethoprim.

c. Before it replicates, the HIV virus builds a DNA template from which to make RNA copies of itself. Azidothymidine so closely resembles thymidine, one of the building blocks of DNA, that the virus tries to use it for the template. AZT doesn't fit in with the other DNA components, however, and the construction of the DNA masque needed for viral replication falls through. This drug strategy arose from the success of acyclovir against herpes viruses. Acyclovir blocks the replication of herpes by mimicking guanosine, a building block of both DNA and RNA.

d. Through recombinant DNA techniques—what the press has labelled genetic engineering—researchers hope to develop chemotherapy techniques that will kill cancerous or virus-infected cells without harming healthy ones. With these selective drugs, for example, your immune cells wouldn't die and your hair wouldn't fall out. Unfortunately the appearance of these drugs on the market is still years in the future.

e. Some other drugs used in KS chemotherapy are actinomycin D, the combination of adriamycin, bleomycin, and vinblastine known as ABV, and etoposide, or VP-16-213 [VePesid].

f. The research team will be headed by Dr. William L. Epstein, chairman emeritus of the Department of Dermatology at UCSF Medical Center and the world's leading expert on DNCB-like reactions; Dr. Marcus Conant, the world-known authority on KS; Dr. Daniel Stites, one of the world's foremost immunologists; and Dr. Bruce Mills, the pioneer researcher on the use of DNCB in AIDS and ARC. In spite of this star-studded roster, the study missed by a hairsbreadth the political axe of personal and professional rivalries. At UCSF, as elsewhere, political control of AIDS research is in the hands of cancer specialists and not immunologists.

g. DNCB is strong stuff. The solution used for treatment contains 2/15 of 1 percent of the substance.

h. These lipids or phosphatides are a neutral phospholipid acting as a carrier, phosphatidylcholine, and phosphatidylethanolamine in a proportion of 7:2:1. Since AL stands for "active lipids," this proportion completes the meaning of AL 721.

i. Lymphocytes lose their capacity to proliferate in response to infection, a function mediated by protein receptors protruding from the lymphocytes' membranes. Since aging affects membrane fluidity, it also affects proper functioning of the protein receptors that trigger lymphocyte proliferation during an infection.

j. Ingesting egg yolks probably doesn't work because the cholesterol in untreated egg–yolk lecithin is likely to counteract membrane fluidization by phosphatides. Until AL 721 is available in this country, you might want to try some of the lecithin preparations with concentrated phosphatidylcholine content available at health food stores.

k. The example is even more significant for someone with AIDS. Certain studies suggest that superficial, or mucocutaneous, candida infections may be held in check by the macrophage–T cell mechanism that is deficient in those with AIDS, while systemic candidiasis may be controlled by the neutrophil phagocytes that still operate in AIDS patients. Appearance of systemic candida infection after antibiotic treatments may indicate that antibiotics somehow dampen neutrophil function.

l. Bacteria do not interchange genetic information through sexual reproduction as do higher organisms like us. Through a process called bacterial conjugation, two bacteria exchange bits of genes and can thus interchange, let's say, the ability to resist an antibiotic.

m. Vitamin C, on the other hand, inhibits the action of PGE2 and PGE2–alpha without inhibiting that of PGE1.

n. Growing up unexposed to the pain of addiction, the alcoholic's grandchildren may often resort to alcohol and drugs.

o. The large number of gay AIDS cases in the U.S. is due to the large homosexual population and not to a higher risk of getting AIDS because one is gay. The Caceres article cites a letter in the British medical journal *The Lancet* that demonstrates, using CDC figures, that 4.2 out of 100 hemophiliacs and 4.6 out of 100 *nongay* IV-users will develop AIDS, whereas only 1 out of 100 gay men will do so.

***

1. Jacques Leibowitch.
   A Strange Virus of Unknown Origin.
   Ballantine Books, 1985.
   Translated from the French by Richard Howard.
2. Kevin M. Cahil.
   Parasitic infections.
   In Kevin M. Cahill, editor, *The AIDS Epidemic*, pages 89–91. St. Martin's Press, 1983.
3. The Burroughs Wellcome Co.
   Protocol for Uncontrolled Trial of the Long Term Safety of AZT™.
   Unpublished paper distributed to physicians and patients interested in AZT.
4. J. Silberner.
   AIDS drug: not cure, but hope.
   Science News 130(13):196, 27 September 1986.
5. Bijan Safai.
   Kaposi's sarcoma.
   In Kevin M. Cahill, editor, *The AIDS Epidemic*, pages 98–112. St. Martin's Press, 1983.
6. Frederick P. Siegal and Marta Siegal.
   AIDS: The Medical Mystery.
   Grove Press, New York, 1983
7. Elinor M. Levy, John C. Beldekas, Paul H. Black, Robert H. Lerman, Martha C. Cottrell, and Lawrence H. Kushi.
   Patients with Kaposi's sarcoma who opt for no treatment.
   The Lancet II(8448):223, 27 July 1985.
8. Leibowitz, *Strange Virus.*
9. Siegal and Siegal, *Medical Mystery.*
10. Bruce Mills
    Stimulation of T-cellular immunity by cutaneous application of dinitrochloro benzene.
    Journal of the American Academy of Dermatology 14 (6):1089, June 1986.
11. John S. James
    DNCB AIDS/ARC Treatment
    SF Sentinel 14(20):9, 26 September 1986.
12. R. C. Gallo, P. S. Sarin, D. I. Scheer, F. Crews, and A. S. Lippa.
    Effects of a novel compound (AL 721) on HTLV-III infectivity in vitro.
    The New England Journal of Medicine 313(20):1289, 14 November 1985.

13. John S. James
AIDS, AL 721, lecithin.
SF Sentinel 14(15):8, 18 July 1986.
14. John S. James
AL 721 update and recipe.
SF Sentinel 14(18):8, 29 August 1986.
15. John S. James
AIDS/ARC treatment: A role for lecithin?
Draft for the article "AIDS, AL 721, Lecithin" in *SF Sentinel* 14(15), 18 July 1986.
For copy write to: JS James, P. O. Box 411256, San Francisco, CA 94141
16. John S. James
Naltrexone for AIDS/ARC.
SF Sentinel 14(22):15, 24 October 1986.
17. Siegal and Siegal, *Medical Mystery*, pages 133–134.
18. Donald B. Louria.
Bacterial and Mycotic Infections, page 75.
In Kevin M. Cahill, editor, *The AIDS Epidemic*, pages 72–85. St. Martin's Press, 1983.
19. Henry G. Bieler.
Food is Your Best Medicine.
Ballantine, 1982.
20. Louria, Bacterial and mycotic infections, page 84.
21. Pauling, *How to Live Longer.*
22. Joel Kaufman, Linda Rabinowitz-Dagi, Joan Levin, Phyllis McCarthy, Sydney Wolfe, Eve Bargmann, and the Public Citizen Health Research Group.
Over-the-Counter Pills That Don't Work.
Pantheon, 1983.
23. Oyle, *The Healing Mind.*
24. Kaufman, et al., *Over-the-Counter-Pills.*
25. Dianna Solis.
Gays band together in workplace to help careers, battle prejudice.
The Wall Street Journal CCVII(49):37, 12 March 1986.
26. Dennis Wholey.
The Courage to Change: Personal Conversations about Alcoholism with Dennis Wholey.
Warner Books, 1984.
27. Katherine Ketcham and L. Ann Mueller.
Eating Right to Live Sober.
New American Library, 1986.
28. Barbara G. Faltz and Scott Madover.
AIDS and substance abuse: Issues for health care providers.
Focus: A Review of AIDS Research 1(9):1, August 1986.
29. Ann Giudici Fettner.
Bringing scientists to their senses: Cesar Caceres vs. selective blindness, pages 15–16.
Christopher Street 9(3):15, 1985.

30. Fettner, Cesar Caceres vs. selective blindness, page 17.

CHAPTER 5. HOW FOOD AFFECTS PEOPLE

a. But there is a point to be made about diet. Not even Buddha, who gone far beyond other people in spiritual awareness, could escape the consequences of food. He died of food poisoning at eighty.

***

1. Anthony J. Sattilaro and Thomas J. Monte.
   Recalled by Life.
   Avon, 1984.

CHAPTER 6. ELEMENTS OF NUTRITION

a. Ketone bodies are certain organic compounds that contain a carbonyl group (a carbon and an oxygen atom joined by a double bond thus: C=O) and that are toxic above certain concentrations.

b. Glucose is also known as dextrose or corn, grape, and blood sugar, fructose as levulose or fruit sugar.

c. About 10 percent of all honey contains spores of the bacterium *Clostridium botulinum,* which has caused botulism in infants and could be harmful to adults with less than ideal immune systems. These spores are not destroyed by cooking. Nan Bronfen, *Nutrition for a Better Life: A Source Book for the Eighties.* Capra Press, 1980.

d. Fatty acids are the basic components of fats, as amino acids are those of proteins. A fatty acid consists of a long chain of carbon and hydrogen atoms. Fatty acids are classified as saturated, unsaturated, and polyunsaturated according to the decreasing amount of hydrogen atoms in the chain.

e. Cholesterol-induced membrane rigidity brought about by alcohol and drug abuse could expose helper T cell receptor molecules to HIV attack. Membrane rigidity also works to HIV's advantage once it infects a helper T cell by isolating the cell from contact with the rest of the immune system. The virus could even be actively altering the cholesterol/phosphatidyl ratio in the membrane to suit its needs. This might well be why suppressor T cells cannot inhibit virus replication in the infected cells of some individuals , as reported by a UCSF research team in December 1987. An infected helper T cell whose receptor molecules are either too rigid or worn down may not be able to induce a suppressor T cell to secrete its HIV-inhibiting substance.

f. Even reputedly low-fat fish, shell fish, and fowl often have too much fat. Codfish has 5 percent fat and shrimp 8, but scallops have 11, lobster 14, crab and skinless light chicken 18, and clams 21. So go light on the chicken and seafood if you feel the need to eat them. Some other foods, like avocados, chocolate, coconut, and olives, are also very high in fat.

g. The *trans* fatty acids. Natural fatty acids are *cis* fatty acids.

h. Low- and very low-density lipoproteins are the lipids whose presence in the blood might cause cholesterol to deposit on arterial walls. High- and very-high density lipoproteins, on the other hand, help reduce cholesterol levels in the blood. Investigators believe that these lipoproteins belong to a large class of substances that regulate and fine-tune the body's immune response.

i. More specifically, cellulose is the principal structural element of a plant's cell walls. Lignin makes up its woody parts, pectin cements its cells together, hemicellulose is found in its cell walls, and mucilage and gum are two of its nonstructural elements.

j. Diverticulosis is a condition characterized by the formation of numerous diverticula, or sac-like protrusions, in the colon. These diverticula may become inflamed and ulcerate, impairing the proper functioning of the colon and bringing about chronic diarrhea and severe loss of weight.

k. IU, or international units, are the most common standard of strength for vitamins A, D, and E. Recommended daily allowances, RDAs, are discussed later in the chapter.

l. The body can also manufacture some niacin from the amino acid tryptophan. *Earl Mindell's Vitamin Bible.*

m. These bacteria are also found in the human intestine but are too far down in the tract for the vitamin to be absorbed by the body.

n. You may ask how humans survived all these years before the advent of vitamin C supplements. The answer is barely or not at all. Up to the twentieth century, disease killed most people at an early age. Vitamin C insufficiency didn't matter unless it was so large as to cause scurvy and kill. During the twentieth century, prescorbutic deficiency is considered the human norm. The two or three yearly colds, the annual flu, the bleeding gums, the cracked lips, and the split nails are seen as a normal part of our lives. Many of these things would change if we took an optimum daily amount of vitamin C.

o. The only established side effect of too large a dose of vitamin C is diarrhea, which according to Cathcart tells you you've reached your body's needs and should cut back around 10 percent. Skin rashes and other allergic reactions have been noted in some individuals but these are usually to traces of raw material the vitamin was obtained from—corn, far example—and not to the vitamin itself. A simple switch of brands often solves the allergy.

Orthodox medicine's big objection to vitamin C megadoses is that these could interfere with some diagnostic tests. In a sense, life also makes diagnosis more difficult; an autopsy is the most unfailing of diagnostics. Medicine should adjust its tests to the patient and not the patients to its tests. In the meantime, if your doctor feels that the amount of vitamin C you take may interfere with a particular test, gradually reduce supplementation a few days before testing and increase it afterwards.

p. Unfortunately, in this case one cannot say without reservations, "Consult your physician." By their own admission, many doctors have only passing knowledge about nutrition and vitamin supplementation.

q. Although some evidence suggests certain bioflavonoids have antiviral properties, the main value of substances such as bioflavonoids and the hesperidin complex may lie in providing a buffer against acid vitamin C. Acidity problems can be avoided at a lower cost by taking calcium or magnesium ascorbates rather than ascorbic acid. These vitamin C salts are already buffered.

r. The craving is usually for magnesium salts, in which the typical American diet tends to be deficient. Magnesium deficiency is a major cause of an enlarged prostate.

s. Contrary to popular belief, lead poisoning had little to do with the fall of Rome. Although the Romans did use lead piping extensively, they lacked faucets and thus had a true running-water system. At no time during the day or night was the cold water from the mountains delayed in its rush to the fountains and gardens of the city. The water did not stand in the pipes. Additionally, the Romans preferred hard, mountain-spring water, rich in calcium carbonates. Recent archeological evidence suggests that these carbonates quickly built thick deposits inside the pipes, thus preventing the water from coming in contact with the lead. Wherever they colonized, the Romans first built an aqueduct, going to great lengths to obtain the pure mountain water they so valued. Thus it might be that the quality of Rome's water was the reason not for its fall but for its rise. A. Trevor Hodge. Siphons in Roman aqueducts. *Scientific American* 252(6):114–119, June 1985.

t. The addition of fluorides to U.S. municipal water supplies is a controversial subject. While authorities claim that fluorides in drinking water help prevent tooth decay, several health experts maintain that whatever antidecay properties flourides might have are offset by the possible formation of carcinogenic fluorocarbons when the fluorides react with organic matter in the water.

* * *

1. Corinne H. Robinson and Marilyn R. Lawler.
   Normal and Therapeutic Nutrition.
   Macmillan, 1982.
2. Gary M. Gray and Michael R. Fogel
   Nutritional aspects of dietary carbohydrates.
   In Robert S. Goodhart and Maurice E. Shils, *Modern Nutrition in Health and Disease,*
   pages 99–112. Lea and Febiger, 1980.

3. William Dufty.
   Sugar Blues, page 46.
   Warner, 1976.
4. Saul Miller and Jo Anne Miller.
   Food for Thought: A New Look at Food and Behavior
   Prentice-Hall, 1979.
5. Dufty, *Sugar Blues*, pages 79, 137–38.
6. Debra Lynn Dadd.
   Nontoxic and Natural: How to Avoid Dangerous Everyday Products and Buy or Make Safe Ones.
   Jeremy P. Tarcher, Los Angeles, California, 1984.
   Distributed by Houghton Mifflin Company.
7. United States, National Academy of Sciences; National Research Council; Committee on Diet, Nutrition, and Cancer.
   Diet, Nutrition, and Cancer: Directions for Research.
   National Academy Press, Washington, D.C., 1983.
8. Alice A. Martin and Frances Tenenbaum.
   Diet against Disease: A New Plan for Safe and Healthy Eating.
   Penguin Books, 1982.
9. Frank L. Iber.
   The gastrointestinal tract: an overview of function.
   In Robert S. Goodhart and Maurice E. Shils, *Modern Nutrition in Health and Disease*, pages 35–50. Lea and Febiger, 1980.
10. Selwyn A. Broitman and Norman Zamcheck.
    Nutrition in diseases of the intestines.
    In Robert S. Goodhart and Maurice E. Shils, *Modern Nutrition in Health and Disease*, pages 912–976. Lea and Febiger, 1980.
11. Robinson and Lawler, *Normal and Therapeutic Nutrition.*
12. *Vegetarian Times* (93):23, May 1985.
    Should you be taking nutritional supplements?
13. Frances Moore Lappé.
    Diet for A Small Planet, page 172.
    Ballantine Books, tenth anniversary edition 1982.
14. Nan Bronfen.
    Nutrition for a Better Life: A Source Book for the Eighties.
    Capra Press, 1980.
15. Michio Kushi and the East-West Foundation.
    The Macrobiotic Approach to Cancer.
    Avery, 1982.
16. National Research Council, *Diet, Nutrition, and Cancer Directions.*
17. Arthur J. Vander, James H. Sherman, and Dorothy S. Luciano.
    Human Physiology: The Mechanisms of Body Function.
    McGraw-Hill, 1975.
18. Bronfen, *Nutrition for a Better Life.*

19. Catherine F. Adams.
Nutritive Value of American Foods in Common Units.
Agriculture Handbook No. 456. United States Department of Agriculture; Agricultural Research Service. Government Printing Office, 1975.
20. Barton, *A Comprehensive Approach to AIDS.*
21. Meir Shinitzky.
Membrane fluidity and cellular functions.
In Meir Shinitzky, editor, *Physiology of Membrane Fluidity,* Volume I, pages 1–52. CRC Press, Boca Raton, Florida, 1984.
22. Keith D. Barton.
Trade secrets: Health improvement considerations in five stages.
SF Sentinel 14(3):8–9, January 31, 1986.
23. Leo D. Galland.
Nutrition in *Candida albicans.*
In Jeffrey Bland, editor, *Second Edition:1986, A Year in Nutritional Medicine,* pages 203–238, Keats Publishing, New Canaan, Connecticut, 1986.
24. Marcia Church, nutritionist at the offices of Richard L. Shames, M.D., Mill Valley, California.
Private communication, 13 March 1986.
25. Bronfen, *Nutrition for a Better Life.*
26. John A. McDougall and Mary A. McDougall.
The McDougall Plan, page 89.
New Century Publishers, Piscataway, New Jersey, 1983.
27. Sattilaro and Monte, *Recalled by Life.*
28. *Scientific American* 253(5): 106, November 1985.
Science and the citizen: Cachectin.
29. Stuart M. Berger.
Dr. Berger's Immune Power Diet.
New American Library, 1985.
30. M. Macy, Y. Okano, A. D. Cardin, E. M. Avila, and J. A. K. Harmony.
Suppression of lymphocyte activation by plasma lipoproteins.
Cancer Research Supplement 43:2496s–2502s, 1985.
31. Michio Kushi and Stephen Blauer.
The new macrobiotic way, page 29.
Macromuse (19):28–33, Spring/Wood 1985.
32. Bronfen, *Nutrition for a Better Life.*
33. McDougall and McDougall.
34. *Medical Abstracts Newsletter,* 4(5): 3, May 1984.
Diet and Cancer: New Findings.
35. McDougall and McDougall.
36. Michael E. Rosenbaum.
Nutrients and the Immune System.
Manuscript in preparation, April 1986.
37. Bronfen, *Nutrition for a Better Life.*

38. Annette Natow and Jo-Ann Heslin.
Megadoses: Vitamins as Drugs.
Pocket Books, 1985.
39. Natow and Heslin, *Megadoses.*
40. William Gottlieb, Carl Lowe, Mark Bricklin, and Susan Zarrow.
The Complete Book of Vitamins.
Rodale Press, 1984.
41. McDougall and McDougall.
42. Emanuel Cheraskin, W. Marshall Ringsdorf, Jr., and Emily L. Sisley.
The Vitamin C Connection.
Bantam Books, 1984.
43. Earl Mindell.
Earl Mindell's Vitamin Bible.
Warner, 1979.
44. Cheraskin, et al., *Vitamin C Connection.*
45. Pauling, *How to Live Longer*, page 78.
46. Pauling, *How to Live Longer.*
47. Cheraskin, et al., *Vitamin C Connection*, page 214.
48. Bronfen, *Nutrition far a Better Life.*
49. Weiner, *Maximum Immunity.*
50. Bronfen, *Nutrition for a Better Life.*
51. Jaques de Langre.
Sea Salt's Hidden Powers: How to Tell Its Integrity and Use It Correctly.
The Grain and Salt Society, P. O. Drawer S–DD, Magalia, California 95954. 1985.
52. Herman Aihara.
Basic Macrobiotics.
Japan Publications, 1985.
53. de Langre, *Sea Salt.*
54. de Langre, *Sea Salt.*
55. Kurt W. Donsbach.
Dr. Donsbach Tells You What You Always Wanted to Know about Water.
The International Institute of Natural Health Sciences, 7422 Mountjoy Drive, Huntington Beach, California 92648. 1983.
56. United States Environmental Protection Agency.
Is Your Drinking Water Safe?
170 35-61-OPA. March 1985.
57. Donsbach.
58. Donsbach, page 20.
59. United States Environmental Protection Agency.
Water Quality Improvement in the Home by Frank Bell, Ervin Bellak, and Joseph Cotruvo.
Typescript. 9 April 1984.

60. San Francisco Water Department, Water Quality Division.
Mineral analysis: Sample collection, September 1984.
San Francisco, after 20 December 1984.
61. Pauling, *How to Live Longer.*

CHAPTER 7. THE COMPONENTS OF A GOOD DIET

a. Some percentages of the minerals eliminated by refining are magnesium, zinc, and chromium, 83 percent; copper, 70 to 90 percent; cobalt, 70 percent; and molybdenum, 50 percent. These are not replaced.

b. More specifically, gluten sensitivity is sensitivity to the protein gliadin, which along with the protein glutenin makes up gluten.

c. Aryl hydroxylases.

d. The kidneylike beans are varieties or close relatives of the common or kidney bean: adzuki, black, great northern, navy, and pinto beans.

e. Garlic's active ingredients, allyl disulphate and other sulphur compounds also found in onions and leeks in smaller amounts, give garlic its characteristic odor.

* * *

1. Lappé, *Diet for A Small Planet.*
2. Bronfen, *Nutrition for a Better Life.*
3. Kushi and Jack, *The Cancer Prevention Diet.*
4. E. Pfeiffer.
Does Bread Nourish?
The Happiness Press, 160 Wycliff, Magalia, California 95954. 1978.
5. Paul M. Newberne.
Naturally occurring food-borne toxicants.
In Robert S. Goodhart and Maurice E. Shils, editors, *Modern Nutrition in Health and Disease*, pages 463–496. Lea and Febiger, 1980.
6. McDougall and McDougall.
7. United States, National Academy of Sciences; National Research Council; Committee on Diet, Nutrition, and Cancer.
Diet, Nutrition, and Cancer.
National Academy Press, 1982.
8. Robinson and Lawler, *Normal and Therapeutic Nutrition.*

9. McDougall and McDougall.
10. Dufty, *Sugar Blues,* page 133.
11. Virginia Livingston-Wheeler and Edmond G. Addeo.
 The Conquest of Cancer: Vaccines and Diet.
 Franklin Watts, 1984.
12. McDougall and McDougall.
13. Kushi and the East-West Foundation, *The Macrobiotic Approach to Cancer.*
14. Bieler, *Food Is Your Best Medicine.*
15. Kushi and Blauer, The new macrobiotic way, page 31
16. Eleanor and John Lewallen.
 Vegetable Gourmet Cookbook and Forager's Guide, page 23..
 Mendocino Sea Vegetable Company,P. O. Box 372, Navarro, California 95463, 1983.
17. Seibin Arasaki and Teruko Arasaki.
 Vegetables from the Sea.
 Japan Publications, 1983.
18. Arasaki and Arasaki, *Vegetables from the Sea.*
19. John A. Mann and Steven William Fowkes.
 Wipe Out Herpes with BHT.
 MegaHealth Society,P. O. Box 1684, Manhattan Beach, California 90266. 1983.
20. Eric Block.
 The chemistry of garlic and onions, page 114.
 Scientific American 252(3): 114–119, March 1985.
21. William G. Crook.
 The Yeast Connection: A Medical Breakthrough.
 Professional Books, P. O. Box 3494, Jackson, Tennesse 38301. Second edition, 1984.
22. Bronfen, *Nutrition for a Better Life.*

CHAPTER 8. THE PITFALLS OF INGESTION

a. AIDS hysteria has prompted some people to avoid restaurants, fearing infection by the HIV virus through food contaminated by an afflicted handler. Little do they realize that it is the person afflicted by AIDS or an AIDS-related condition that should avoid them and their restaurants because they could be the source of a fatal opportunistic infection.

b. The *afla* in aflatoxins comes from a(spergillus) fla(vus).

c. Many restaurants and food establishments use peanut oil in food preparation.

d. These toxic chemicals include the carcinogenic fumigants Vapam and pentachlorobenzene, the herbicides 1,4-2 and dicambia, the fungicides

Mer-Tec and Captan (banned in Canada), and the pesticide Temik, best known for causing the 1985 California watermelon scare.

e. "Nearly 500 of these ingredients are not required to be identified on labels.This inconsistency in labeling goes so far that an additive may have to be listed on the label of one food but not on that of another. For example, monosodium glutamate (MSG) must be noted on soup labels but not on mayonnaise or salad dressing." John McDougall and Mary McDougall, *The McDougall Plan,* page 145.

f. A 1976 test tried to determine the extent of the additive interaction problem: "When three additives were treated one at a time on rats, the animals stayed well: two at a time, the rats became ill; and with a three-additive combination, all the animals died within fourteen days." Ruth Winter, *A Consumer's Dictionary of Food Additives,* page 4. Crown Publishers, New York, 1984.

g. "Pesticide contaminants and other organic chemicals are being found at an ever-increasing rate in underground drinking-water supplies." California State Assembly Bill 2027.

h. Sold to farmers as Temik.

i. Many chemical and drug manufacturers have bought into seed companies in order to produce strains of plants which will allow farmers to use more chemicals more frequently. Farmers will buy the new seeds and the chemicals as a package, thereby husbanding new growth in the profits of the chemical manufacturers. The tragedy of such profit-grabbing efforts is that they have added little to the efficiency of our agricultural efforts. According to leading pest control researchers, crop loss due to insects is today the same as it was in 1900, about 20 percent.

j. Environmental medicine covers the study of allergies and of poisonous or toxic materials.

k. Food-induced immune complexes have damaged the blood-brain barrier in animals, inducing behavioral changes and possibly affecting the barrier's capacity to keep out large molecules, such as certain toxins, and submicroscopic particles, such as certain viruses.

l. I recommend the exclusion of animal products for health rather than religious reasons.

m. These antibiotics also kill many of the beneficial intestinal bacteria that help retard candida growth.

n. *Escherichia coli* is a lactose-fermenting bacteria commonly present in the human intestine. Although *E. coli* is usually nonpathogenic, under certain conditions it can cause urogenital infections and diarrhea in children.

o. Cheese tends to be low in lactose—only 2 percent of its calories come from milk sugar—and causes less problems to those with lactose intolerance. MacDougall and MacDougall.

p. I have not, however, come across any evidence that acidophilus is harmful, so I take one teaspoon three times a day hoping it will promote beneficial bacteria and suppress harmful yeast (candida) in the bowel. There are soy-based acidophilus cultures available for those allergic to milk.

q. The bovine C-type virus.

r. The monoamine oxidase inhibitors such as furazolidone, isocarboxacid, pargyline, phenelzine, procarbazine, and tranylcypromine.

s. Produced by the pancreas to help digest proteins.

t. Known as triterpenoid saponins.

u. Although it is true that we process most food to one degree or another as we prepare it for eating, when I say prepared or processed food I am talking about food whose original makeup has been radically altered by an industrial or commercial process.

v. The portions of vitamins lost are as follows: thiamine or B1, 90 percent; riboflavin or B2, 70 percent; niacin or B3, 70 percent; pyridoxine or B6, 80 percent; vitamin E, 50 percent. The loss of minerals is just as devastating: iron and calcium, 80 and 50 percent, respectively. Iron is usually replaced, but calcium only occasionally is. Minerals like copper, magnesium, zinc, chromium, manganese, and cobalt are never replaced. Their losses range from 60 to 90 percent.

w. Low dosages consist of up to 100 kilorads delivered by cobalt 60, cesium 137, or a beam of high-energy electrons from an electron accelerator. This radiation is 1,000 times greater than that delivered by the usual chest x-ray. Medium dosages are up to 1,000 kilorads, or 10,000 times those of chest x-rays.

x. Irradiated food is often euphemistically labeled as "picowaved," perhaps so the buyer associates the name with the convenience of the friendly home microwave. Since *pico-* indicates something a million times smaller than *micro-*, what harm could such a tiny little wave do? In the real universe, however, the smaller an energy wave, the more powerful it is. A picowave is a million times deadlier than a microwave.

y. San Francisco currently requires fast-food establishments to list, where the public can see them, the ingredients and nutrients in their products.

z. Published by the Center for Science in the Public Interest. You might want to join this organization in order to keep abreast of the latest nutritional findings. For address, see Nutrition Information in appendix H.

* * *

1. Robinson and Lawler, *Normal and Therapeutic Nutrition.*
2. Block, The chemistry of garlic and onions.
3. Bronfen, *Nutrition for a Better Life.*
4. Newberne, Naturally occurring food-borne toxicants.
5. Louria, Bacterial and mycotic infections.
6. Newberne, Naturally occurring food-borne toxicants, page 472.
7. Newberne, Naturally occurring food-borne toxicants.
8. Natow and Heslin, *Megadoses.*
9. Robinson and Lawler, *Normal and Therapeutic Nutrition.*
10. Herbert M. Shelton.
    Food Combining Made Easy.
    Willow Publishing , San Antonio, Texas. second edition 1982.
11. Lynn Ludlow.
    Toxic seeds lurking under Central Valley.
    San Francisco Examiner 1985(32):B1, 11 August 1985.
12. William F. Allman.
    Pesticides: An unhealthy dependence?
    Science 85 6(8): 14, October 1985.
13. R. E. Taylor.
    Pesticide Aldicarb causes suppression of immunity in lab mice, study shows.
    Wall Street Journal CCVI(34):8, 16 August 1985.
14. Lappé, *Diet for a Small Planet.*

15. Robert F. Cathcart, III.
Vitamin C in the treatment of aquired immune deficiency syndrome (AIDS). *Medical Hypotheses* 14: 423, 1984.
16. Weiner, *Maximum Immunity.*
17. Robert A. Good.
Immunologic aberrations: The AIDS defect.
In Kevin M. Cahil, editor, *The AIDS Epidemic*, pages 41–59. St. Martin's Press, 1983.
18. Iris R. Bell.
Clinical Ecology: A New Medical Approach to Environmental Illness.
Common Knowledge Press, Bolinas. California, 1982.
19. George T. Lewith and Julian N. Kenyon.
Clinical Ecology: A Therapeutic Approach to Understanding and Treating Food and Chemical Sensitivities.
Thorsons Publishers, Wellingsborough, Northamptonshire, England, 1985.
20. United States, National Academy of Sciences; National Research Council's Commission on Life Sciences; Food and Nutrition Board.
What Is America Eating? Proceedings of the December 1984 Symposium, page 89. National Academy Press, 1986.
21. Berger, *Dr. Berger's Immune Power Diet.*
22. Weiner, *Maximum Immunity.*
23. Bronfen, *Nutrition for a Better Life*, page 36.
24. *Vegetarian Times* (93):849, May 1985.
News Digest.
25. McDougall and McDougall.
26. Harry D. Fein.
Nutrition in diseases of the stomach, including related areas in the esophagus and duodenum.
In Robert S. Goodhart and Maurice E. Shils, editors, *Modern Nutrition in Health and Disease*, pages 892–952. Lea and Febiger, 1980.
27. Robinson and Lawler, *Normal and Therapeutic Nutrition.*
28. Louria, Bacterial and mycotic infections.
29. McDougall and McDougall,page 43.
30. Bronfen, *Nutrition for a Better Life.*
31. McDougall and McDougall, page 43.
32. Louis V. Alvioli.
Calcium and phosphorus.
In Robert S. Goodhart and Maurice E. Shils, editors, *Modern Nutrition in Health and Disease*, pages 294–309. Lea and Febiger, 1980.
33. Miller and Miller, *Food for Thought.*
34. Rudolph Ballentine.
Nasal function and energy.
In Swami Rama, Rudolph Ballentine, and Alan Hymes, *Science of Breath: A Practical Guide*, pages 57–87. Himalayan International Institute of Yoga Science and Philosophy, Honesdale, Pennsylvania, 1979.

35. Gray and Fogel, Nutritional aspects of dietary carbohydrates.
36. Iber, The gastrointestinal tract.
37. *Medical Self-Care* (28):17, Spring 1985.
Vital signs: yogurt and yeast infections.
38. C. Orion Truss.
The Missing Diagnosis.
The Missing Diagnosis., P. O. Box 26508, Birmingham, Alabama 35226. 1983.
39. McDougall and McDougall, page 51.
40. Kushi and the East-West Foundation, *The Macrobiotic Approach to Cancer.*
41. Gary Null and Steve Null.
Protein for Vegetarians.
Pyramid Books, 1975.
42. Newberne, Naturally occurring food-borne toxicants.
43. Mindell, *Vitamin Bible.*
44. Kushi and the East-West Foundation, *The Macrobiotic Approach to Cancer.*
45. Newberne, Naturally occurring food-borne toxicants.
46. Miller and Miller, *Food for Thought.*
47. Robinson and Lawler, *Normal & Therapeutic Nutrition.*
48. Bronfen, *Nutrition for a Better Life.*
49. McDougall and McDougall.
50. Bieler, *Food Is Your Best Medicine.*
51. Barton, A comprehensive approach to AIDS.
52. *Tufts University Diet and Nutrition Letter* 3(12):2, February 1986.
Is ginseng the root to good health?
53. Ben A. Franklin
Carcinogens: A review of twenty major controversies.
New York Times CXXXIII(45):.C12, 20 March 1984.
54. Miller and Miller, *Food for Thought.*
55. Bell, *Clinical Ecology.*
56. Miller and Miller, *Food for Thought.*
57. Sally Hayhow.
Behind the glowing reports on irradiation.
Vegetarian Times (81) : 52, May 1984.
58. National Research Council, *Diet, Nutrition, and Cancer.*
59. *Nutrition Action Healthletter* 12(5): 10, June 1985.
Eater's digest. Fast food: what's in the stuff?
60. *Nutrition Action Healthletter* 12(3): 3, April 1985.
In the public interest: Bill calls for limited sulfite ban.
61. *Nutrition Action Healthletter* 12(2): 10, March 1985.
In the public interest: Panel calls for sulfite ban.
62. *Wall Street Journal* CCVI(34):21, 16 August 1985.
Television bureau of advertising broadcast advertisers' reports.
63. McDougall and McDougall, page 143.
64. Miller and Miller, *Food for Thought.*

65. McDougall and McDougall.
66. McDougall and McDougall.
67. John Cairns.
The treatment of diseases and the war against cancer.
Scientific American 253(3):51, November 1985.
68. *The Washington Post National Weekly Edition* 2(37):26, 15 July 1985.
A lipstick you can live with.

CHAPTER 9. MAKING THE CHANGE

a. There are people for whom food has become a true addiction. If you feel you have a problem with compulsive eating, you might want to consider counseling or one of the various support groups such as Overeaters Anonymous (OA).

b. This is not to say that you must eat when you are ill even if you don't feel like it. Loss of appetite can be part of the body's strategy against illness. Digestion takes energy. By forcing you to eat lightly, your body can use most of its energy to fight disease.

⁂ ⁂ ⁂

1. Dadd, *Nontoxic and Natural.*
2. Catharine Osgood Foster.
The Organic Gardener.
Alfred A. Knopf, 1972.

CHAPTER 10. LIVING WITH FOOD

a. However, the following soaking method is recommended by physician James O'Shea for his candida patients to remove fungi, bacteria, insecticides and certain chemicals from suspect food: Treat fruits and vegetables separately. Soak in a solution of 1/2 teaspoon Clorox® per gallon of water (use stainless-steel measuring spoons and no other brand than Clorox®). Soak frozen, leafy vegetables and thin rind fruits fifteen minutes, heavy rind fruits and root vegetables twenty minutes and thick-skinned vegetables like squash twenty-five. Discard solution after each use. Now soak the treated fruit or vegetables in clean water for fifteen minutes. Discard water after each use. Once treated, vegetables can be stored in freezer bags in the refrigerator. (Crook, *The Yeast Connection*)

❊ ❊ ❊

1. *S.F. Macronews* (4):1, February 1987.
   Macronews interview: Susan Broad Stokes.
2. Kushi and Jack, *The Cancer Prevention Diet*.
3. Theron G. Randolph, M.D.
   The "inner tube" (the gastrointestinal tract) in food allergies.
   Unpublished manuscript, August 1976.
   Available through the American Academy for Environmental Science.
   See Environmental Medicine in appendix H.
4. Livingston-Wheeler and Addeo, *The Conquest of Cancer*.
5. Fritz Perls.
   Ego: Hunger and Aggression.
   Vantage Books, 1969.

CHAPTER 12. DETOXIFYING THE BODY: OFFENDERS

a. The unsanitary conditions of the Third World also exist in the slums and refugee communities of the United States. Poverty pays no heed to nationality, race, sex, creed, or sexual orientation.

b. The studies do not indicate how these parasites are transmitted. Yet unsafe sex practices such as oral-anal contact and anal sex without a condom are the most likely culprits.

c. Don't ship your cat to the SPCA tomorrow, however. Because toxoplasma is contracted mainly from cat feces and not from the cat, avoid contact with the litter box. Have someone else clean the tray for you, or, if this isn't possible, get plastic tray liners that you can throw out without touching the litter.

d. Under check, candida is a commensal, an organism that, like a customary mealtime companion, eats at your table but doesn't really harm you.

e. Because of lactose, the sugar in milk.

1. John S. James.
   On guard: The parasitic connection.
   San Francisco Sentinel 14(13):8, 20 June 1986.
2. Cathcart, Vitamin C in AIDS.
3. Walker, et al., CD8 lymphocytes can control HIV infection.
4. James, The parasitic connection.
5. Richard B. Pearce.
   Parasites and AIDS.
   New York Native 3(20):26, 20 August - 11 September 1983.
6. Edward K Markell and Marietta Voge.
   Medical Parasitology.
   W.B. Saunders, 1981.
7. Pearce, Parasites and AIDS.
8. Erica Allanson-Jones, Adrian Mindell, Peter Sargeaunt, and Peter Williams.
   Entamoeba histolytica as a commensal intestinal parasite in homosexual men.
   The New England Journal of Medicine 315(6): 356, 7 August 1986.
9. Pearce, Parasites and AIDS.
10. William A. Petri and Jonathan I. Ravdin.
    Treatment of homosexual men infected with *Entamoeba histolytica.*
    The New England Journal of Medicine 315(6): 393, 7 August 1986.
11. J. Laurence and H. J. Kunkel.
    Soluble suppressor factors in patients with acquired immune deficiency syndrome.
    Clinical Research 31(2):347A, April 1983.
12. Pearce, Parasites and AIDS, page 27.
13. Allanson-Jones et al., *Entamoeba histolytica.*
14. Markell and Voge, *Medical Parasitology.*
15. Cahill, Parasitic infections, page 94.
16. Cahill, Parasitic infections.
17. *Physician's Desk Reference.*
    Medical Economics Company, Oradell, New Jersey, 1985.
18. Markell and Voge, *Medical Parasitology.*
19. Cahill, Parasitic infections.
20. Louria, Bacterial and mycotic infections.
21. Siegal and Siegal, *Medical Mystery.*
22. United States, National Academy of Sciences; Institute of Medicine.
    Mobilizing against AIDS: The Unfinished Story of a Virus, by Eve K. Nichols.
    Harvard University Press, 1986.
23. Cahill, Parasitic infections, p. 86.
24. Louria, Bacterial and mycotic infections.
25. Institute of Medicine, *Mobilizing against AIDS.*
26. Crook, *The Yeast Connection.*
27. Weiner, *Maximum Immunity.*
28. David J. Fletcher.
    Allergy self-care.

Medical Self-Care 33:25, March/April 1986.
29. Louria, Bacterial and mycotic infections.
30. Truss, *The Missing Diagnosis.*
31. Crook, *The Yeast Connection.*
32. Weiner, *Maximum Immunity.*
33. Crook, *The Yeast Connection.*
34. Weiner, *Maximum Immunity.*
35. Weiner, *Maximum Immunity.*
36. Crook, *The Yeast Connection*, page 244.
37. Truss, *The Missing Diagnosis.*
38. *1985 Physician's Desk Reference.*
39. Weiner, *Maximum Immunity.*
40. *1985 Physician's Desk Reference.*
41. *Mosby's Medical & Nursing Dictionary.*
    C. V. Mosby Company, St. Louis, Missouri, 1983.
42. Donald Armstrong.
    Viral infections.
    In Kevin M. Cahill, editor, *The AIDS Epidemic*, pages 63–71. St. Martin's Press, 1983.
43. Siegal and Siegal, *Medical Mystery.*
44. Institute of Medicine, *Mobilizing against AIDS.*
45. Jacques Leibowitch, *Strange Virus.*
46. Nicholas Sampsidis.
    Herpes: Something Can Be Done about It.
    Sunflower Publishing, Glenwood Landing, New York, 1984.
47 Armstrong, Viral infections.
48. Siegal and Siegal, *Medical Mystery.*
49. Institute of Medicine, *Mobilizing against AIDS.*
50. Jacques Leibowitch, *Strange Virus.*
51. *Physician's Desk Reference: Supplement A.*
    Medical Economics Company, Oradell, New Jersey, 1985.
52. Sampsidis, *Herpes: Something Can Be Done about It.*
53. A. E. Friedman-Kien, F. L. Lafleur, E. Gendler, N. P. Hennessey, R. Montagna, S. Halbert, P. Rubenstein, K. Krasinski, E. Zang, and B. Poiesz.
    Herpes zoster: A possible early clinical sign of acquired immunodeficiency syndrome in high-risk individuals.
    Journal of the American Academy of Dermatology 14(6):1023–28, June 1986.
54. Michael Castleman.
    Colds.
    Medical Self-Care (32): 46, January/February 1986.

CHAPTER 13. DETOXIFYING THE BODY: METHODS

1. McDougall and McDougall, page 263.

2. Robert Gray.
The Colon Health Handbook: New Health through Colon Rejuvenation.
Rockridge Publishing, 1982..
3. Ken Coupland.
Life after AIDS, part IV. The new medicine: getting results.
SF Sentinel 12(22):7, 28 February 1985
4. Richard Miles.
The holistic view.
In Larry Geis, Alta Picchi Kelly and Aidan Kelly, editors, *The New Healers: Healing the Whole Person,* pages 5–17. And/Or Press, Berkeley, California, 1980.
5. Shirley McLaine.
Dancing in the Light, page 360.
Bantam, 1985.

CHAPTER 14. BREATH AND EXERCISE

1. Castleman, Colds.
2. Dorothy Luciano, James S. Sherman, and Arthur J. Vander.
Human Physiology: The Mechanisms of Body Function.
McGraw-Hill, 1975.
3. Swami Rama, Rudolph Ballentine, and Alan Hymes.
Science of Breath.
The Himalayan International Institute of Yoga Science and Philosophy, Honesdale, Pennsylvania, 1981.
4. Bronfen, *Nutrition for a Better Life.*
5. Rama, et al., *Science of Breath.*
6. Bronfen, *Nutrition for a Better Life.*
7. Donald Roy Morse and M. Lawrence Furst.
Stress for Success: A Holistic Approach to Stress and Its Management.
Van Nostrand Reinhold, 1979.
8. O. Carl Simonton, Stephanie Matthews-Simonton, and James L. Creighton.
Getting Well Again: A Step-by-Step, Self-Help Guide to Overcoming Cancer for Patients and Their Families.
Bantam, 1980.
9. Morse and Furst, *Stress for Success.*
10. Simonton, et al., *Getting Well Again.*
11. Morse and Furst, *Stress for Success.*
12. Peter Jaret.
Our immune system: The wars within.
National Geographic 169(6):702, June 1986.
13. Bronfen, *Nutrition for a Better life.*
14. Selye, *Stress without Distress,* pages 137–38.

15. Shirley S. Lorenzani.
Candida: A Twentieth Century Disease, pages 99–100.
Keats Publishing, New Canaan, Connecticut, 1986.
16. T.T. Liang.
T'ai Chi Ch'üan for Health and Self-Defense: Philosophy and Practice.
Vintage, 1977.
17. *Medical Self-Care* (28):8 Spring 1985.
Vital Signs: Jogging and Injuries.

CHAPTER 15. BODY MANIPULATION

1. Neshama Franklin.
Bodywork.
In Sheperd Bliss, editor, *The New Holistic Health Handbook: Living Well in a New Age*, pages 332–337. The Stephen Greene Press, Lexington, Massachusetts, 1985.
2. Ilana Rubenfield.
Alexander: The use of the self
In Leslie J. Kaslof, editor, *Wholistic Dimensions in Healing: A Resource Guide*, pages 222–224. Doubleday & Company, 1978.
3. Moshe Feldenkrais and Will Schutz.
Movement and the mind.
In Larry Geis, Alta Picchi Kelly, and Aidan Kelly, editors, *The New Healers: Healing the Whole Person*, pages 40–47. And/Or Press, Berkeley, California, 1980.
4. Kathryn L. Goldman and Barbara M. White.
Everyday miracles: Understanding the Feldenkrais method.
Association for Transpersonal Psychology Newsletter, Winter 1984.
5. Weil, *Health and Healing*.
6. G. F. Rickeman.
Chiropractic.
In Sheperd Bliss, editor, *The New Holistic Health Handbook: Living Well in a New Age*, pages 348–350. The Stephen Greene Press, Lexington, Massachusetts, 1985.
7. T. A. Vondarhaar.
Chiropractic in theory and practice.
In Sheperd Bliss, editor, *The New Holistic Health Handbook: Living Well in a New Age*, pages 349–350. The Stephen Greene Press, Lexington, Massachusetts, 1985.
8. George J. Goodheart and Walter H. Schmitt.
Applied kinesiology.
In Leslie J. Kaslof, editor, *Wholistic Dimensions in Healing: A Resource Guide*, pages 77–79. Doubleday & Company, 1978.
9. Weil, *Health and Healing*.
10. Ida P. Rolf.
Rolfing.
In Leslie J. Kaslof, editor, *Wholistic Dimensions in Healing: A Resource Guide*, pages 225–228. Doubleday & Company, 1978.

11. Neshama Franklin.
My favorite bodywork.
In Sheperd Bliss, editor, *The New Holistic Health Handbook: Living Well in a New Age*, page 334. The Stephen Greene Press, Lexington, Massachusetts, 1985.
12. Richard Hoff.
Overview of Reichian therapy.
In Sheperd Bliss, editor, *The New Holistic Health Handbook: Living Well in a New Age*, pages 338–343. The Stephen Greene Press, Lexington, Massachusetts, 1985.
13. Alexander Lowen.
Bioenergetics, page 44.
Penguin Books, 1975.
14. Franklin, Bodywork.
15. Michael O. Smith and Naomi Rabinowitz.
Acupuncture Treatment of AIDS.
Unpublished manuscript obtainable from Lincoln Hospital Acupuncture Clinic, 349 E. 140th St., Bronx, NY. (212) 993-3100.
16. William Rodarmor.
How to find a good acupuncturist.
Medical Self-Care (35):21, July-August 1986.
17. Michael Reed Gach and Elizabeth Rosner.
Acupressure: Age-old therapy for tension release.
Yoga Journal (67):7, March–April 1986.
18. Pierre Pannetier.
Polarity therapy.
In Leslie J. Kaslof, editor, *Wholistic Dimensions in Healing: A Resource Guide*, pages 216–218. Doubleday & Company, 1978.
19. Crook, *The Yeast Connection*.
20. Dolores Krieger.
The potential use of therapeutic touch in healing.
In Leslie J. Kaslof, editor, *Wholistic Dimensions in Healing: A Resource Guide*, pages 182–191. Doubleday & Company, 1978.

* * *

APPENDIX D. FOOD ADDITIVES

1. Ruth Winter.
A Consumer's Dictionary of Food Additives.
Crown Publishers, New York, 1984.

APPENDIX E. FOOD ALLERGY TESTS

a. Former National Institutes of Health researcher Russell M. Jaffe has developed what could be a major improvement over cytotoxic testing. Though still experimental, the advanced cell test (ACT) promises results with allergies to over 186 foods and chemicals. For more information contact Advanced Cell Technologies at the address listed for Russell M. Jaffe in the appendix H.

* * *

1. Doris J. Rapp.
   Questions and Answers about Allergies and Your Child.
   Drake Publishers, New York, 1974.
2. Lewith and Kenyon, *Clinical Ecology.*
3. Fletcher, Allergy self-care, page 35.
4. Lewith and Kenyon, *Clinical Ecology.*
5. Lewith and Kenyon, *Clinical Ecology.*
6. Bell, *Clinical Ecology.*
7. Lewith and Kenyon, *Clinical Ecology.*

APPENDIX F. HERBS IN AIDS AND ARC

a. In Chinese medicine, meridians are pathways used by the *qi*, or energy, that flows through the body. While there are many meridians, the main ones are associated with the organ systems of the kidney, lungs, heart, liver, urinary bladder, stomach, large intestine, and small intestine. There are two other energetic organ systems not recognized as anatomical organs by Western medicine: the pericardium and the triple burner. For a more extensive explanation of Chinese medicine, I recommend *The Web That Has No Weaver* by Ted Kaptchuk.

b. Weissbuch claims alcohol is the best vehicle for this particular herb combination.

c. *Qi*, or *ch'i* in the older system of transliterating Chinese, is the vital energy—literally the breath—that animates a person. It manifests itself variously throughout the body.

d. *Jing* is the life essence stored in the kidney at birth and replenished through correct diet, herbs, and moderate lifestyle. Because *jing* can also be translated as sperm, a weakness of the sperm is a deficiency in kidney *jing*. *Yin* can be loosely translated as material substance and a person lacking kidney *yin* may become emaciated or manifest symptoms such as constipation, urinary difficulty, nightsweats, afternoon or night fever, and fatigue accompanied by restlessness and insomnia.

e. Serum glutamic pyruvic transaminase, a liver enzyme whose high levels in the blood indicate liver dysfunction.

* * *

1. Barton, *A Comprehensive Approach to AIDS.*
2. Steven Foster.
   Echinacea exalted.
   Ozark Beneficial Plant Project, HCR Box 3, Brixey, MO 656618. 1985
3. Brian Weissbuch.
   Notes for herb classes taught in San Francisco and San Anselmo from 1984 to 1986.
   In the author's possession.
4. Subhuti Dharmananda.
   A new herbal combination for the treatment of immunodeficiency syndromes.
   Pacific Journal of Oriental Medicine 3(1):20, Spring 1986.
5. John S. James.
   Licorice for AIDS/ARC.
   SF Sentinel 14(23):13, 7 November 1986.
6. Other works used as general references in this article are:

   Dan Bensky, Andrew Gamble, and Ted Kaptchuk.
   Chinese Herbal Medicine: Materia Medica.
   Eastland Press, Seattle, 1986.

   Misha Cohen.
   Acupuncture, AIDS, and natural healing.
   Pacific Journal of Oriental Medicine 3(2):54, Fall 1986.

Further reading

The following books are essential reading material for anyone with AIDS or ARC:

Herbert Benson.
Beyond the Relaxation Response.
Berkley Books, 1985.

Viktor E. Frankl.
Man's Search for Meaning.
Washington Square Press, 1985.

Louise L. Hay.
You Can Heal Your Life.
Coleman Publishing, 99 Milbar Blvd., Farmingdale, New York 11735. 1984.

Arnold A. Hutschnecker.
The Will to Live.
Simon and Schuster, 1983.

M. Scott Peck.
The Road Less Travelled: A New Psychology of Love, Traditional Values, and Spiritual Growth.
Simon and Schuster, 1978.

Garrett Porter and Patricia A. Norris.
Why Me? Harnessing the Healing Power of the Human Spirit.
Stillpoint Publishing, Walpole, New Hampshire, 1985.

O. Carl Simonton, Stephanie Matthews-Simonton, and James L. Creighton.
Getting Well Again: A Step-by-Step, Self-Help Guide to Overcoming Cancer for Patients and Their Families.
Bantam, 1980.

The following books, intended as additional—and optional—reading material, are listed in the order and under the chapter title in which they appear in the text:

CHAPTER 1. LEARNING ABOUT HEALTH

Jacques Leibowitch.
A Strange Virus of Unknown Origin.
Ballantine, 1985.
Translated from the French by Richard Howard.

Steven B. Mizel and Peter Jaret.
In Self-Defense.
Harcourt Brace Jovanavich, 1985.

Barbara Peabody.
The Screaming Room: A Mother's Journal of Her Son's Struggle with AIDS.
Oaktree Publications, San Diego, California, 1986.

CHAPTER 2. NURTURING HEALTH

Norman Cousins.
Human Options.
Berkley Books, 1983.

Martha Friedman.
Overcoming the Fear of Success.
Warner, 1982.

Lawrence LeShan.
You Can Fight for Your Life: Emotional Factors in the Treatment of Cancer.
M. Evans and Company, 1980.

Robert J. McKain, Jr.
Realize Your Potential.
Amacom, New York, 1975.

Frieda Porat.
Creative Procrastination: Organizing Your Own Life.
Harper and Row, 1980.

John Renesch.
Setting Goals.
Context Publications, 20 Lomita Ave., San Francisco, California 94122. 1983.

CHAPTER 3. OTHERS AND YOUR HEALTH

Michael Lerner.
Integral Cancer Therapy.
Commonweal, P. O. Box 316, Bolinas, California 94924. 1984.

Judith Glassman.
The Cancer Survivors.
Dial Press, 1983.

Robert S. Mendelsohn.
Confessions of a Medical Heretic.
Warner Books, 1980.

Stephanie Matthews-Simonton and Robert L. Shook.
The Healing Family: The Simonton Approach for Families Facing Illness.
Bantam, 1984.

Andrew Weil.
Health and Healing: Understanding Conventional and Alternative Medicine.
Houghton Mifflin, 1983.

CHAPTER 4. THE HARD CHOICES OF DRUGS

Neville Hodgkinson.
Will to Be Well: The Real Alternative Medicine.
Samuel Weiser, 1984.

Joel Kaufman, Linda Rabinowitz-Dagi, Joan Levin, Phyllis McCarthy, Sidney Wolfe, Eve Bargmann, and the Public Citizen Health Research Group.
Over-the-Counter Pills That Don't Work.
Pantheon, 1983.

Katherine Ketcham and L. Ann Mueller.
Eating Right to Live Sober.
New American Library, 1986.

Physicians' Desk Reference.
Medical Economics Company, Oradell, New Jersey 07649. 1987

Phyllis Saifer and Merla Zellerbach.
Detox: A Successful and Supportive Program for Freeing Your Body from the Physical and Psychological Effects of Chemical Pollutants (at Home or at Work), Junk-Food Additives, Sugar, Nicotine, Drugs, Alcohol, Caffeine, Prescription and Nonprescription Medications, and Other Environmental Toxins.
Jeremy P. Tarcher, Los Angeles, 1984.

CHAPTER 6. ELEMENTS OF NUTRITION

Paavo Airola.
The Miracle of Garlic.
Health Plus Publishers, P. O. Box 22001, Phoenix, Arizona 85028. 1978.

William Gottlieb, Carl Lowe, Mark Bricklin, and Susan Zarrow, editors.
The Complete Book of Vitamins.
Rodale Press, 1984.

Frances Moore Lappé.
Diet for a Small Planet.
Ballantine, tenth anniversary edition 1982.

Earl Mindell.
Earl Mindell's Vitamin Bible.
Warner, 1979.

Linus Pauling.
How to Live Longer and Feel Better.
W. H. Freeman and Company, New York, 1986.

CHAPTER 8. PITFALLS OF INGESTION

Iris R. Bell.
Clinical Ecology: A New Medical Approach to Environmental Illness.
Common Knowledge Press, Bolinas, California, 1982.

John Heinerman.
The Complete Book of Spices: Their Medical, Nutritional, and Cooking Uses.
Keats Publishing, New Canaan, Connecticut, 1983.

Paul Schauenberg and Ferdinand Paris.
Guide to Medicinal Plants.
Keats Publishing, New Canaan, Connecticut, 1977.

CHAPTER 10. LIVING WITH FOOD

Annemarie Colbin.
The Book of Whole Meals: A Seasonal Guide to Assembling Balanced Vegetarian Breakfasts, Lunches, and Dinners.
Ballantine, 1983.

East-West Journal.
Whole World Cookbook.
Avery Publishing Group, Wayne, New Jersey, 1984.

Wendy Esko.
Introducing Macrobiotic Cooking.
Japan Publications, 1979.

Dennis Nelson.
Food Combining Simplified: How to Get the Most from Your Foods.
Plan, P. O. Box 872B, Santa Cruz, California 95061. 1983.

Herbert M. Shelton.
Food Combining Made Easy.
Willow Publishing, San Antonio, Texas, second edition 1982.

CHAPTER 12. DETOXIFYING: OFFENDERS

William G. Crook.
The Yeast Connection: A Medical Breakthrough.
Professional Books, P. O. Box 3494, Jackson, Tennessee 38301. 1984.

C. Orion Truss.
The Missing Diagnosis.
The Missing Diagnosis, P. O. Box 26508, Birmingham, Alabama 35226. 1983

CHAPTER 13. DETOXIFYING: METHODS

Fred Rohé.
Metabolic Ecology: A Way to Win the Cancer War.
Wedgestone Press, Winfield, Kansas, 1982.

CHAPTER 14. BREATH AND EXERCISE

Bob Anderson.
Stretching.
Shelter Publications, Bolinas, California, 1980.

Richard Hittleman.
Richard Hittleman's Introduction to Yoga.
Bantam, 1969.

Swami Rama, Rudolph Ballatine, and Alan Hymes.
Science of Breath: A Practical Guide.
Himalayan International Institute of Yoga Science and Philosophy, Honesdale, Pennsylvania, 1979.

CHAPTER 15. BODY MANIPULATION

Michael Reed Gach and Carolyn Marco.
Acu-Yoga: Self-Help Techniques to Relieve Tension.
Japan Publications, 1981.

Richard Gordon.
Your Healing Hands: The Polarity Experience.
Wingbow Press, Berkeley, California, 1984.

Dolores Krieger.
The Therapeutic Touch: How to Use Your Hands to Help or Heal.
Prentice Hall, 1979.

Felix Mann.
Acupuncture: The Ancient Chinese Art of Healing and How It Works Scientifically.
Vintage Books, 1972.

Iona Marsaa Teeguarden.
Acupressure Way of Health: Jin Shin Do.
Japan Publications. 1978.

John F. Thie.
Touch for Health.
De Vorss and Company, 1046 Princeton Drive, Marina del Rey, California 90291.
1979.

APPENDIX F. HERBS IN AIDS AND ARC

Ted J. Kaptchuk.
The Web That Has No Weaver: Understanding Chinese Medicine.
Congdon and Weed, 1984.

Index

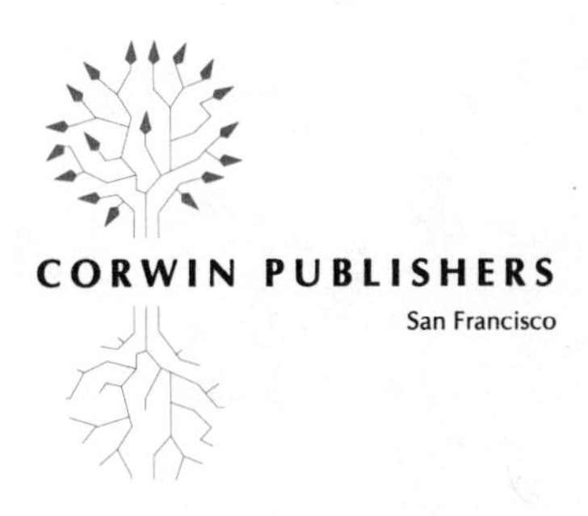

LIVING WITH AIDS: REACHING OUT

This book was designed and produced by Ahmed González-Núñez.
It was typeset at The Copy Network, San Francisco, California.
The text type, 11 on 14 Palatino, and display type, Optima,
were set on a Linotronic 300 laser imagesetter.
Printing and binding were done by Haddon Craftsmen, Inc.,
Scranton, Pennsylvania.
Text paper is Miami Book Smooth, 50 lb.
The cover was designed by Mark Ong.

This book is also available for $18.95 plus $1.00 for postage and handling
from Corwin Publishers, P. O. Box 2806, San Francisco, CA 94126.
California residents please include sales tax.